Recent Advances in Dentistry

(Volume 2)

(Pediatric Orthodontics: Theory and Practice)

Authored by

George Litsas
Private Practice, Limited to Orthodontics, El. Venizelou 2,
Kozani 501 00, Greece

Recent Advances in Dentistry

Volume # 2

Pediatric Orthodontics: Theory and Practice

Author: George Litsas

ISSN (Online): 2468-5046

ISSN (Print): 2468-5038

ISBN (Online): 978-1-68108-609-5

ISBN (Print): 978-1-68108-610-1

BENTHAM SCIENCE PUBLISHERS LTD.

End User License Agreement (for non-institutional, personal use)

This is an agreement between you and Bentham Science Publishers Ltd. Please read this License Agreement carefully before using the ebook/echapter/ejournal (**"Work"**). Your use of the Work constitutes your agreement to the terms and conditions set forth in this License Agreement. If you do not agree to these terms and conditions then you should not use the Work.

Bentham Science Publishers agrees to grant you a non-exclusive, non-transferable limited license to use the Work subject to and in accordance with the following terms and conditions. This License Agreement is for non-library, personal use only. For a library / institutional / multi user license in respect of the Work, please contact: permission@benthamscience.org.

Usage Rules:

1. All rights reserved: The Work is the subject of copyright and Bentham Science Publishers either owns the Work (and the copyright in it) or is licensed to distribute the Work. You shall not copy, reproduce, modify, remove, delete, augment, add to, publish, transmit, sell, resell, create derivative works from, or in any way exploit the Work or make the Work available for others to do any of the same, in any form or by any means, in whole or in part, in each case without the prior written permission of Bentham Science Publishers, unless stated otherwise in this License Agreement.
2. You may download a copy of the Work on one occasion to one personal computer (including tablet, laptop, desktop, or other such devices). You may make one back-up copy of the Work to avoid losing it. The following DRM (Digital Rights Management) policy may also be applicable to the Work at Bentham Science Publishers' election, acting in its sole discretion:

- 25 'copy' commands can be executed every 7 days in respect of the Work. The text selected for copying cannot extend to more than a single page. Each time a text 'copy' command is executed, irrespective of whether the text selection is made from within one page or from separate pages, it will be considered as a separate / individual 'copy' command.
- 25 pages only from the Work can be printed every 7 days.

3. The unauthorised use or distribution of copyrighted or other proprietary content is illegal and could subject you to liability for substantial money damages. You will be liable for any damage resulting from your misuse of the Work or any violation of this License Agreement, including any infringement by you of copyrights or proprietary rights.

Disclaimer:

Bentham Science Publishers does not guarantee that the information in the Work is error-free, or warrant that it will meet your requirements or that access to the Work will be uninterrupted or error-free. The Work is provided "as is" without warranty of any kind, either express or implied or statutory, including, without limitation, implied warranties of merchantability and fitness for a particular purpose. The entire risk as to the results and performance of the Work is assumed by you. No responsibility is assumed by Bentham Science Publishers, its staff, editors and/or authors for any injury and/or damage to persons or property as a matter of products liability, negligence or otherwise, or from any use or operation of any methods, products instruction, advertisements or ideas contained in the Work.

Limitation of Liability:

In no event will Bentham Science Publishers, its staff, editors and/or authors, be liable for any damages, including, without limitation, special, incidental and/or consequential damages and/or damages for lost data and/or profits arising out of (whether directly or indirectly) the use or inability to use the Work. The entire liability of Bentham Science Publishers shall be limited to the amount actually paid by you for the Work.

General:

1. Any dispute or claim arising out of or in connection with this License Agreement or the Work (including non-contractual disputes or claims) will be governed by and construed in accordance with the laws of the U.A.E. as applied in the Emirate of Dubai. Each party agrees that the courts of the Emirate of Dubai shall have exclusive jurisdiction to settle any dispute or claim arising out of or in connection with this License Agreement or the Work (including non-contractual disputes or claims).
2. Your rights under this License Agreement will automatically terminate without notice and without the need for a court order if at any point you breach any terms of this License Agreement. In no event will any delay or failure by Bentham Science Publishers in enforcing your compliance with this License Agreement constitute a waiver of any of its rights.
3. You acknowledge that you have read this License Agreement, and agree to be bound by its terms and conditions. To the extent that any other terms and conditions presented on any website of Bentham Science Publishers conflict with, or are inconsistent with, the terms and conditions set out in this License Agreement, you acknowledge that the terms and conditions set out in this License Agreement shall prevail.

Bentham Science Publishers Ltd.
Executive Suite Y - 2
PO Box 7917, Saif Zone
Sharjah, U.A.E.
Email: subscriptions@benthamscience.org

BENTHAM SCIENCE

CONTENTS

PREFACE

Pediatric Orthodontics: Theory and Practice seeks to answer clinical questions and to provide the reader with knowledge to solve daily orthodontic problems. I have written this book for three different parts of dental community: dentists, residents and specialists. It is the intent of this book to provide the dentist with an easily available and readable source of information for dealing with a specific clinical problem in pediatric orthodontics or to assist in diagnosing a clinical finding. Second, it is intended to supplement the post-graduate student's dental curriculum in order to provide the proper pediatric orthodontic knowledge. Finally, the busy orthodontist who is interested in the specific topic will find this review helpful.

Chapter 1 is a review of craniofacial growth and development. Chapter 2 emphasized the importance on frontal and lateral facial esthetics in pediatric orthodontic diagnosis and treatment planning. Chapter 3 focuses on skeletal and dental relationships and their contributions to orthodontic treatment. Chapter 4 provides in depth the relationship between tooth eruption pattern and dental arches changes during transition from mixed to permanent dentition. Moreover, through clinical examples and problem based approach, a thorough knowledge of tooth eruption sequence as well as tooth eruption abnormalities and arch space loss is provided. Chapter 5 emphasizes the principles for proper occlusal guidance, prevention of developing malocclusions and proper interceptive orthodontic treatment during the mixed dentition period. A series of clinical examples and pediatric orthodontic intervention treatment were also presented. Chapter 6 addresses the etiology, diagnosis and treatment of maxillary transverse discrepancy in the mixed dentition period. Chapter 7 approaches the early diagnosis and appropriate orthodontic intervention of dental anomalies and tooth impaction. Chapter 8 focuses on the diagnosis and orthodontic management of class II, III malocclusions during the mixed dentition period.

With the help of visual aid and the unique question-answer format, the reader can quickly focus on a specific area of interest to answer the question. The problem-based approach allows the clinicians to test and improve their knowledge in Pediatric Orthodontics. The topics are covered with figures, cases, diagrams and references.

George Litsas, D.D.S., M.Sc., Ph.D,
Private Practice, Limited to Orthodontics,
Kozani, Greece

CONFLICT OF INTEREST

The author declares no conflict of interest, financial or otherwise.

ACKNOWLEDGMENTS

To my family and especially to my parents and my wife, Katerina, and my children Melas and Maria whose love, encouragement and support have helped make this book a reality.

A great deal of thanks goes to the Dental School of Aristotle University, to the entire staff of the Department of Orthodontics, Dental Faculty, Marmara University as well as to the Department of Pediatric Dentistry, TUFTS University, School of Dental Medicine. I owe a great deal of appreciation to professors Dr. Nejat Erverdi, Dr. A.E. Athanasiou and Dr. A. Pappas.

CHAPTER 1

Craniofacial Growth

Abstract: The biologic process that has an underlying control system at the cellular and tissue levels is called Morphogenesis. Two mechanisms combine to form the skeleton: intramemebranous ossification and endochondral ossification. It is in the latter that the vertebrae and long bones are formed, while intramembranous ossification is responsible for the cranial bones. While somatic and craniofacial development have been shown clearly to be associated, the growth of the craniofacial region – involving, as it does, interaction between growth sites adjacent to each other, each of which has a different pattern and grows at different times and at different rates, is highly complex. The purpose of this chapter with the question-answer format is to provide the basic concepts on craniofacial growth and development.

Keywords: Cranial bones, Craniofacial growth, Mandibular condyle.

INTRODUCTION

Craniofacial growth is a complicated interaction between hormones function and genes. In dentofacial orthopedics, in depth understanding of craniofacial morphogenesis is essential for determining treatment goals and predicting stability during the retention period. Furthermore, general principle of orthodontic and orthopaedic treatment is to utilize growth of the child considering the amount of growth remaining and the direction in which the forces are to be applied to stimulate growth in the desired direction. The histogenic functioning of the cells and tissues carries out their individual roles, but the control signals that selectively activate the composite of them are now clinically manipulated.

1. Provide the Definition of the Terms

a. Growth vs. Development

What we call ***"growth"*** is the process by which the size of the whole organism and the size of organs, tissues and cells are increased. Growth usually refers to an increase in size and number [1 - 3].

Development refers to an increase in tissue organization and specialization. Development is a progress towards maturity [1 - 3]. The two processes rely on

George Litsas

each other. Growth is basically anatomic and quantitative phenomenon whereas development is physiologic and qualitative phenomenon.

b. Growth Centre vs. Growth Site

Growth centers are primary bone growth regions, as in the cartilaginous growth plates of long bones, that have intrinsic growth potential and tissue-separating capabilities [4, 5]. The epiphysis of a growing long bone is the commonest example of a bone growth centre, lengthening the long bones by way of proliferation of cartilage as well as hypertrophy. When this region has been lengthened, stabilisation and strengthening through replacement with bone follow [5]. The newly lengthened region is then stabilized and strengthened by replacement with bone. All centers of growth are sites as well.

Growth site is a secondary, adaptive region where the remodelling of bone occurs with no cartilage as an intermediate stage. Until stimulated by an external signal, bone growth sites remain dormant [4, 5]. For example, expansion of the brain and lengthening of the cranial base synchondroses cause the sutures to add intra-membranous bone at the bone front edges in such a way that the sutures retain their width and there is an increase in the size of the cranial vault to accommodate the brain as it enlarges. This growth can be seen, for example, in synchondrosis of the basicranium, maxillary tuberosity, mandibular condyle, sutures and the alveolar process [6 - 8].

c. Endochondral Ossification vs. Intramemebranous Ossification

In **endochondral ossification,** bone develops from a cartilaginous precursor which is responsible for elongation of individual bone (cranial base, mandibular condyle) [8 - 12]. Bones formed in this matter are less susceptible to environmental influences during growth and are under direct genetic control. In **intramembranous ossification,** bone is formed by osteoblasts present in mesenchymal tissue. The formation of bone is not preceded by formation of a cartilage but bone is laid down directly in a fibrous membrane. Example of intramemebranous bone formation is the cranial vault, body of the mandible and the maxilla [1, 2, 7].

d. Synchondrosis

Except that growth is bipolar, synchondrosis resembles long bone growth plate. We can think of it as two back-to-back growth plates sharing a common zone in which chondroblasts proliferates actively (the "rest zone") [6, 12]. Structurally, it resembles all primary cartilages, at least in basic plan. There are three zones (**Fig. 1**):

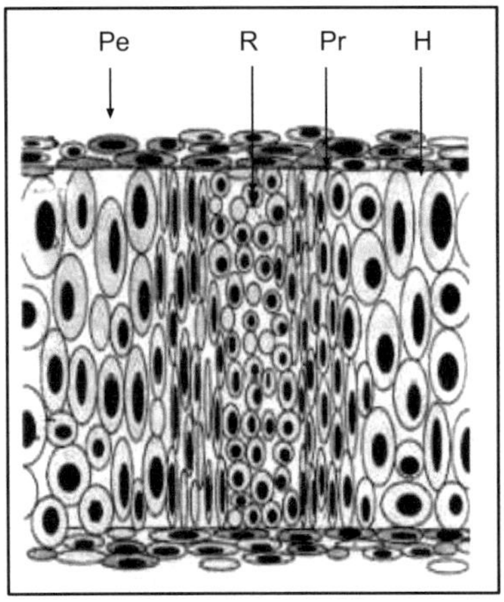

Fig. (1). Synchondroses are present in the basicranium's midline part.

a. A resting zone comprising chondrocytesprecursors tasked with directing the synchondrosis formation and organisation.
b. A proliferation zone.
c. A hypertrophic zone without active growth.

e. Primary Displacement vs. Secondary Displacement

Primary displacement occurs in combination with bone's own growth.As the maxilla at the tuberosity region grows, the maxilla is pushed against the cranial base so that is displaced forwards and downwards. This should be distinguished from secondary displacement, which results from the enlargement of adjacent bones and soft tissue (*e.g.* forward and downward displacement of the maxilla also results from the cranial base's growth) [1, 2].

f. Remodeling and Relocation

The process by which the shape of a bone changes through time is called ***remodeling***. It could be characterized as the differential growth activity which includes the simultaneous deposition and resorption on all the surfaces of the bone [6]. The remodeling of a bone occurs during the growth because its regional parts move from one location to another as well as the whole bone is enlarged. The inner and outer surfaces of a bone are covered with fields of growth, which are either appository or repository. The apposition and resorption combination is responsible for the relocation of the bone in space and for the enlargement of the [1, 2, 13]. *For example*, ramus moves posterior by a combination of resorption & deposition.

The relative movement in space of a bony structure, due to bone deposition on one side and resorption on the other side called ***relocation***. It is a key concept in the remodeling process [1, 2], for example the whole ramus is thus relocated the posterior part of the lengthening corpus becomes relocated into the area previously occupied by the ramus.

2. What is the Following Growth Curve?

According to this growth curve (Fig. **2**), different tissue in body grows at different times and different rates. Neural tissues complete 90% of growth at 6 years and 98% by 10 years of age [14]. Lymphoid tissues-proliferates rapidly in late childhood and reaches almost 200% of adult size. Height and most body measurements follow the "general" curve. Genital tissues grow rapidly at puberty leading adult size after which growth ceases. Furthermore, the maxilla located closer to the brain, grows earlier and follows a pattern closer to that of neural tissues whereas the mandible grows later and exhibits more characteristics of a growth spurt paralleling the general tissue growth spurt in body height [1, 2, 15, 16].

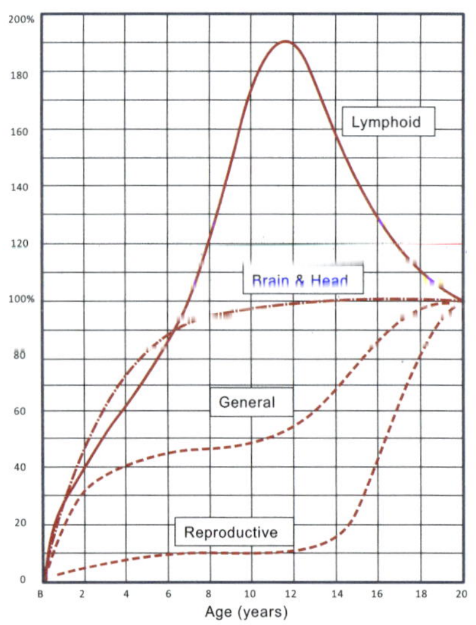

Fig. (2). Scammon's growth curve.

3. Which is the Important Growth Process for Normal Cranial Vault Growth?

Sutural Growth and Surface Remodeling (Fig. **3**). As the brain expands the cranial vault bones are displaced **(a, b)**. Displacement causes tension at cranial sutures **(c)** with bone resorption and new bone deposition on the internal and the external surface **(d)** [1]. Surface remodeling occurs near sutures and causes flattening of the vault. 90% of cranial vault growth completed by 5-6 yrs of age [14].

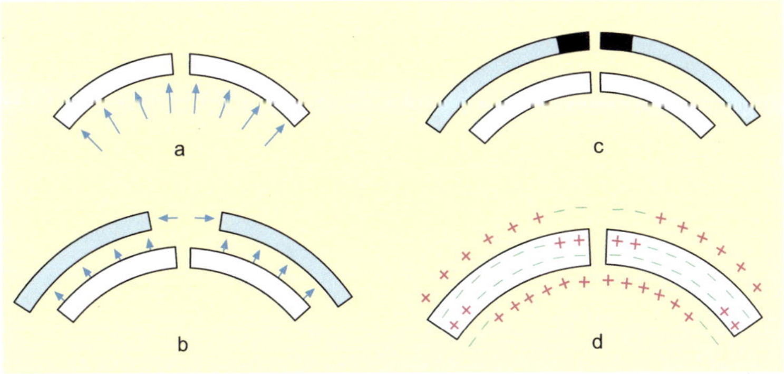

Fig. (3). Sutural growth and surface remodeling.

4. How the Cranial Base is Growth?

For the most part, it is endochondral osteogenesis that completes the cranial base's ossification. Intra-membranous ossification, on the other hand, is conducted in limited areas such as sphenoidal wings and part of the sella turcica. Postnatal growth of the cranial base is the result of a complex interaction involving:

- ***An intrinsic component***, arising from the synchondrosis potential for growth. A synchondrosis will usually be temporary; it is present during the growing phase until the point where the intervening cartilage becomes progressively thinner as the skeleton matures and ultimately converts to bone [15 - 18].
- ***An extrinsic component***, which corresponds to the functional matrix, derives from the interaction between the intrinsic sutural growth at their growth sites, and the thrust of the brain, which is expressed at the sutural and at the periosteal level. The growth of the cerebral hemispheres, especially the frontal lobes and the temporal lobes, expands the medial and anterior cranial fossa [15 - 18].

5. Which are the Cranial Base Synchondroses? Describe their Functions

There are three basic synchondroses (Fig. **4**) along the cranial base's midline [6, 12].

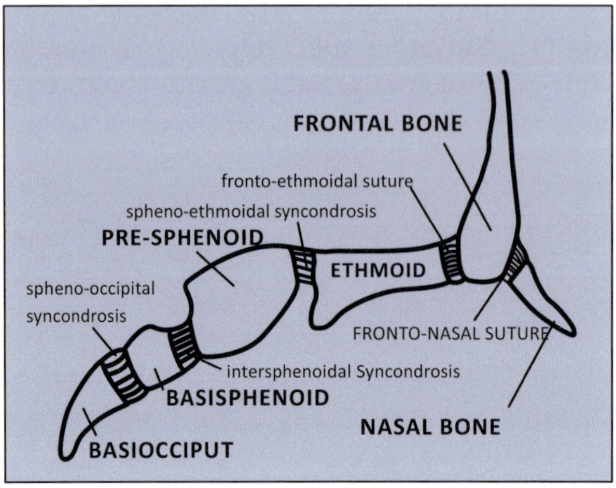

Fig. (4). Cranial base synchondroses.

Spheno-ethmoidal synchondrosis is located between sphenoid and ethmoidal bones. It ceases at the age of six, as a result of which the anterior cranial base has been used (wholly or in part) to refer to a number of cephalometric analyses.

Inter-sphenoid synchondrosis (cartilaginous band), which is ossified by the time of birth, is located between two parts of the sphenoid bone.

Spheno-occipital synchondrosis is located between sphenoid and basio-occipital bones. The spheno-occipital synchondrosis because of its late ossification and its location has an important influence on the relationship between these bones [19]. Excessive growth can lead to an increase in cranial base length and development of a skeletal Class II relationship whereas deficient growth is more likely to result in a skeletal Class III relationship [20 - 22]. Intrinsic genetic factors are mostly responsible for this Chondrocranial growth [3].

6. Explain the Relationship between Anterior Cranial Base Growth and the Upper Facial Growth

Elongation of the anterior cranial base proceeds in parallel with growth in the brain's frontal lobes. By the age of six years (the end of the neural growth period), it will have reached about 95% of its adult size [14].

There are the following elements of the anterior cranial base which are incorporated in the upper face:

a. Ethmoid
b. Parts of the sphenoid
c. A significant portion of the frontal bone.

Expansion of the eyes leads to a similar expansion in the orbital cavity and this takes place anteriorly, inferiorly and laterally by means of rotation and translation. In this way, the upper face grows away from the remainder of the cranial base. As the orbit's is part of the anterior cranial fossa's floor, growth in the frontal lobes and anterior cranial fossa affects the orbital roof's shape, orientation, and position [7, 8].

7. Explain the Relationship between Cranial Base Growth and Maxilla-Mandible Position?

During development, the anterior and posterior cranial base flexes at the sella turcicain the middle sagittal plane and thus constitutes an angle in the cranial base, termed the cranial base angle or saddle angle. This angle consists of two lines. The anterior line, where the maxilla is attached, extends from the sella turcica **(S)** to the frontal-nasal suture **(N).** The posterior line, where the mandible is attached, extends from the sella turcica **(S)** to the anterior border of the foramen magnum, defined as the basion **(Ba).** Therefore, any change in the cranial base angle can affect the relationships of the maxilla and mandible and influence the type of malocclusion. General speaking, a large cranial base angle contribute to a skeletal class II relationship whereas a small cranial base angle to a skeletal class III relationship [1, 20 - 23].

8. Name the Basic Nasomaxillary Growth Sites? Summarize the Mechanisms of Maxillary Growth in a Horizontal, Vertical and Transverse Direction

a. Sutures - Nasal septum - Zygomatic arch - Orbital remodeling - Palatal remodeling and Vertical drift of teeth.
b. General speaking, it is *via* intra-membranous ossification except nasal septum growth. **Cranial base growth** pushes the maxilla forward which occurs up to 7 years [6]. After that, tension placed across the **circum-maxillary sutures** leads to bone deposition by intra-membranous ossification and primary displacement of the maxilla. **Nasal septum growth and surface remodeling**, by bone deposition and resorption can produce additive and subtractive changes in the maxilla [24, 25].

i. Horizontal

Posterior bone deposition at the tuberosity region will cause primary anterior displacement of the maxillary complex. It is a major- depository site of maxillary growth. The extent of forward displacement is matched by the amount of backward bone growth (Fig. **5**) [26].

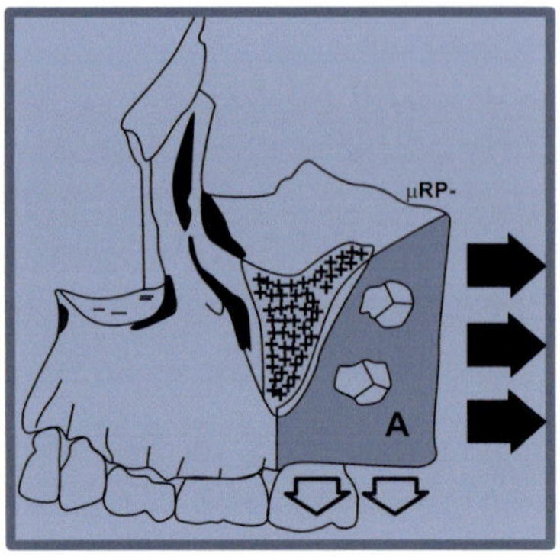

Fig. (5). Posterior bone deposition at the tuberosity region.

Secondary anterior displacement: Increase in the size of middle cranial fossa result in a marked displacement movement of the whole maxillary complex anteriorly and inferiorly. This is quite independent of the enlargement of maxilla itself (Fig. **6**) [27].

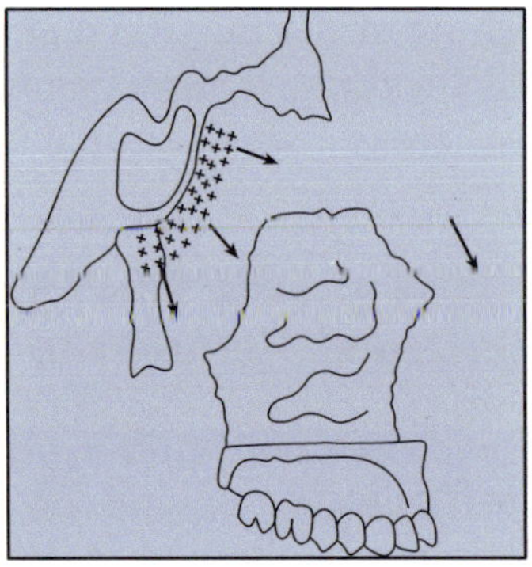

Fig. (6). Secondary anterior displacement.

ii. Vertical

Growth of the palatine process of the maxilla results from surface deposition on the entire oral side of the palatal cortex, resorptive removal from the opposite nasal side as well as from periosteal labial surfaces of the anterior maxillary arch. The direction is generally down. Following the V principle of growth, inferior growth is carried out by remodelling. It follows the V principle of growth and hence grows inferiorly by later alremodeling and expansion (Fig. **7**) [1, 2].

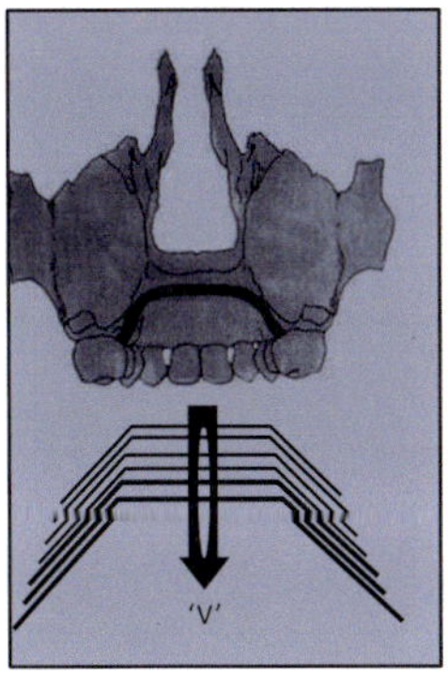

Fig. (7). Growth of the palatine process of the maxilla.

The maxillary arch's downward growth is produced by:

- The nasomaxillary complex's downward displacement as a result of bone apposition on the site of the sutures (Fig. **8**).
- A sutural growth mechanism that is responsible for half of the maxillary arch and palate's total downward movement.
- Remodelling through resorption and deposition processes acting together to bring about a direct inferior relocation of the palate and maxillary arch (Fig. **9**).

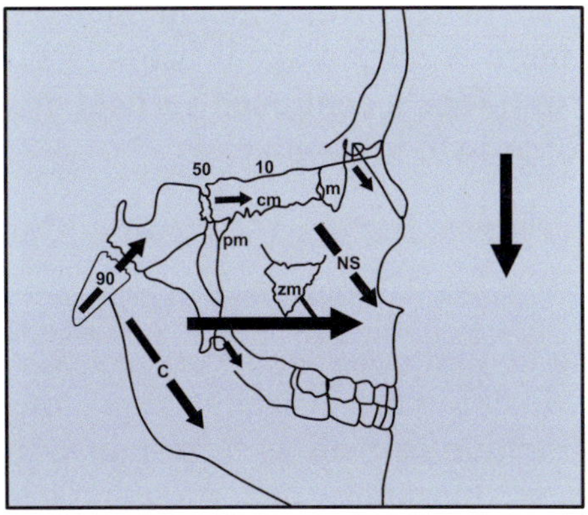

Fig. (8). Nasomaxillary complex's downward displacement.

iii. Transverse

Transverse Growth in the midpalatal suture: Remodelling at the alveolar process's lateral surface and the palatal vault contribute to widen the maxilla [27]. In the same way, the downward movement of teeth is a two-part process:

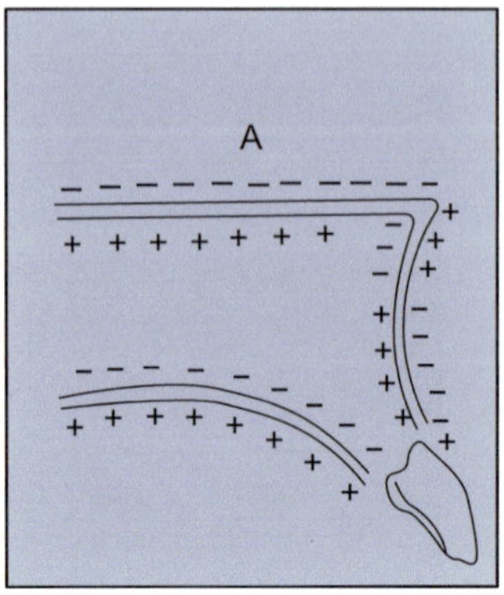

Fig. (9). Direct inferior relocation of the palate and maxillary arch.

- Remodelling growth of the alveolar bone.
- Displacement of the maxilla as a whole, with no participation by the alveolar bone.

9. Name the Main Growth Sites of Postnatal Mandibular Growth

Condylar cartilage, ramus and alveolar bone [10, 11]. These areas account for increases in the mandibular height, length, and width respectively. The width of the mandible completes its growth first (before the growth spurt). The length of the mandible continues to increase throughout puberty. Until the length has reached its final point, there is only a small height increase; this subsequently carries on the match the mid-face's continued vertical growth. Bi-condylar width shows small increase until growth in length ends.

10. Describe the Differences Between Primary Cartilage and Condylar Cartilage

Condylar cartilage which is designated as secondary cartilage differs from other primary cartilage in histological organization, modes of proliferation, differentiation and calcification as well as to response in environmental factors (*e.g.*, biomechanical stress, hormones and growth factors, Fig. **10**) [28, 29]. *Primary cartilage*, such as articular cartilage and growth plates in a long bone, synchondrosis in the cranial base, and nasal septum cartilage, consists of a chondrocytes population whereas condylar cartilage is a heterogeneous tissue containing fibroblasts, osteochondral progenitor cells, and chondrocytes [30]. In addition, condylar cartilage contains chondroid bone (a specialized calcified tissue with morphological properties intermediate between those of bone and cartilage) which plays an important role in regulating different rates of bone formation in intramembranous and endochondral ossification. In contrast, only a single cartilage, the mandibular condylar cartilage, exists in the mandible throughout life, and plays roles in articulating function and growth. Therefore, the condylar cartilage is an "all-in-one type tissue".

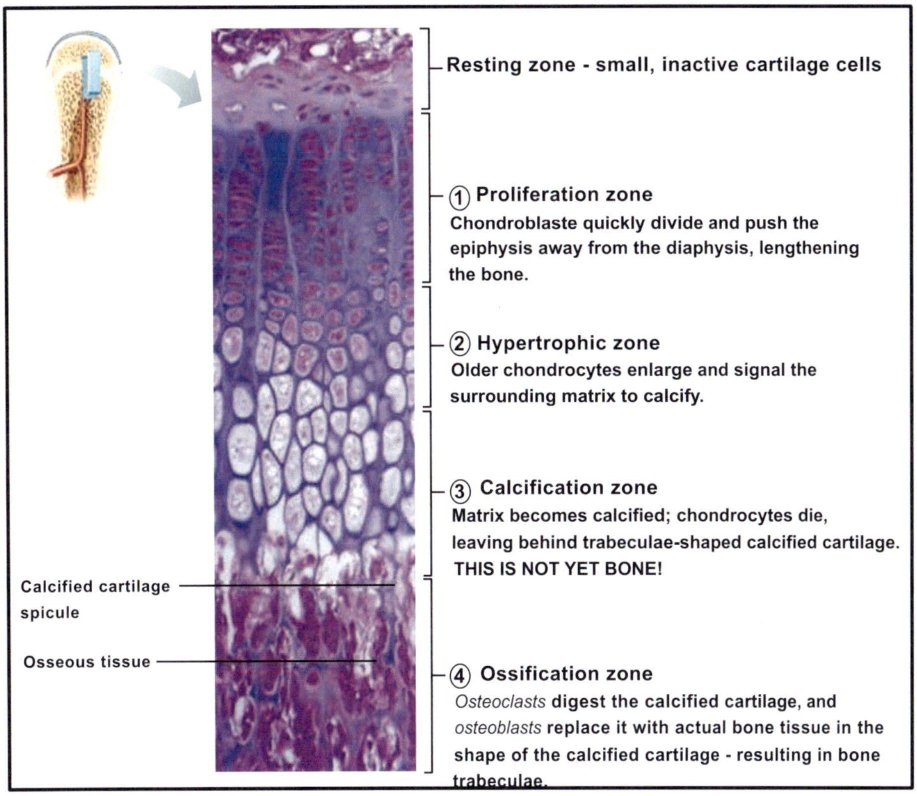

Fig. (10). Condyle growth plate.

11. Give the Main Functions of the Mandibular Condyle

The condyle's main function is provision of multi-dimensional bone growth where intramemebranous growth would not be possible, and to act as a pressure-tolerant articular contact. For many years thought to be the main mandibular growth center, but it is now seen as a regional growth field with a genetic potential for growth that seems to be restricted to a capacity for continued cellular proliferation. Upward and backward growth movement results from proliferation, but endochondral growth is seen only at the condyle's articular contact part [1 - 4, 30, 31].

12. Summarize the Growth Process of Mandibular Ramus, Corpus, Condylar Neck and Mandibular Coronoid Process

Mandibular Ramus

Resorption occurs on the ramus's anterior part, while bone deposition occurs on the posterior region. Greater amount of resorption occurs inferiorly than superiorly whereas a greater amount of bone additions occurs on the inferior than the superior part of the posterior region. The consequence is that the ramus drifts in a posterior and more vertical direction. As anterior border of ramus resorbs, the body of the mandible lengthens making room for the molar teeth (Fig. **11**).

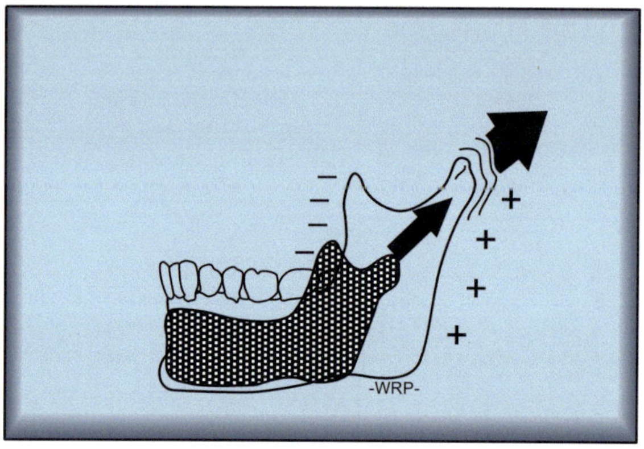

Fig. (11). Mandibular Ramus.

Mandibular Corpus

Ramus displacement leads to what was the ramus being converted into the mandible body's posterior body. So the corpus lengthens by the posterior molar region is becoming relocated anteriorly into premolar and canine regions (Fig. **11**). At the same time, it accommodates the vertical dimension of the face giving space for permanent molar to be erupted. An increase in the vertical length is necessary to keep pace with growth in the pharynx and middle cranial fossa. Moreover, provides an attachment base for the increasing mass of masticatory muscles.

Mandibular Condylar Neck

The condylar neck relocates progressively into areas that previously were held by the much wider condyle. As one is remodelled from the other, what was condyle turns into neck through a combination of periosteal resorption and endosteal deposition. Superior, posterior and medial growth results from deposits of bone on the lingual surface.

Coronoid Process

It follows V principle: Deposition on lingual side and resorption on buccal surface. Deposits of bone on the lingual surface bring about growth superiorly, posteriorly and medially [1, 2, 7, 10, 11].

13. Describe the role of Fibroblast Growth Factor Receptor (FGFR), Sonic Hedgehog (Shh), SOX 9 and Cbfa1 in Craniofacial Development?

Fibroblast growth factor receptor (FGFR), Sonic Hedgehog (Shh), SOX 9 and Cbfa1 are examples of genes that play critical roles in craniofacial development. Mutations in genes encoding FGFRs have been identified as causes of Apert syndrome, Crouzon syndromes and Pfeiffer syndromes. Where SOX 9 is absent, severe skeletal dwarfism may result. Mutations involving Cbfa1 lead to cleidocranial dysplasia. Shh belongs to the vertebrate Hedgehog gene family and plays an important part in the establishment of craniofacial midline structures as well as in the regulation of cranial suture development [32, 33].

14. Summarize the Following Craniofacial Growth Theories

- *Sutural theory (Weinmann and Sicher)*
- *Cartilaginous theory (Scott)*
- *The functional matrix (Moss)*
- *The Servo-system theory (Petrovic)*
- *Enlow's V principal*

Sutural Theory (Weinmann and Sicher) [34]

Cranio-facial growth occurs mainly at the sutures which have the growth potential. Genetically regulated primary bone growth takes place at the craniofacial skeleton's connective tissue and cartilaginous joints. The cranial vault's growth results from the intrinsic sutural growth forcing the vault's bones away from each other, while sutural connective tissue proliferation in the circumaxillary suture system forces downward and forward growth in the mid-face. Sutures between the frontal process of maxilla and the frontal bone, between the zygomatic bone and the maxilla, and between the pyramidal process of the palatine bone and the pterygoid process of the sphenoid bone may be important contributors to maxillary growth. These sutures are all parallel with downward and forward slant (Fig. **12**). Although it was earlier thought that the mandible was a bent long bone, with the mandibular condylar cartilage fulfilling the role of the epiphyseal plates of long bones whose growth forces the mandible downward and forward, it is now clear that there is no independent growth potential to sutures and that these respond to external influences.

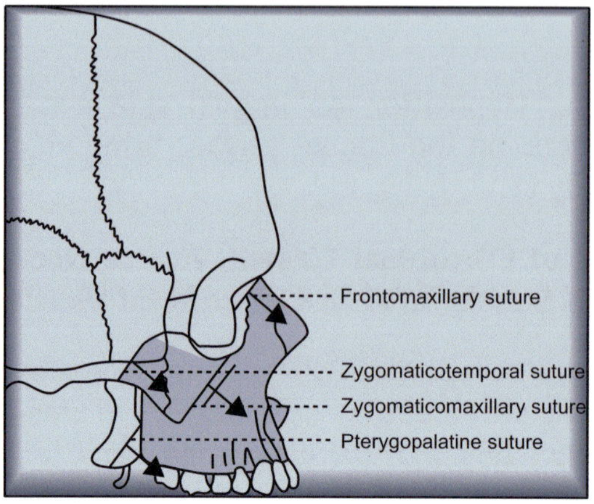

Fig. (12). Sutural theory.

Cartilaginous Theory (Scott) [24, 25]

Cartilage and periosteum both possess growth factors, and the role of sutures is secondary. Growth of the maxilla stems from growth of the nasal septum cartilage – a theory that backs up the idea that the nasal septum cartilage's anterior-inferior growth, buttressed against the cranial base posterior, needs to downward and forward growth in the mid-face (Fig. **13**). On the other hand, the growth of the mandible is attributed to the cartilage of the mandibular condyle. However, transplantation experiments demonstrate that not all skeletal cartilage in acts the same way when transplanted. When the epiphyseal plate of a long bone is transplanted, it will continue to grow in a new location whereas, little growth was observed when the cartilage of the mandibular condyle was transplanted.

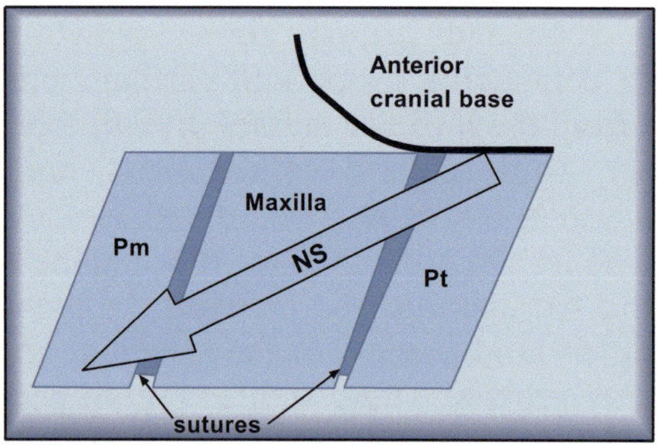

Fig. (13). Cartilaginous theory.

The Functional Matrix [35, 36]

The functional matrix hypothesis says that the initial development and the growth of the craniofacial skeleton are direct responses to its extrinsic, epigenetic environment. Functional cranial components consist of two elements: a functional matrix and a skeletal unit. The functional matrix is the soft tissue and spaces that perform given functions, while the skeletal unit is the bony structures supporting the functional matrix which could not function without them. There are two types of functional matrices: *The periosteal matrix* (muscles, blood vessels and nerves) and the *capsular matrix* (brain, globe of eyes, nasopharynx and oropharynx). There are also two types of skeletal units: *The macroskeletal units and the microskeletal units*. Growth of the face occurs as a response to functional needs and is mediated by the soft tissue in which the jaws are embedded. Primary growth of the capsular matrix (brain) results in a stimulus for secondary growth of the sutures and synchondrosis leading to overall enlargement of the neurocranium.

The Servo-System Theory (Petrovic) [10]

According to the servo-system theory, growth of the mid-face and the cranial base affected directly and indirectly by systemic hormones. Growth of the mandibular condyle is highly adaptive and responds to both systemic and local functional factors. According to this theory, the anterior and inferior growth of the mid-face under the primary influence of the cartilaginous cranial base and nasal septum, results in a slight occlusal deviation between the maxillary and mandibular dentitions. Perception of this occlusal deviation by proprioceptors (periodontal regions and temporomandibular joint) triggers the muscles of the mandible which are responsible to reposition the mandible anterior. The muscle activity and the protrusion in the presence of appropriate hormonal factors stimulate growth at the mandibular condyle.

Enlow's V Principal [1]

Many facial and cranial bones or parts of bones have a V-Shaped configuration. Bone deposition occurs on the inner side of the "V" and resorption occurs on the outer side of the "V". The direction of movement is toward the wide end of the "V". The counterpart Enlow'sprinciple of craniofacial growth states that the growth of any facial and cranial part relates specifically to other structural and geometric counterparts in the face and cranium. According to this theory, the naso-maxillary complex relates to the anterior cranial fossa whereas the horizontal dimension of the pharyngeal space relates to the middle cranial fossa. Maxillary and mandibular dental arch, maxillary bone and corpus of the mandible as well as maxillary tuberosity and the lingual tuberosity are mutual counterparts.

CONCLUDING REMARKS

No part is growth and development independent and self-contained. The growth process works toward an ongoing state of composite functional and structural equilibrium. For example, in the mandible, the middle cranial fossa determine the placement of the temporomandibular joints and, if asymmetric one will be lower or higher.

REFERENCES

[1] Enlow DH, Hans MG. Essentials of facial growth. Philadelphia: W.B. Saunders Company 1996.

[2] Carlson DS. Theories of craniofacial growth in the postgenomic era. Semin Orthod 2005; 4: 172-83. [http://dx.doi.org/10.1053/j.sodo.2005.07.002]

[3] Kohn LA. The role of genetics in craniofacial morphology and growth. Annu Rev Anthropol 1991; 20(1): 261-78. [http://dx.doi.org/10.1146/annurev.an.20.100191.001401]

[4] Baron R. General principles of bone biology.Favus MJ, ed Primer on the metabolic bone diseases and disorders of mineral metabolism 5th end American Society for Bone and Mineral Research: Washington DC. 2003; pp. 1.1-8.

[5] Nilsson O, Baron J. Fundamental limits on longitudinal bone growth: growth plate senescence and epiphyseal fusion. Trends Endocrinol Metab 2004; 15(8): 370-4. [http://dx.doi.org/10.1016/j.tem.2004.08.004] [PMID: 15380808]

[6] Roberts GJ, Blackwood HJ. Growth of the cartilages of the mid-line cranial base: a radiographic and histological study. J Anat 1983; 136(Pt 2): 307-20. [PMID: 6682850]

[7] Proffit WR, Fields HW, Sarver DM. Contemporary orthodontics 5th. St. Louis, Mo, USA: Mosby 2013.

[8] Buschang PH, Baume RM, Nass GG. A craniofacial growth maturity gradient for males and females between 4 and 16 years of age. Am J Phys Anthropol 1983; 61(3): 373-81. [http://dx.doi.org/10.1002/ajpa.1330610312] [PMID: 6614151]

[9] Litsas G. Gh and craniofacial tissues. An Update. Open Dent J 2015; 9: 1-8. [http://dx.doi.org/10.2174/1874210601509010001] [PMID: 25674165]

[10] Petrovic A. Control of postnatal growth of secondary cartilages of the mandible by mechanisms regulating occlusion. Cybernetic model. Trans Eur Orthod Soc 1974; 69-75. [PMID: 4534981]

[11] Petrovic A, Stutzmann JJ, Oudet CL. Control processes in the postnatal growth of the condylar cartilage of the mandible.Determinants of mandibular form and growth, monograph 4, craniofacial growth series. Ann Arbor: Center for Human Growth and Development, The University of Michigan 1975.

[12] Bjork A. Cranial base development. Am J Orthod 1955; 41: 198-225. [http://dx.doi.org/10.1016/0002-9416(55)90005-1]

[13] Rakosi T, Jonas I, Graber T. Color atlas of dental medicine. Orthodontic Diagnosis. Stuttgart: Thieme Medical Publishers 1993.

[14] Scammon RE. The measurement of the body in childhood. The measurement of man. Minneapolis: University of Minnesota Press 1930.

[15] Stramrud L. External and internal cranial base. A cross sectional study of the growth and association in form. ActaOdontoScand 1959; 17: 239-66.

[16] Nie X. Cranial base in craniofacial development: developmental features, influence on facial growth, anomaly, and molecular basis. Acta Odontol Scand 2005; 63(3): 127-35.

[http://dx.doi.org/10.1080/00016350510019847] [PMID: 16191905]

[17] VandeBerg JR, Buschang PH, Hinton RJ. Absolute and relative growth of the rat craniofacial skeleton. Arch Oral Biol 2004; 49(6): 477-84. [http://dx.doi.org/10.1016/j.archoralbio.2003.12.007] [PMID: 15099805]

[18] Vandeberg JR, Buschang PH, Hinton RJ. Craniofacial growth in growth hormone-deficient rats. Anat Rec A Discov Mol Cell Evol Biol 2004; 278(2): 561-70. [http://dx.doi.org/10.1002/ar.a.20051] [PMID: 15164344]

[19] Thilander B, Ingervall B. The human spheno-occipital synchondrosis. II. A histological and microradiographic study of its growth. Acta Odontol Scand 1973; 31(5): 323-34. [http://dx.doi.org/10.3109/00016357309002520] [PMID: 4520245]

[20] Houston WJ. A cephalometric analysis of Angle class II, division II malocclusion in the mixed dentition. Dent Pract Dent Rec 1967; 17(10): 372-6. [PMID: 5229343]

[21] James GA. Cephalometric analysis of 100 class II div 1 malocclusions with special reference to the cranial base. Dent Pract 1962; 14: 35-46.

[22] Nanda SK. Growth patterns in subjects with long and short faces. Am J Orthod Dentofacial Orthop 1990; 98(3): 247-58. [http://dx.doi.org/10.1016/S0889-5406(05)81602-6] [PMID: 2403077]

[23] Anderson D, Popovich F. Relation of cranial base flexure to cranial form and mandibular position. Am J Phys Anthropol 1983; 61(2): 181-7. [http://dx.doi.org/10.1002/ajpa.1330610206] [PMID: 6881319]

[24] Scott JH. The cartilage of the nasal septum (a contribution to the study of facial growth). Br Dent J 1953; 95: 37-43.

[25] Scott JH. Dentofacial development and growth. Oxford: Pergamon Press 1967.

[26] Melsen B, Melsen F. The postnatal development of the palatomaxillary region studied on human autopsy material. Am J Orthod 1982; 82(4): 329-42. [http://dx.doi.org/10.1016/0002-9416(82)90467-5] [PMID: 6961805]

[27] Dixon AD, Hoyte DA, Ronning O. Fundamentals of craniofacial growth. Boca Raton: CRC Press 1997.

[28] Silbermann M, Reddi AH, Hand AR, Leapman RD, Von der Mark K, Franzen A. Further characterisation of the extracellular matrix in the mandibular condyle in neonatal mice. J Anat 1987; 151: 169-88. [PMID: 3308801]

[29] Solem RC, Eames BF, Tokita M, Schneider RA. Mesenchymal and mechanical mechanisms of secondary cartilage induction. Dev Biol 2011; 356(1): 28-39. [http://dx.doi.org/10.1016/j.ydbio.2011.05.003] [PMID: 21600197]

[30] Winter RM. What's in a face? Nat Genet 1996; 12(2): 124-9. [http://dx.doi.org/10.1038/ng0296-124] [PMID: 8563748]

[31] Cobourne MT. Construction for the modern head: current concepts in craniofacial development. J Orthod 2000; 27(4): 307-14. [http://dx.doi.org/10.1093/ortho/27.4.307] [PMID: 11099568]

[32] Schell-Apacik C, Rivero M, Knepper JL, Roessler E, Muenke M, Ming JE. SONIC HEDGEHOG mutations causing human holoprosencephaly impair neural patterning activity. Hum Genet 2003; 113(2): 170-7. [PMID: 12709790]

[33] Cendekiawan T, Wong RW, Rabie AB. Temporal expression of SOX9 and type II collagen in spheno-occipital synchondrosis of mice after mechanical tension stimuli. Angle Orthod 2008; 78(1): 83-8.

[http://dx.doi.org/10.2319/012507-36.1] [PMID: 18193955]

[34] Weinmann JP, Sichefr H. Bone and bones Fundamentals of bone biology. 2nd ed., St. Louis: CV Mosby Comp 1955.

[35] Moss ML, Salentijn L. The capsular matrix. Am J Orthod 1969; 56(5): 474-90. [http://dx.doi.org/10.1016/0002-9416(69)90209-7] [PMID: 5261161]

[36] Moss ML, Salentijn L. The primary role of functional matrices in facial growth. Am J Orthod 1969; 55(6): 566-77. [http://dx.doi.org/10.1016/0002-9416(69)90034-7] [PMID: 5253955]

CHAPTER 2

Soft Tissue Evaluation

Abstract: Orthodontic diagnosis and treatment planning is based on three important components: facial, skeletal and dental diagnoses. In the last years, the impact of facial/dental appearance, the malocclusion, and treatment for these conditions on psychological and functional well-being have drawn increasing attention from clinicians and researchers. Emphasis has been placed on frontal and lateral aesthetics, keeping in mind that facial proportions are more important than absolute numerical values. The most common photo evaluation in orthodontic diagnosis includes the facial frontal, facial profile facial smile, and oblique smile photo. Facial concavity or convexity, lips dimension and position, smile arc, gingival display and over all facial balance should be considered in the overall treatment plan. This chapter, with the question-answer format and clinical examples, describes the surface markings of the face, soft-tissue cephalometric points, facial planes and facial angles.

Keywords: Facial angles, Facial planes, Orthodontic diagnosis, Soft-tissue cephalometric points.

INTRODUCTION

The facial appearance is usually an area of significant concern for the individual because it draws the most attention from other people in interpersonal interactions and is the primary source of vocal, physical, and emotional communication. Both the children and their parents view the orthodontic treatment not only as a treatment to improve the occlusion, mastication, and speech but also as a means to achieving a better quality of life. The discipline of orthodontic aesthetics involves micro and macro aesthetics, gingival, and facial aesthetics. For this reason, one of the main components of the orthodontic diagnosis and treatment planning should be the frontal and profile facial evaluation.

George Litsas

PART A. FRONTAL FACIAL ANALYSIS

1. Describe the Angle's Theory *Versus* Soft Tissue Theory for Goals of Orthodontic Treatment [1, 2]

	Angle Theory	Soft Tissue Theory
Goal of Treatment	Ideal dental occlusion and skeletal relationships	Ideal soft tissue proportions and functional occlusion
Hard *vs.* Soft tissue relationships	Ideal skeletal and dental relationships produce ideal soft tissue proportions	Ideal soft tissue proportions define ideal skeletal and dental relationship
Diagnosis	Dental casts and radiographs	Clinical examination of soft tissues
Treatment	Obtain ideal dental and skeletal relationships	Determine ideal soft tissue proportions and then treat the jaws and teeth as needed to obtain them

2. Describe the Three Essential Outcomes of the First Clinical Examination

The essential outcomes of the first clinical examination [1 - 5] are:

- The facial and dental health,
- The facial and dental aesthetics,
- Function (TMJ)

3. Provide Some Parameters of "Facial Health and Aesthetics" During the First Visual Examination

a. Face and expression
b. Facial symmetry and proportions
c. Lips and smile evaluation
d. Genetic defects (cleft patients)
e. Profile evaluation [1 - 5].

4. Why is the Frontal Facial Analysis Required?

Frontal facial photographs empower a two-dimensional soft tissue examination in horizontal and vertical planes for the reasons of assessing facial asymmetries and soft tissue attributes. The position of the maxilla and the mandible has a large influence on the relationship between the maxillary and mandibular dentitions. A little level of bilateral facial asymmetry exists in all normal individuals, and this has been termed **"ordinary asymmetry"** [6 - 8].

5. Which Are the Important Soft Tissue Points in the Frontal Facial Analysis?

The **forehead** possesses the upper face, from the hairline to the eyebrows (Fig. **1**). It is usually convex, and its shape is dictated by the shape of the frontal bone and conveyance of subcutaneous and sub-muscular fat cushions. There is a prominence between the eyebrows called the **glabella.** The root of the nose lies inferior to the glabellain the midline, over the **frontonasal** suture. The nose projects anteriorly and inferiorly from the **nasion,** or deepest part at the root, to the **pronasale**. The widest part of the nose consists of the **alae, or nostrils**, which lead into the nasal vestibule. Between the alae of the nose and the lateral borders of the lip, the **nasiolabial groove or fold** separates the upper lip from the cheek. The **columella** connects the nose to the **philtrum** of the cutaneous upper lip. The junction of the red part of the lips with the skin is the **vermillion border**. The **labiomental groove** passes between the lower lip and the chin [9, 10].

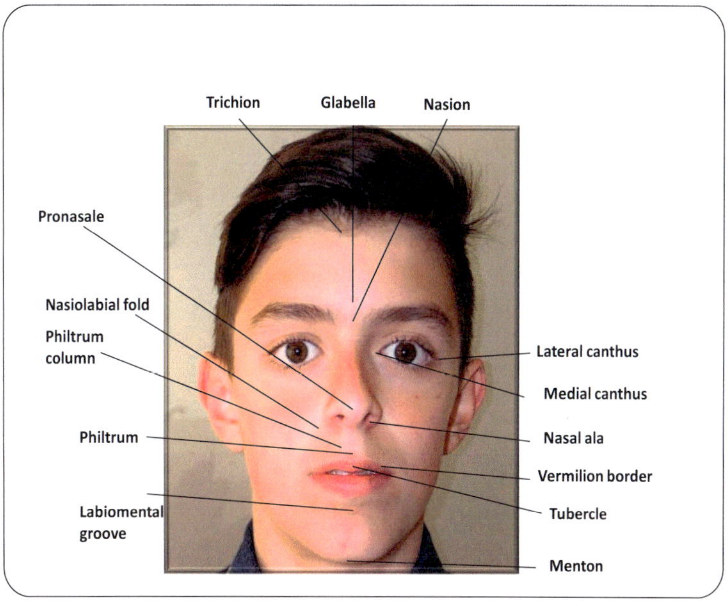

Fig. (1). Soft tissue points in the frontal facial view.

6. Describe the Assessment of the Transverse Dimension in the Frontal Facial Figures

Assess the Facial Asymmetry (Fig. **2**). A line drawn through from the trichion (**Tr**) through glabella (**G**), pronasale (**Pn**), midpoint of the upper lip filtrum (**F**) and the soft tissue menton (**Me**). The maxillary and the mandibular dental midlines should be evaluated in relation to the facial midline and whether they are coincident each other [5 - 7, 9]. The discrepancy between the right and left sides could be due to an asymmetry:

a. In the dentition
b. In the skeleton
c. Both

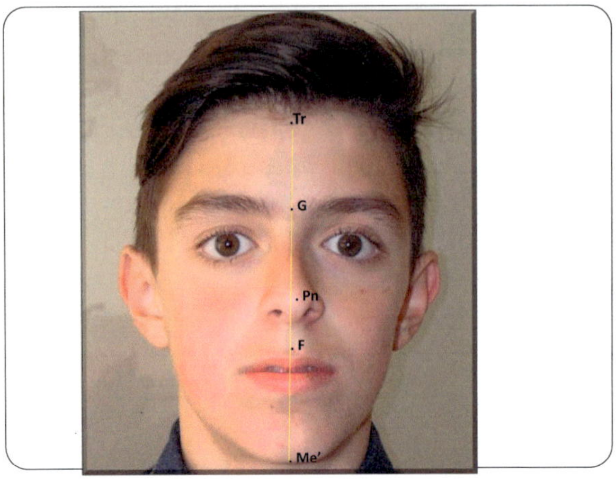

Fig. (2). Facial asymmetry.

Frontal Facial Analysis (Fig. **3**). This method analyses the height **(**Trichion to soft tissue Menton) relative to the bizygomatic (Za-Za) or bigonial width (Go-Go) of the face. Ideally, the facial height to bizygomatic widthshould be **1.35:1 in males** and **1.3:1 to females**. The bigonial width should be approximately 30% less than the bizygomatic width [5, 11].

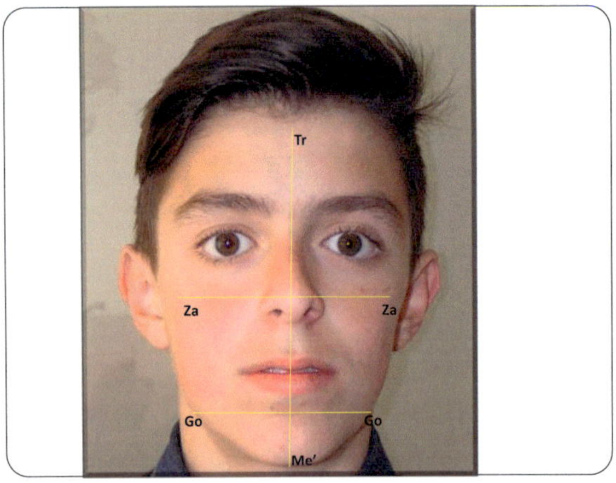

Fig. (3). Frontal facial analysis.

'Rule of fifths' (Fig. **4**) to evaluate the transverse facial proportions; the face is divided into five equal parts, and each of the parts should be approximately the width of the eye [5, 10, 11]. Prominent ears have an important effect on facial proportions and the width of the alar base is influenced by ethnic characteristics [7].

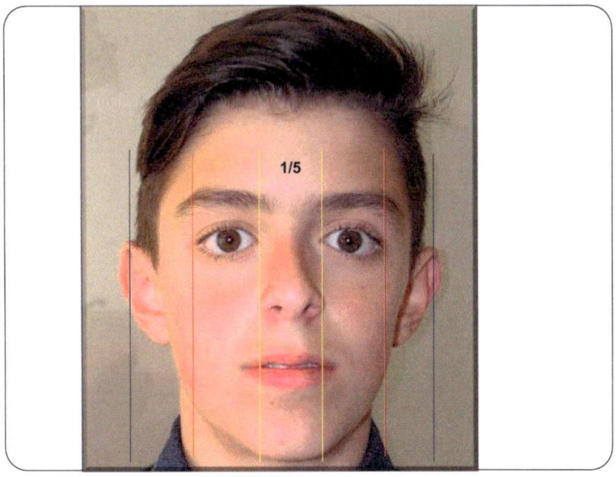

Fig. (4). Rule of fifths.

Table 1. Ideal proportions based on the 'rule of fifths'.

Vertical lines drawn through the outer canthus of the eyes should coincide with the gonial angles of the mandible
Vertical lines drawn through the medial canthus should coincide with the alar base of the nose and
The inter-pupillar distance should be equal to the width of the mouth

7. Describe the Vertical Assessment in the Frontal Facial Figures

'Rule of thirds' to evaluate the vertical facial proportions (Fig. **5**). The ideal face is divided into equal thirds by drawing horizontal lines through the trichion (Tr), glabella (G), subnasale (Sn) and soft tissue menton (Me). The middle face (glabella-subnasale) should be approximately equal to the lower third (subnasale-menton). The lower third can be subdivided into an upper third (commisure/lip height) and lower two-thirds [1, 2, 5, 11].

An ideally proportioned face can be divided into central, medial, and lateral equal fifths, and superior, middle, and inferior facial thirds.

8. Explain the Upper Lip Position in the Next Figures

The upper lip length (**Sn to Ls**) should be almost equal to the commissure's height. The philtrum height should be 2 to 3mm less than the commissure's height because the lip lengthening continues even after vertical skeletal growth is completed [12 - 14]. The upper lip length is 20 ± 2mm for females and 22 ± 2mm for males (Sn to Ls). However, the clinical significant part is not the linear measurement but the relationship of the upper lip length or the philtrum height to the commissure's height of the mouth (Fig. **6**). An extremely short upper lip relative to the commissure height results in a reverse-resting upper lip line (Fig. **7**) [14].

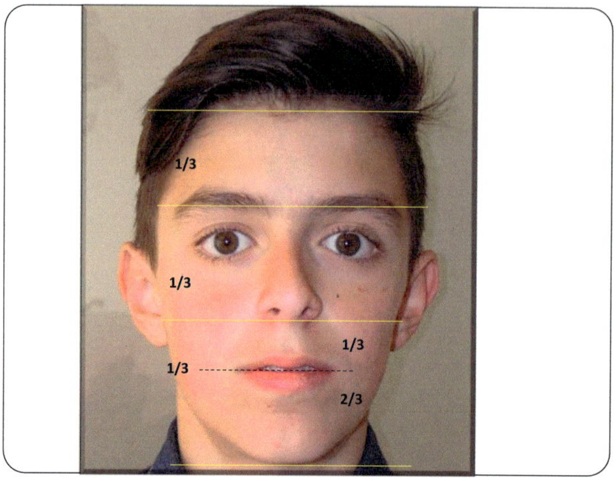

Fig. (5). Rule of thirds.

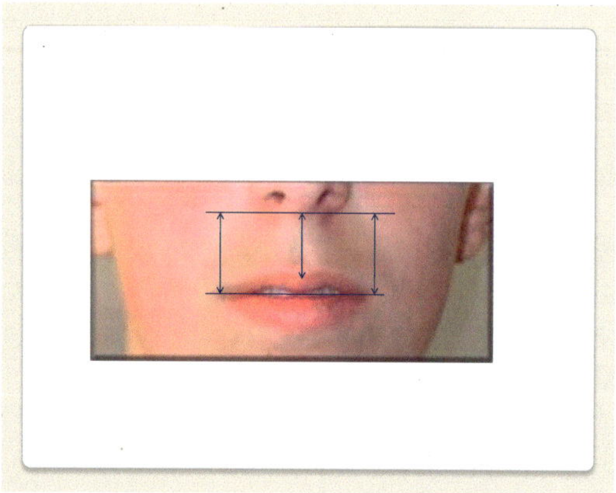

Fig. (6). Normal upper lip length (Sn to Ls).

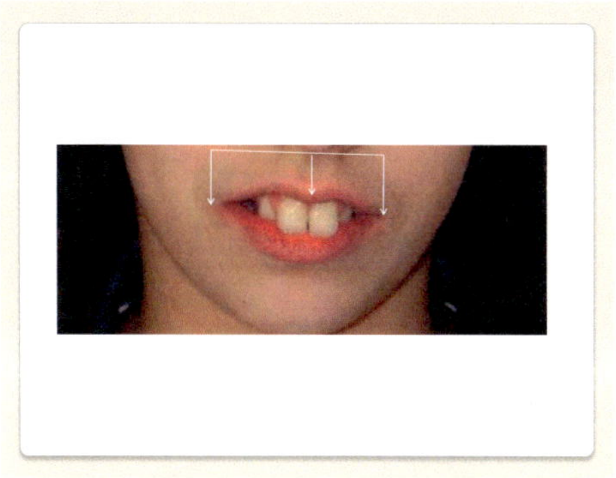

Fig. (7). Short upper lip length.

9. Describe the Three Basic Parameters to Evaluate when Analysing the Smile Photograph

a. Smile arc or smile line
b. Gingival/tooth display
c. Transverse smile.

10. What exactly is The Smile Arc? Could you Describe the Smile Arc in the Following Pictures?

Smile arc is the relationship of the curvature of the incisal edges of the maxillary teeth to the curvature of the lower lip in the smile. The smile arc could be consonant (Fig. **8**), flat (Fig. **9**) or reverse (Fig. **10**) [14 - 16].

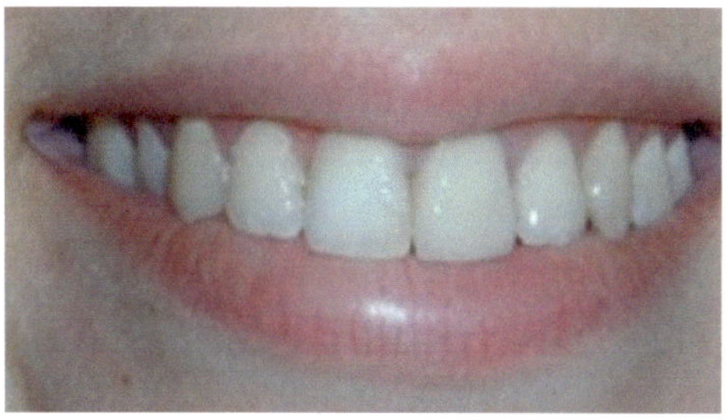

Fig. (8). The *consonant smile arc* is defined by the parallel curvature of the maxillary incisal edges and the curvature of the lower lip.

11. What is the Ideal Gingival- Upper Tooth Display Ratio? Which Factors Determine the Amount of Tooth Exposure?

The ideal tooth exposure when smiling is the full tooth crown to 2mm of gingiva.

The amount of upper tooth display is influenced by many factors [14 - 16] such as:

a. Upper lip length
b. Vertical maxillary length
c. Lip thickness
d. Crown height
e. Torque value of the upper teeth.

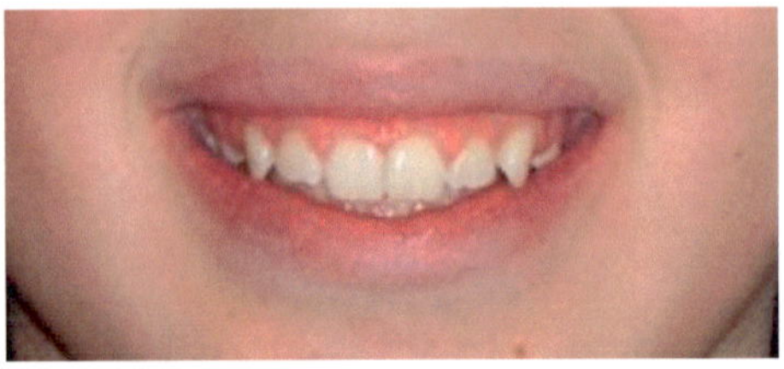

Fig. (9). *The flat smile arc* is characterized by the flat maxillary incisor curvature relative to the curvature of the lower lip.

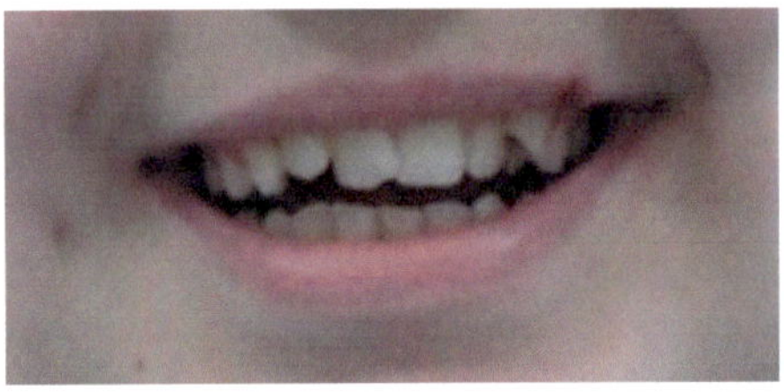

Fig. (10). *The* reverse smile arc is characterized by the concave maxillary incisor curvature relative to the curvature of the lower lip.

12. Which Factors Determine Anexcessive Amount of Gingival Display in "Gummy Smiling" and "Low" Smiling Line?

An excessive amount of gingival display during smiling (Fig. **11**) could be the result of *vertical maxillary excess, short upper lip and/or philtrum, lingual tipped incisors and excessive upper lip animation.*

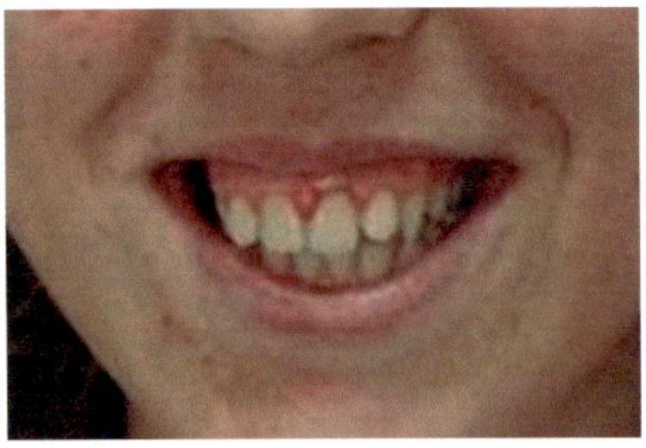

Fig. (11). Gummy smile.

Conversely, a low smiling line with no upper incisor display during smiling (Fig. **12**) *is "skeletal" and associated with inadequate lower facial height due to a vertically deficient maxilla* [14 - 16].

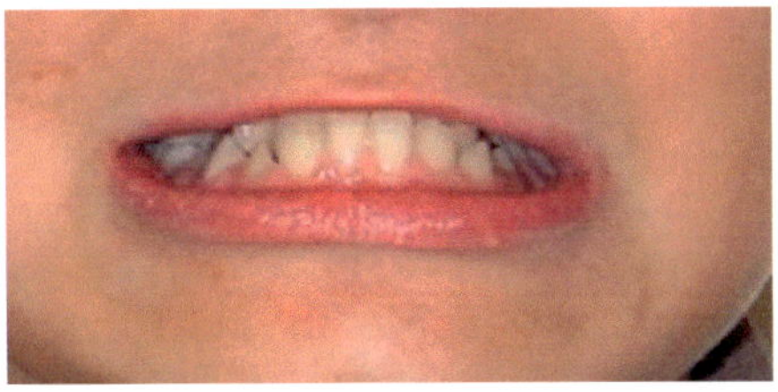

Fig. (12). Low smiling line.

13. Why is the Lower Lip Line Important?

Because the lower lip line describes the vertical relationship between the lower lip and maxillary incisors at rest. Ideally, the lower lip is seated to the middle third of the maxillary incisor [15 - 18]. The lips could be characterised as:

- **Competent** if a lip seal is produced with minimum effort in the rest position.
- **Potential competent** if a lip seal could be produced after correction of the position of the maxillary incisors.
- **Incompetent** when a lip seal could be produced after excessive mentalis contraction and flattening of the labiomental fold.

14. Which Factors Influence the Lip Competency?

- Increased lower anterior facial height
- Mandibular retrognathic position
- Proclined maxillary incisors
- Short upper lip [15 - 18].

15. What Factors Affect the Transverse Smile?

In smiling, the width of the mouth increases by as much as 30%; therefore, an excessive transverse lip extension in smiling would theoretically produce a wider buccal corridor [14 - 16].

Several factors affect the transverse smile such as:

a. Arch form and arch width. Increasing arch width will decrease the dark corridors.
b. Anteroposterior position of the maxilla. The more forward the maxilla, the less the dark corridors.
c. Transverse cant of the maxillary occlusal plane (inclination of molars/premolars).
d. Thickness of the buccal soft tissues.

PART B. PROFILE FACIAL ANALYSIS

1. Why is the Facial Profile Analysis Required?

Profile facial photos enable two-dimensional soft tissue analysis in horizontal and vertical planes for the purposes of evaluating facial asymmetries and soft tissue characteristics. The facial profile analysis gives the clinician an immediate impression of the patient's facial harmony and aesthetics as well as the underlying dental and skeletal structure [19 - 22]. It is important to assess the patient in the natural head position. The relationship of the mandible relative to the maxilla can be classified (Fig. **13**) as:

- **Class I**. When the mandible lies 2-3mm behind the maxilla.
- **Class II**. When the mandible is retrusive relative to the maxilla.
- **Class III**. When the mandible is protrusive relative to the maxilla.

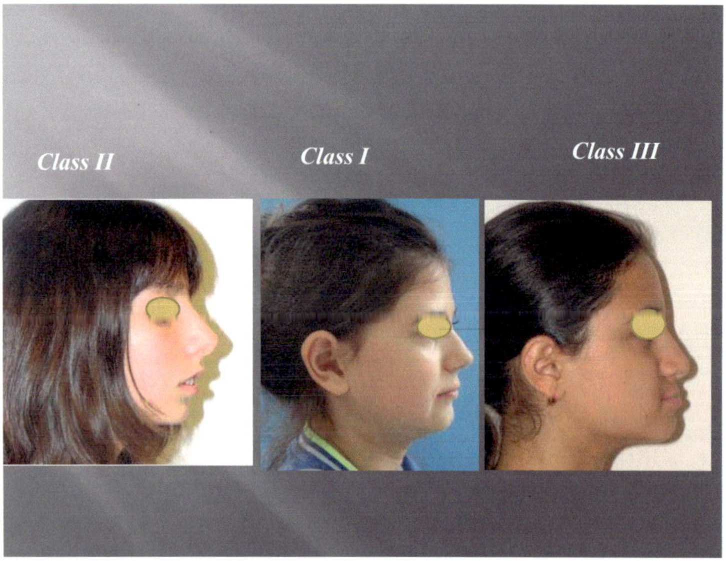

Fig. (13). Profile facial photos.

2. Which Arc thc Important Soft Tissue Points in Profile Analysis?

The important soft tissue landmarks (Fig. **14**) [5, 10] are:

- The glabella (G) is the most prominent part in the midline between the brows.
- The soft tissue nasion (N′) lies at the root of the nose in the midline.
- The pronasale (Pn) is the most anterior part of the nose.
- The subnasale (Sn) is the junction of the columella and upper cutaneous lip.
- The labrale superior labrum (Ls) is the junction of the red and cutaneous parts of

the lip at the vermilion border in the midline.

- The stomion (St) is the point where the lips meet in the midline.
- The inferior labrum (Li) is the point in the midline of the lower lip at the vermilion border.
- The supramentale (Sm) is the midpoint of the labiomental crease between the lower lip and chin.
- The soft tissue pogonion (Pog') is the most anterior point of the chin.
- The soft tissue menton (Me') is the most inferior point of the chin.

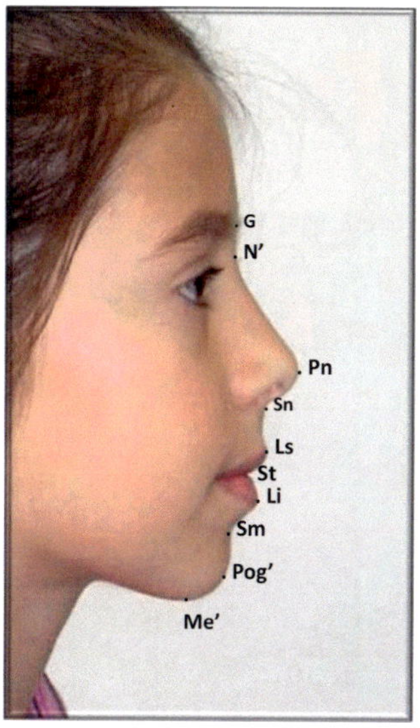

Fig. (14). Facial profile landmarks.

3. Describe the Soft Tissue Planes

The facial planes (Fig. **15**) [5, 10, 17] are:

- Facial plane: Extends from soft tissue nasion to soft tissue pogonion
- Upper facial plane: Extends from glabella to subnasale
- Lower facial plane: Extends from subnasale to soft tissue pogonion
- Aesthetic plane (E-line): Extends from the soft tissue pogonion to pronasale.

4. Describe the Soft Tissue Sagittal Angles in the Following Pictures

Angle of Facial Contour (Fig. **16**) (facial convexity or facial concavity, Fig. **17**) is formed by the line from glabella (**G**) to subnasale (**Sn**) and by the line from subnasale (**Sn**) to soft tissue pogonion **Pog′** [19 - 24]. The facial contour measurement *does not reveal* the localization of the deformity.

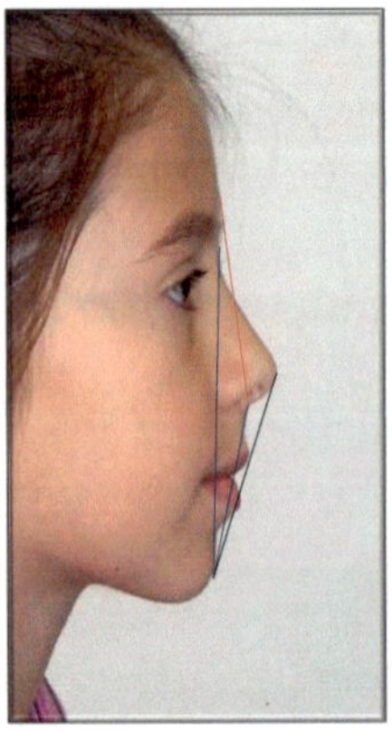

Fig. (15). Facial profile planes.

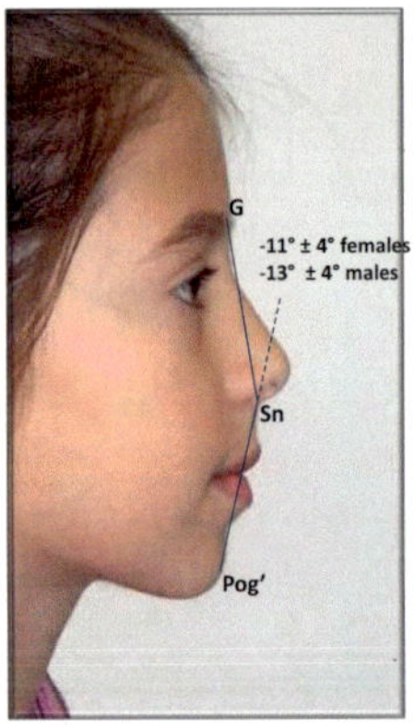

Fig. (16). Angle of Facial Contour.

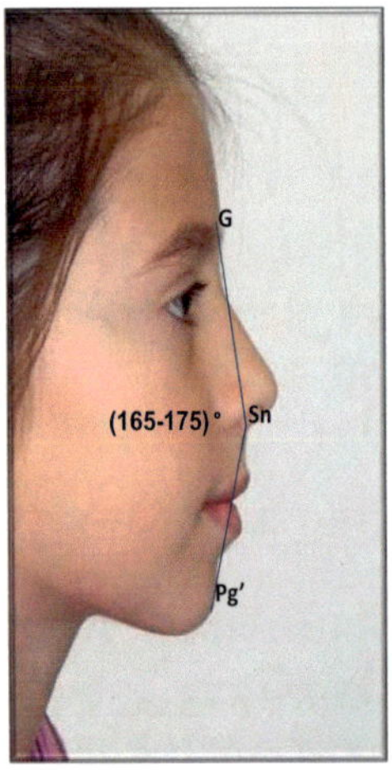

Fig. (17). Angle of Facial Convexity.

a. The line **G— Sn** is known as **upper facial plane.**
b. The line **Sn — Pog′** is Known **as lower facial plane**.
c. The facial contour angle is (-11 ± 4)° for males and (-13 ± 4)° for females.

- Class I profile: (165–175)°
- Class II profile: ≤ 165 °
- Class III profile: ≥ 175°

Nasiolabial angle. It is measured between the inclination of the upper lip and the columella (Fig. **18**). The angle is more acute in males and incisor protruded cases. Where crowding necessitates upper premolar extraction, the nasiolabial angle could determine the decision to extract first *versus* second [14, 23, 25].

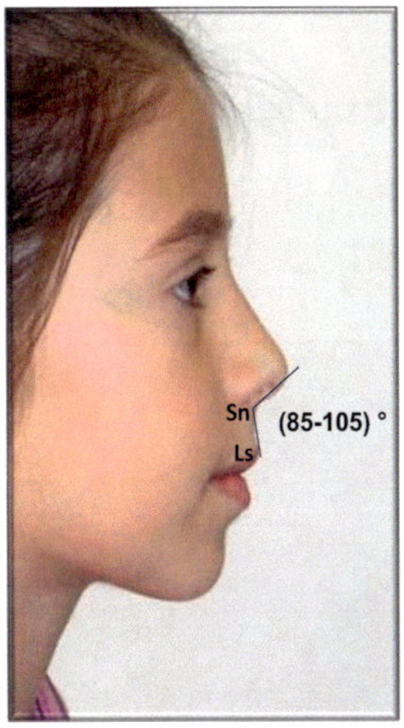

Fig. (18). Nasiolabial angle.

The nasiolabial angle is influenced by:

a. Maxillary incisor-upper lip support
b. Inclination of the columella
c. Lip thickness. Thick lips respond less than thin lips to tooth movement
d. Strained lips. Move posterior once tension has been released
e. Magnitude of the dental overjet

Merrifield's Z-angle. Merrifield's Z-angle is formed (Fig. **19**) by the intersection of Frankfort Horizontal (**FH**) and a line connecting the soft tissue pogonion (**Pg ′**) and the most prominent lip [10]. A Z-angle greater than 80° indicates an excessive mandible whereas a Z-angle less than 80° indicates a deficient mandible [26].

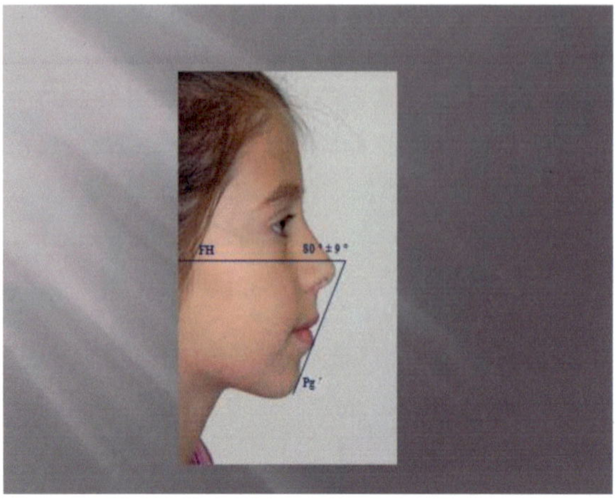

Fig. (19). Merrifield's Z-angle.

5. Describe the Soft Tissue Sagittal Measurements in the Next Pictures

A vertical line drawn through the glabella (**G′**). Subnasale (**Sn**) should be 6 ± 3 mm ahead of this line. Soft tissue pogonion (**Pog′**) should be 1 ± 4mm behind this line (Fig. **20**).

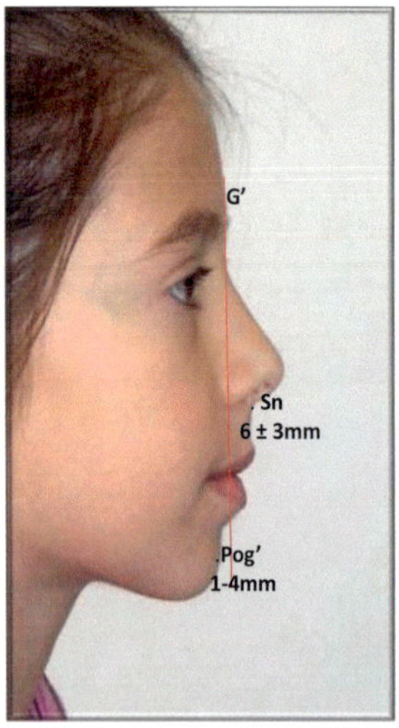

Fig. (20). Maxillary and mandibular anteroposterior position.

Lower facial plane (Fig. **21**): Subnasale (**Sn**) - soft tissue Pogonion (**Pog′**) line. The distance of the labrale superior (**Ls**) and the labrale inferior (**Li**) to this line should be 3 ± 1mm and 2 ± 1mm, respectively (Fig. **9**). These measurements determine the lip prominence. A change in soft tissue Pogonion (**Pog′**) position results in a change in the lip position relative to the Sn-Pog′ line. The labrale inferior (**Li**) could be more forward of the lower facial plane in an individual with mandibular anterior-posterior deficiency and more behind the lower facial plane line in an individual with mandibular prognathism [21 - 23, 27].

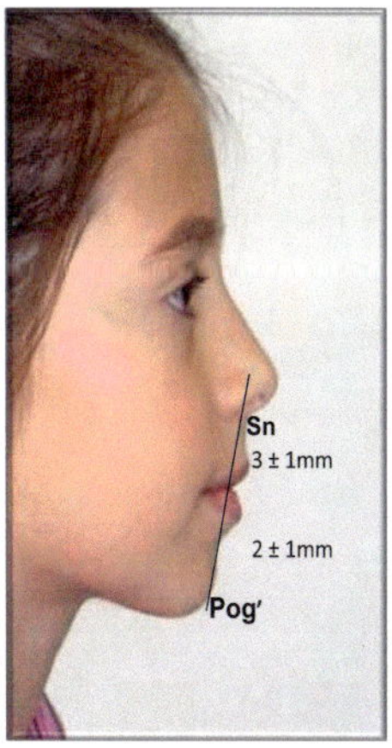

Fig. (21). Lower facial plane.

E-line (Ricketts). Pronasale (**Pn**) to soft tissue pogonion (**Pg′**). The Labrale superior (**Ls**) should lie behind the line about 4mm and the Labrale inferior (**Li**) should be behind about 2mm (Fig. **22**) [17].

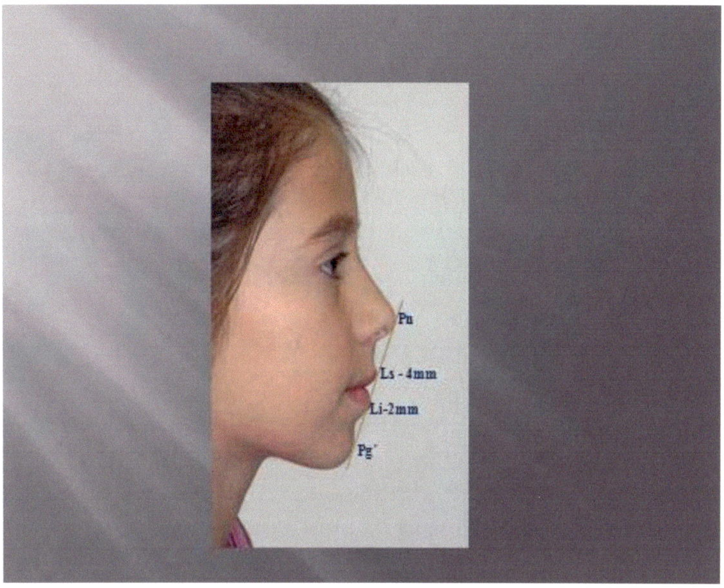

Fig. (22). E-line.

6. Describe the Soft Tissue Vertical Profile Evaluation in the Following Figures

- Soft tissue Nasion (**Na′**) to Subnasale **(Sn)**: **Middle third facial height.**
- Subnasale (**Sn**) to soft tissue Menton (**Me′**)**: Lower third facial height**.

The ratio should be approximately 45/55%. In most orthognathic cases, abnormalities are in the lower third of the face [5, 14] (Fig. **23**).

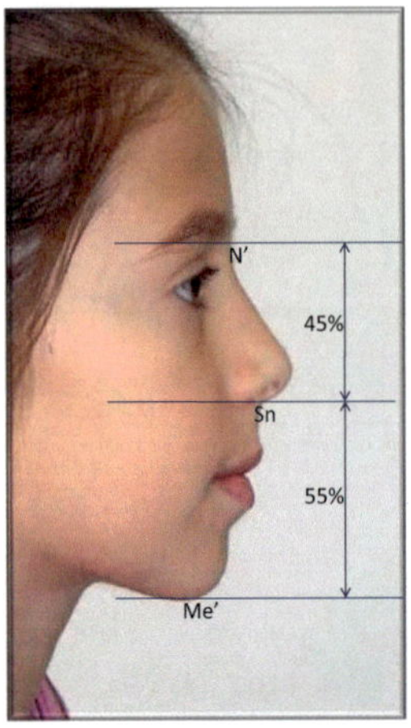

Fig. (23). Vertical profile evaluation.

The lower third face (Fig. **24**) increased in:

a. Vertical maxillary excess
b. Mandibular anterior height excess.

The lower third face decreased:

a. Vertical maxillary deficiency
b. Vertical deficiency of the anterior mandibular height
c. Dental deep-bite
   - The upper lip length (ULL): Subnasale (**Sn**) to labrale superior (**Ls**).
   - The lower lip and chin length (LLL): Labrale inferior **(Li)** to soft tissue Menton (**Me′**).
   - The ratio of the ULL/LLL should be approximately **½.**
   - When the patients' lips are relaxed, 0-4mm should be visible under the upper lip.

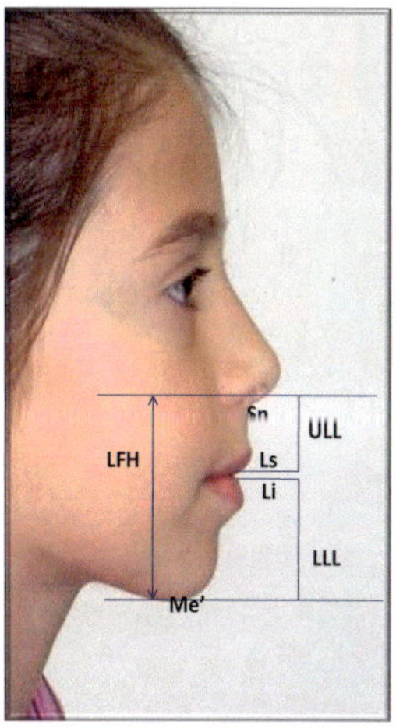

Fig. (24). Lower *third* profile evaluation

PART C. CLINICAL EXAMPLES

Assess the Extra-Oral Features (Figs. 25-29)

Patient 1

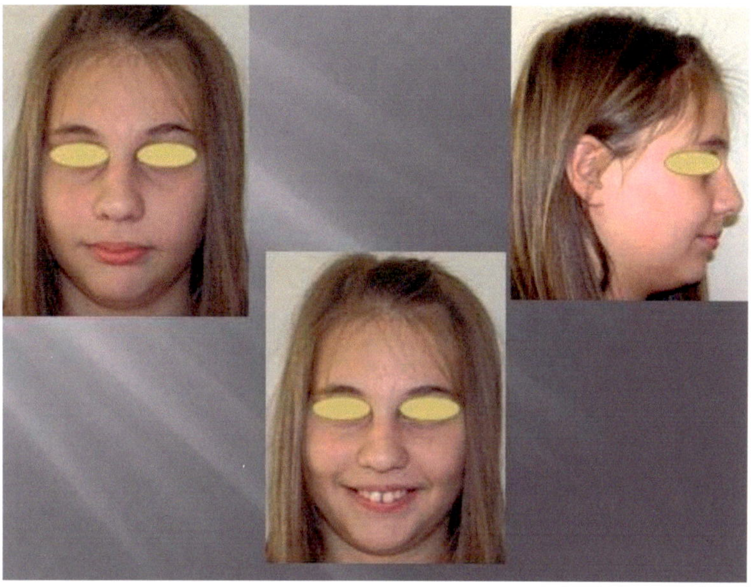

Fig. (25). Frontal, Smiling, Profile.

Frontal View

- Symmetrical face
- Broad alar base and nostrils
- An everted lower lip
- A deep labiomental fold
- A week (double) chin
- Sub-mental fat deposition

Smiling Evaluation

- Consonant smile arc with dark corridors
- 100% of the maxillary incisors was exposed on smile, so there was no vertical maxillary deficiency

Profile View

- A convcx profilc
- Normal nasiolabial angle
- A curled lower lip
- An acute labiomental fold
- A deficient chin
- A short chin to throat length
- An obtuse lower lip to chin-throat angle

Patient 2

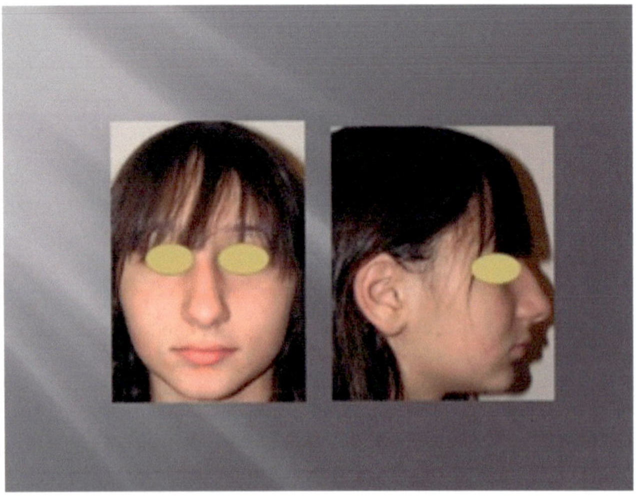

Fig. (26). Frontal, Profile.

Frontal View

- Short lower face
- Broad mandible
- Accentuated mentiolabial sulcus
- Everted lower lip
- Well-developed elevator muscles

Profile View

- Prominent nose
- Strong chin
- Short lower facial height and low mandibular plane angle
- Deep labiomental fold
- Curled lower lip

Patient 3

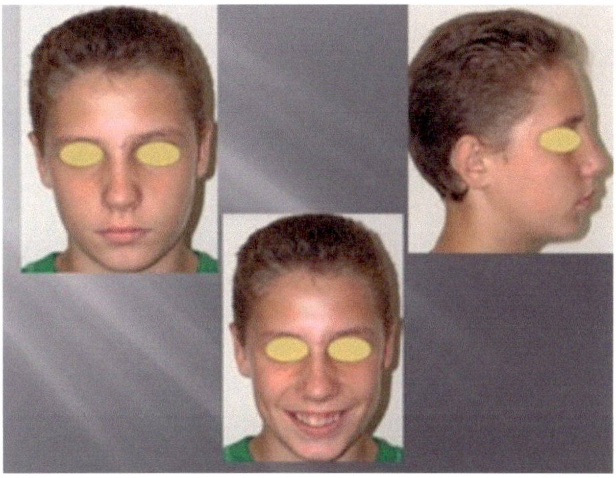

Fig. (27). Frontal, Smiling, Profile.

Frontal View

- Symmetrical face
- Competent lips
- Short lower facial height
- Deep labiomental sulcus
- Slightly everted lower lip

Smile Evaluation

- Gummy smile

Profile View

- Normal nose
- Obtuse nasiolabial angle
- Short lower third of the face
- Retruded mandible
- Slightly everted lower lip

Patient 4

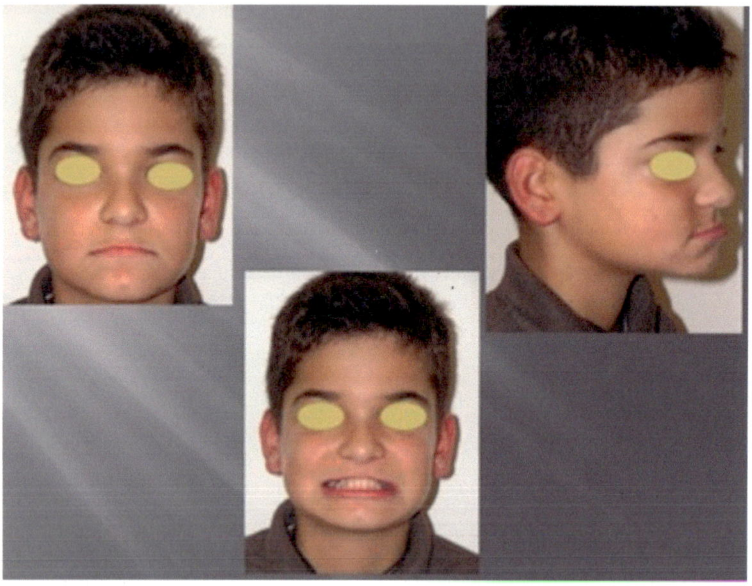

Fig. (28). Frontal, Smiling, Profile.

Frontal View

- Square face with exaggerated masseter muscles
- Midface deficiency
- Vertical deficient maxilla
- Para-nasal flattening
- Flat and thin upper lip. Thin vermillion.
- Corners of the mouth turned down
- Mandible appears excessive

Smiling Evaluation

- Short upper lip
- Allow lip line with no upper incisor display (vertically deficient maxilla)

Profile

- Concave profile
- Short lower and middle third of the face
- Lack of upper lip support
- Chin appears excessive
- Lower lip in front of the upper lip
- Acute nasiolabial angle
- Obtuse labiomental angle

Patient 5

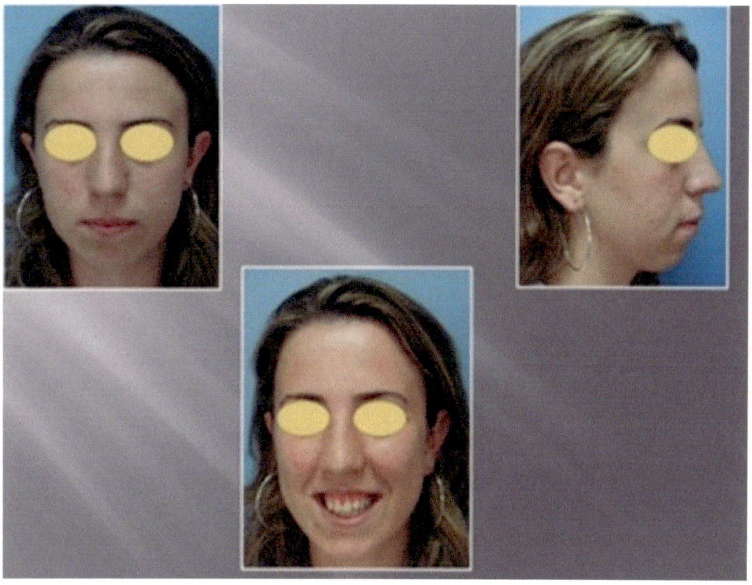

Fig. (29). Frontal, Smiling, Profile.

Frontal View

- Narrow alar base
- Long face because of the excessive lower third of the face
- Lip strain (better seen on the profile view)

Smile Evaluation

- Vertical maxillary excess
- Gummy smile
- Dark corridors

Profile View

- Increase facial height
- Convex profile
- Mandible rotated downward and backward
- Lip strain
- Protruded both lips relative to chin

CONCLUDING REMARKS

If we accept that dental and facial attractiveness represents an important element of quality of life for patients seeking orthodontic treatment, facial analysis plays an important role in orthodontic diagnosis as it shows vertical and horizontal facial proportions, the position of jaws, lip posture and prominence, tooth position and gingiva appearance, nose prominence and mandibular/maxilla relationship. Although facial proportions and contours vary with age, sex, and race, the clinical assessment of the face is probably the most important of all the diagnostic procedures.

REFERENCES

[1] Arnett GW, Bergman RT. Facial keys to orthodontic diagnosis and treatment planning. Part I. Am J Orthod Dentofacial Orthop 1993; 103(4): 299-312. [http://dx.doi.org/10.1016/0889-5406(93)70010-L] [PMID: 8480695]

[2] Arnett GW, Bergman RT. Facial keys to orthodontic diagnosis and treatment planning--Part II. Am J Orthod Dentofacial Orthop 1993; 103(5): 395-411. [http://dx.doi.org/10.1016/S0889-5406(05)81791-3] [PMID: 8480709]

[3] Bell WH. Modern practice in orthognathic and reconstructive surgery. WB Saunder 1992; 3: 2439-88.

[4] Biller JA, Kim DW. A contemporary assessment of facial aesthetic preferences. Arch Facial Plast Surg 2009; 11(2): 91-7. [http://dx.doi.org/10.1001/archfacial.2008.543] [PMID: 19289680]

[5] Sarver DM, Proffit WR, Ackerman JL. Evaluation of facial soft tissues.Contemporary Treatment of Dentofacial Deformity. St Louis, Mo: CV Mosby 2004; pp. 92-126.

[6] Farkas LG, Hreczko TA, Kolar JC, Munro IR. Vertical and horizontal proportions of the face in young adult North American Caucasians: revision of neoclassical canons. Plast Reconstr Surg 1985; 75(3): 328-38. [http://dx.doi.org/10.1097/00006534-198503000-00005] [PMID: 3883374]

[7] Iglesias-Linares A, Yáñez-Vico RM, Moreno-Manteca B, Moreno-Fernández AM, Mendoza-Mendoza A, Solano-Reina E. Common standards in facial esthetics: craniofacial analysis of most attractive black and white subjects according to People magazine during previous 10 years. J Oral Maxillofac Surg 2011; 69(6): e216-24. [http://dx.doi.org/10.1016/j.joms.2010.12.052] [PMID: 21470749]

[8] Riolo ML, Moyers RE, Ten Have TR, Mayers CA. Facial soft tissue changes during adolescencein Craniofacial Growth during Adolescence, D S Carlson and K A Ribbens, Eds, Monograph 20, Craniofacial Growth Series, Center for Human Growth and Development, University of Michigan, Ann Arbor, Mich, USA. 1987.

[9] Grummons DC, Kappeyne van de Coppello MA. A frontal asymmetry analysis. J Clin Orthod 1987; 21(7): 448-65.
[PMID: 3476493]

[10] Arnett GW, Jelic JS, Kim J, *et al.* Soft tissue cephalometric analysis: diagnosis and treatment planning of dentofacial deformity. Am J Orthod Dentofacial Orthop 1999; 116(3): 239-53.
[http://dx.doi.org/10.1016/S0889-5406(99)70234-9] [PMID: 10474095]

[11] Baker BW, Woods MG. The role of the divine proportion in the esthetic improvement of patients undergoing combined orthodontic/orthognathic surgical treatment. Int J Adult Orthodon Orthognath Surg 2001; 16(2): 108-20.
[PMID: 11482289]

[12] Burstone CJ. Lip posture and its significance in treatment planning. Am J Orthod 1967; 53(4): 262-84.
[http://dx.doi.org/10.1016/0002-9416(67)90022-X] [PMID: 5227460]

[13] Zachrisson BU. Esthetic factors involved in anterior tooth display and the smile: Vertical dimension. J Clin Orthod 1998; 32: 432-45.

[14] Proffit WR, Fields HM, Sarver DM. Contemporary Orthodontics. 5th ed., St Louis, Missouri, United States: Mosby 2013.

[15] Sarver DM. The importance of incisor positioning in the esthetic smile: the smile arc. Am J Orthod Dentofacial Orthop 2001; 120(2): 98-111.
[http://dx.doi.org/10.1067/mod.2001.114301] [PMID: 11500650]

[16] Sarver DM, Ackerman MB. Dynamic smile visualization and quantification: Part 2. Smile analysis and treatment strategies. Am J Orthod Dentofacial Orthop 2003; 124(2): 116-27.
[http://dx.doi.org/10.1016/S0889-5406(03)00307-X] [PMID: 12923505]

[17] Ricketts RM. Esthetics, environment, and the law of lip relation. Am J Orthod 1968; 54(4): 272-89.
[http://dx.doi.org/10.1016/S0002-9416(68)90278-9] [PMID: 5238879]

[18] Riedel RA. Esthetics and its relation to orthodontic therapy. Angle Orthod 1950; 20(3): 168-78.
[PMID: 14790327]

[19] Legan HL, Burstone CJ. Soft tissue cephalometric analysis for orthognathic surgery. J Oral Surg 1980; 38(10): 744-51.
[PMID: 6932485]

[20] Spradley FL, Jacobs JD, Crowe DP. Assessment of the anteroposterior soft-tissue contour of the lower facial third in the ideal young adult. Am J Orthod 1981; 79(3): 316-25.
[http://dx.doi.org/10.1016/0002-9416(81)90079-8] [PMID: 6938139]

[21] Holdaway RA. A soft-tissue cephalometric analysis and its use in orthodontic treatment planning. Part I. Am J Orthod 1983; 84(1): 1-28.
[http://dx.doi.org/10.1016/0002-9416(83)90144-6] [PMID: 6575614]

[22] Holdaway RA. A soft-tissue cephalometric analysis and its use in orthodontic treatment planning. Part II. Am J Orthod 1984; 85(4): 279-93.
[http://dx.doi.org/10.1016/0002-9416(84)90185-4] [PMID: 6585146]

[23] Burstone CJ. The integumental profile. Am J Orthod 1958; (44): 1-25.
[http://dx.doi.org/10.1016/S0002-9416(58)90178-7]

[24] Jacobson A. The “Wits” appraisal of jaw disharmony. Am J Orthod 1975; 67(2): 125-38.
[http://dx.doi.org/10.1016/0002-9416(75)90065-2] [PMID: 1054214]

[25] Chaconas SJ. A statistical evaluation of nasal growth. Am J Orthod 1969; 56(4): 403-14.
[http://dx.doi.org/10.1016/S0002-9416(69)80007-2] [PMID: 5258936]

[26] Merrifield LL. The profile line as an aid in critically evaluating facial esthetics. Am J Orthod 1966; 52(11): 804-22.

[http://dx.doi.org/10.1016/0002-9416(66)90250-8] [PMID: 5223046]

[27] Chaconas SJ, Bartroff JD. Prediction of normal soft tissue facial changes. Angle Orthod 1975; 45(1): 12-25.
[PMID: 1054930]

CHAPTER 3

Hard Tissue Evaluation and Dental Relationship Assessment

Abstract: It is important to understand the aetiology of malocclusion so that orthodontic treatments can focus on the prevention of these conditions. Angle was the first to develop a simple dental relationship assessment based on the sagittal relationship between the upper and lower permanent molars. Since the introduction of cephalometric radiographs, hard tissue evaluation through cephalometric analysis has become an integral part of orthodontic treatment planning because it provides information such as the skeletal size, position, proportion and symmetry of the individual by which it is possible to assess skeletal disharmonies. The diagnosis of skeletal and dental relationships and their contributions to orthodontic treatment will be addressed in this chapter.

Keywords: Cephalometric analysis, Cone beam computed tomography, Dental relationships, Linear and angular measurements.

INTRODUCTION

Lateral cephalometric analysis is used on many occasions for clinical diagnosis, treatment and teaching purposes. Linear and angular measurements performed on lateral cephalometric radiographs are important for the evaluation of severe skeletal malocclusions and for the planning of orthodontic appliances; they remain the standard method in clinical routine until today. Although the real value of cephalometric analysis for the diagnosis and planning of orthodontic treatment remains uncertain, many authors agree that an adequate orthodontic diagnosis and treatment plan could not be performed without comparing a lateral cephalometric radiograph before and after orthodontic treatment. Moreover, by assessing skeletal and dental relationships, it allows for the diagnosis and monitoring of various growth and development abnormalities.

George Litsas

PART A. CEPHALOMETRIC ANALYSIS

1. List the Goals of Cephalometric Analysis in Paediatric Orthodontics

The goals of cephalometric analysis [1 - 3] are:

a. To evaluate dentofacial proportions and clarify the anatomic basis of diagnosis of malocclusion,
b. To evaluate the horizontal and vertical relationship of cranial base, maxilla, mandible, maxillary and mandibular dentition,
c. To identify the growth pattern and direction of growth,
d. To guide in treatment planning possibilities and limitations,
e. To predict the consequences of treatment plan in the hard and soft tissues

According to our opinion, the most important purpose of the cephalometric analysis is to differentiate between skeletal and dento-alveolar malocclusions in order to apply the proper treatment planning.

2. Which Are the Four Types of Cephalometric Landmark Points?

The four types of cephalometric landmark points [1, 3] are:

- *Anatomic:* Represent actual anatomic structures.
- *Derived:* Construct points from anatomical structures.
- *Single:* From structures fall in the Midsagittal plane (*e.g*. Sella).
- *Double:* From structures occurring in both sides of the face (*e.g*. Orbitale, Porion, Articulare)

3. Describe the Cephalometric Hard Tissue Landmark Points

The most frequently hard tissue landmarks (Fig. **1**) [1, 3, 5 - 10] are:

- Sella (**S**): The point representing the midpoint of the pituitary fossa or sella turcica. It is a constructed point.
- Nasion (**N**): The most anterior point of the junction of the nasal and frontal bones.
- Orbitale (**Or**): Lowest point in the inferior margin of the orbit.
- Porion (**Po**): The midpoint of the upper contour of the external auditory canal (Anatomic Porion).
- Articulare (**Ar**): A point at the intersection of mandibular ramus with the basilar portion of the occipital bone.
- Anterior Nasal Spine (**ANS**): The most anterior point on the maxilla at the nasal base.
- Posterior Nasal Spine (**PNS**): The junction of the anterior wall of the

pterygomaxillary fissure and the nasal flore.

- A-point (**A**): The deepest point in the midline between anterior nasal spine and the crest of the maxillary alveolar process.
- (**U1A**): Maxillary central incisor root tip.
- B-point (**B**): The innermost curvature from chin to alveolar junction. It is located on the anterior bony curvature of the mandible.
- (**L1A**): Mandibular central incisor root tip
- Pogonion (**Pg**): The most anterior point of the mandibular symphysis
- Menton (**Me**): The lowest point on the mandibular symphysis.
- Gnathion (**Gn**): Located midway between pogonion and menton. The most outward point on the curvature of the mandibular symphysis.
- Gonion (**Go**): Constructed point at the junction of ramus and the mandibular plane.
- Basion (**Ba**): The median point of the anterior margin of the foramen magnum.
- Pterygomaxillary fissure (**Ptm**): The posterior border of the tuberosity of the maxilla.

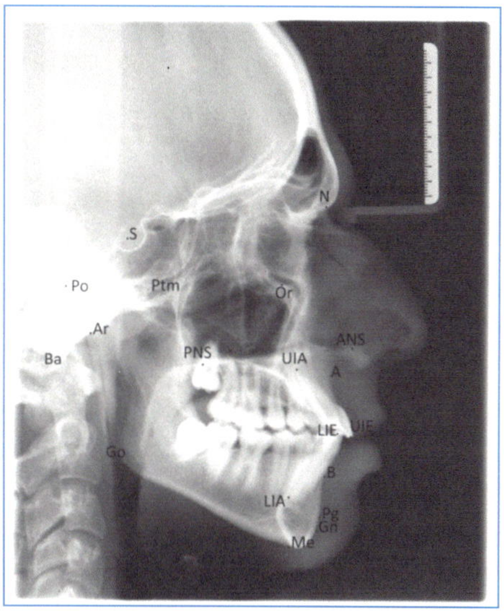

Fig. (1). Hard tissue landmarks.

4. What is the Reference Plane in the Lateral Cephalometric Radiograph? Provide the Most Frequently Used Reference Planes in the Cephalometric Analysis

The reference planes (Fig. **2**) are defined as a straight line connecting two landmarks.

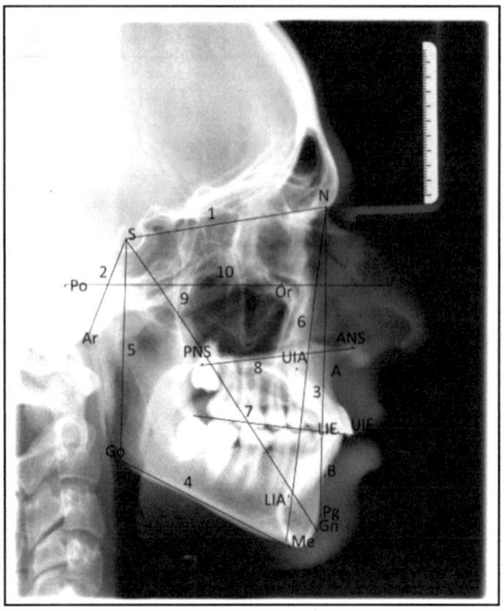

Fig. (2). Reference planes.

The most frequently reference planes [1, 3, 5 - 10] are:

1. *Anterior cranial base*: a line connecting sella **(S)** to nasion **(Na)**.
2. *Lateral cranial base*: a line connecting sella **(S)** to articulare **(Ar)**.
3. *Facial depth*: a line connecting nasion **(Na)** to Pogonion **(Pg)**.
4. *Mandibular plane*: a line connecting gonion **(Go)** to menton **(Me)**.
5. *Posterior facial height*: a line connecting sella **(S)** to gonion **(Go)**.
6. *Anterior facial height*: a line connecting nasion **(Na)** to menton **(Me)**.
7. *Occlusal plane*: a line connecting the midpoint of the anterior overbite and the most distal point of contact between the most posterior molars in occlusion.
8. *Palatal plane (PP)*: a line connecting anterior nasal spine **(ANS)** to posterior nasal spine **(PNS)**.
9. *Y-axis (Y)*: a line connecting sella **(S)** to pogonion **(Pg)** or gnathion **(Gn)**.
10. *Frankfort Horizontal*: a line connecting Porion **(Po)** to Orbitale **(Or)**.

5. Could You Name the Main Sources of Cephalometric Analysis Errors?

- **Landmark Identification:** The generation of 2D images from three-dimensional (3D) structures and the superimposition of the right and left sides on the median sagittal plane make the identification of cephalometric landmarks in lateral cephalograms a challenging problem [12, 13]. Certain anatomical landmarks, such as the porion **(Po)**, condylion **(Co),** orbitale **(Or),** gonion (**Go**), anterior nasal spine (**ANS**), posterior nasal spine (**PNS**), and lower inferior apex (**LIA**) may be more prone to error due to overlapping structures superimposed on the landmark and its location. It seems that when landmarks are located on a curve, the error is larger, whereas landmarks placed in anatomically formed edges are easier to identify [14]. Finally, dental landmarks tend to have poorer validity than skeletal landmarks.

- **Magnification:** It should be known that the head position as well as the distance between the X-ray source and the image receptor will always cause a degree of magnification, enlargement or a possible distortion [11].
- **Tracing and Measurements:** Cephalometric analyses provide angular and linear measurements useful for diagnostic purposes and planning orthodontic treatment. Inaccurate landmark identification may lead to erroneous diagnoses and treatment plans. However, landmark identification errors of less than 1 mm or less than 2° would most likely not make a significant difference in the treatment plan [14, 15].

6. Describe the Two Basic Methods of Cephalometric Analysis

Metric method: Using selected linear and angular measurements. It is preferable to use *angular rather than linear measurements*, as angular measurements vary little due to size and age differences between individuals. The use of linear parameters should always be accompanied by a respect for the wide individual variability. *Graphic method.* Overlay an individual's radiograph on a reference template and inspect the degree of variation [5].

7. Which is the Reference Plane in Down's and Steiner's Cephalometric Analyses?

In Down's cephalometric analysis [5], the *Frankfort horizontal.* From this plane the *facial angle* was defined (*Frankfort horizontal to facial depth* Fig. **2**). Analysis of the *facial angle* defined the relative position of the mandible to the maxilla as retrognathic, normal or prognathic.

In Steiner's cephalometric analysis [8, 9], the *anterior cranial base*, sella to nasion **(SN)**, it is the plane of reference (Fig. **2**). Riedel [4] highlighted difficulties in accurate location of the porion **(Po)** point, which affected the orientation of *Frankfort Horizontal plane* (Down's analysis). Another advantage of sella **(S)** and nasion **(Na)** points is that the anterior cranial base **(SN)** undergoes very little change after the age of 6-7 years. From nasion **(Na)**, Reidel drew a line to points **A** and **B,** creating the angles **SNA** and **SNB**.

8. Describe the SNA, SNB, ANB, Mandibular Planes

SNA Angle: 82°± 3

It is used to assess the anteroposterior position of the maxilla relative to the anterior cranial base. Higher values indicate the relative forward positioning of maxilla, whereas lower values indicate the recessive location of the maxilla [8 - 10].

SNB Angle: 80°± 3

It is used to assess the anteroposterior position of the mandible relative to the anterior cranial base. Values less than 80° indicate a recessive mandible, whereas angles greater than 80° suggest a prognathic mandible [8 - 10].

ANB Angle: 2°

Indicate the magnitude and not the absolute discrepancy between the maxilla and mandible [30 - 31].

Mandibular Plane Angle, SN-GoGn: 32°

Steiner focused on the mandibular plane angle (SN-GoGn) as the center piece of his analysis. Excessively high or low mandibular plane angles suggest unfavorable growth patterns in individuals [8 - 10].

9. Describe the Limitations of SNA, SNB and ANB Measurements

In order to effectively implement these variables, the inclination of the *anterior cranial base* (**SN**) relative to the *Frankfort horizontal* (**FH**) level should be normally 6°. If, for example, the **SN** forms with a **FH** an angle of 10 degrees, the difference of 4 degrees should be added to each of Stciner's measurements. Otherwise, it will lead to the wrong diagnostic results [6].

10. Mention Another Cephalometric Method that can Reliably Identify the Relationship Between Maxilla, Mandible and the Anterior Cranial Base

- **Maxilla:** *The nasion Na perpendicular (McNamara)* [6] is usually a reliable line of orientation for determining the maxillary position except:
    a. The Class III malocclusion with short anterior cranial base and
    b. The Class II/II malocclusion when there is excessive lingual tipping of the crown of the upper incisors.

The point **A** to the nasion **Na** perpendicular is 0 mm in the mixed-dentition and 1 mm in adults (Fig. **3**).

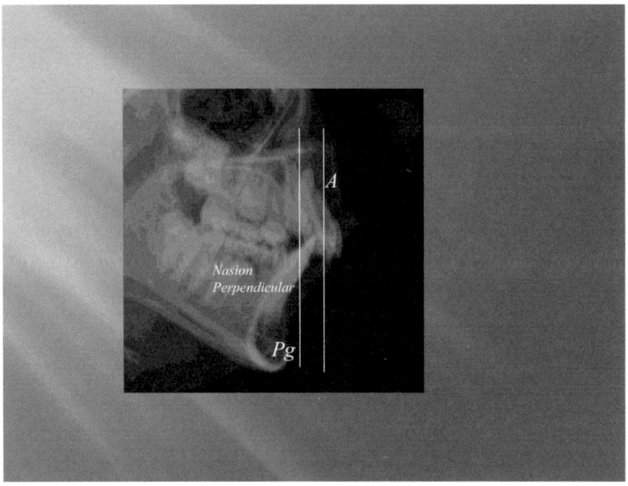

Fig. (3). The Nasion perpendicular.

- **Mandible:** The relationship of the mandible to the cranial base could be determined by measuring the distance from pogonion **Pg** to the nasion **Na** perpendicular (Fig. **3**). In children with a balanced face, pogonion **Pg** lies posterior **(– 8 mm to – 6 mm)** to the nasion **Na** perpendicular. In adults, the measurement of the chin position is usually – 2 mm to 2 mm relative to the nasion **Na** perpendicular.

11. What Do You See in the Following Picture?

Steiner emphasized the value of interpreting all aspects of the analysis and not simply reading the numbers (Fig. **4**) [10]. He devised ways to alter incisor positions to achieve normal occlusions even when the ideal **ANB** angle couldn't be achieved. His analysis took into account that it may not be possible to reach ideal proportions and relationships in all cases, but there are ways to maximise aesthetics. Thus, he created **chevrons** representing the ideal and acceptable compromises (*e.g.* ANB: 2°, Maxillary central incisor to NA: 4mm and 22°, Mandibular central incisor to NB: 4mm and 25°).

12. Which Biological Phenomenon is Behind Steiner's Chevrons?

Dento-alveolar Compensation: This biological mechanism often masks the actual skeletal deviations and must be considered during treatment planning. It is necessary to reduce or remove the compensation in order to achieve a skeletal correction, especially in growing patients who are planned for growth modification treatment correction. In other words, it may be desirable to maintain the compensatory changes or even accentuate them to achieve an acceptable treatment result [10].

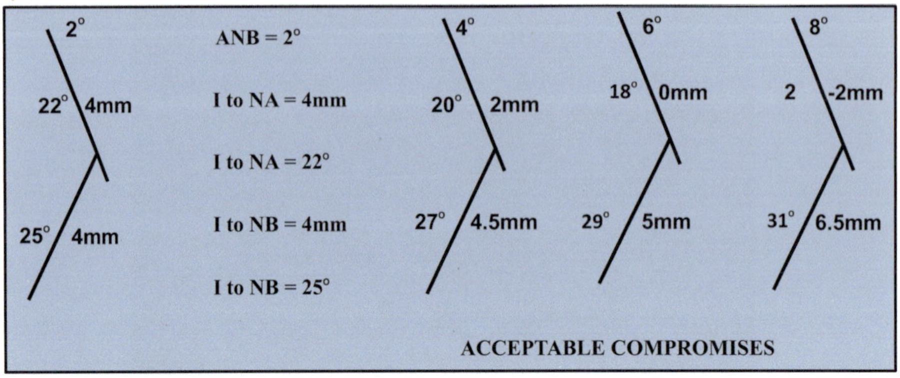

Fig. (4). Steiner's chevrons.

13. What Do You See Here? Interpret the Clinical Importance in Paediatric Orthodontics

Holdaway Lower Incisor Ratio (Fig. **5**) [16, 17]: It is the ratio thatevaluates the relative prominence of the mandibular incisors compared to the size of the bony chin. According to Holdaway, the distance of the labial surface of the mandibular central incisor to the **NB** line and the linear distance of the pogonion **Pg** to the same line should be equal.

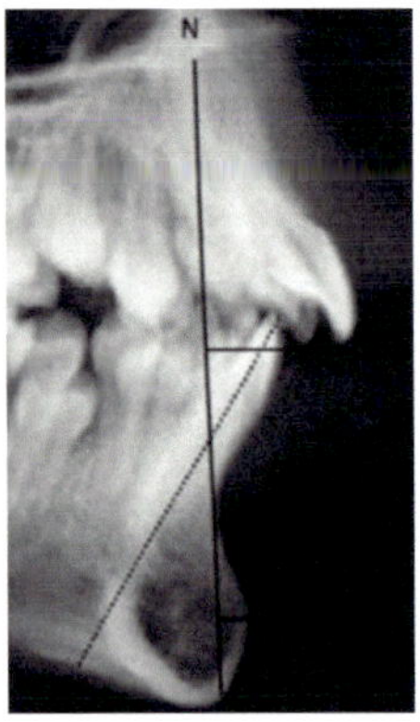

Fig. (5). Holdaway ratio.

- If the ratio is 2:1 (acceptable), it means that the lower incisors are more proclined compared to chin prominence.
- If the discrepancy is more than 3mm (unacceptable), orthodontic intervention is indicated,such asteeth extraction or growth modification treatment.

14. a. Which Analysis is This?
b. Why is it Very Useful in Paediatric Orthodontics?

a. Bjork-Jarabak's Polygon analysis (Fig. **6**) [18]. The basis of this analysis is two-fold:
   i. The sum of the Saddle angle (**N-S-Ar**), Articulare angle **(S-Ar-Go)** and Gonial Angle **(Ar-Go-Me)** predicts the direction of growth change in the lower face.
   ii. A polygon is used to assess the relationships between the anterior and posterior facial height, anterior cranial base to mandibular body length and posterior cranial base length to ramus height.

b. It is very useful in paediatric orthodontics because:
   i. The facial components are highly correlated to each other and changes in their sagittal and vertical position influence the dento-alveolar relationships and thereby the occlusion of the teeth. If the sum total of the three angles exceeds 396º, there would be a tendency towards "clockwise" growth rotation, indicating that the anterior facial height is increasing more rapidly than the posterior facial height. If the sum total of three angles is less than 396 degrees, there is a tendency for counter-clockwise growth rotation of the mandible [7, 19].
   ii. We can predict early the growth direction of patients with an abnormal growth pattern. *We should always remember the importance of developing a differential diagnosis for each patient in order to correctly address the problems at hand* [6, 23].

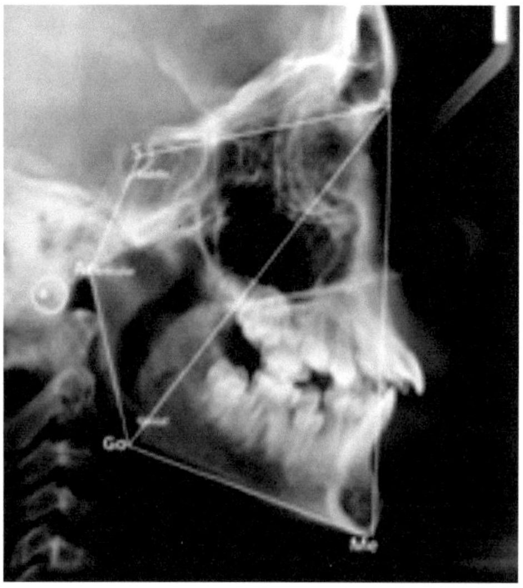

Fig. (6). Bjork-Jarabak's Polygon analysis.

15. a. Describe the Relationship between the Saddle Angle and the Location of Glenoid Fossa in Bjork-Jarabak's Polygon Analysis
b. Provide the Differences between High and Low Values of the Articular Angle
c. Provide the Differences between High and Low Values of the Gonial Angle

a. Low values of the Saddle angle indicate more vertical posterior cranial base results in more downward displacement of the glenoid fossa and forward position of the mandible (brachyphacial growth pattern). High values of the Saddle angle indicate the downward and backward displacement of the glenoid fossa, resulting in a more distal position of the mandible (dolichophacial growth pattern) [3, 18, 19].

b. High values indicate a dolichophacial growth pattern, mandibular retrognathism and short ramus. A low value indicates a brachyphacial growth pattern and possible mandibular prognathism.

c. High values indicate a dolichophacial growth pattern, retrognathic profile, whereas low values indicate a brachyphacial growth pattern, orthognathic profile and square mandible.

16. What Are the Angles of the "Triangle of Tweed" and What Are their Measurements?

- *Frankfort plane to mandibular plane angle* (FMA 25°). It indicates the direction of lower facial growth, both horizontally and vertically. FMA: ≤ 25° indicates the horizontal growth pattern whereas FMA: ≥ 25° indicates the vertical growth pattern (Fig. 7) [20].
- *Frankfort plane-mandibular incisor angle* (FMIA 65°).
- *Lower incisor axis- mandibular plane angle* (IMPA (85°- 95°).

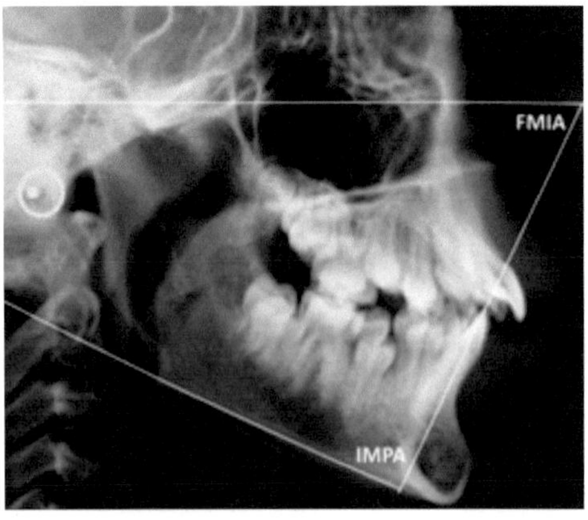

Fig. (7). Triangle of Tweed.

17. In Steiner's Analysis the Location and the Axial Inclination of the Maxillary Incisors are Determined by Relating the Teeth to N-A Line (4mm, 22°)

a. What is the Possible Skeletal Relationship if the Distance is > 4mm, < 4mm, or the Angle is > 22°, < 22°?

b. What is the Possible Skeletal Relationship if the Angle of the Lower Incisor with N- B line is: i) > 25°, ii) < 25°?

a. If the distance is > 4mm: Class II/ I or bimaxillary protrusion
  - If the distance is < 4mm: Class II/II malocclusion
  - If the angle is > 22°: Class II/I or Class III with dental compensation
  - If the angle is < 22°: Class II/II

b. Class II/I malocclusion

Class II/II or Class III malocclusion

*The cephalometric analysis in general must be used as a guide to what area or structure an occlusal problem may be related and the numbers serve only as guides — **not as a target**.*

18. Is it Important to Determine How Much the Skeletal Pogonion Will Grow?

It is very important to determine how much the Pogonion will grow because we need to predict the final position of the lower incisors. If the lower incisor to Pogonion is at least a 1:1 ratio, this will usually result in a stable dentition and pleasant facial appearance [10, 16, 17].

19. Could you Determine the Crowding Cephalometrical?

- Check the age of the patient.
- Look at the expected Pogonion growth chart.
- Decide where to place the lower incisor.

For every 1 mm you decrease or increase, the lower incisor to the NB line, you decrease or increase the arch length double [10].

Age	Males	Females
10	-	*0 - 3-4mm*
11	-	*0 - 2-3mm*
12	*0 - 3-5mm*	*0 - 1-2mm*
13	*0 - 2-4mm*	*0 - ½-1mm*

Contd.....

Age	Males	Females
14	*0 - 1-2mm*	*0mm*
15	*0 -½-1½mm*	-
16	*0mm*	-

20. Which Other Radiographs Are Most Commonly Used in Paediatric Orthodontics?

a. Dental Panoramic Radiograph.
b. Posterior-Anterior Cephalometric radiograph.
c. Periapical/Occlusal radiograph.
d. Three dimension hard and soft tissue scans.

21. Why is the Panoramic Radiograph Useful in Paediatric Orthodontics?

- To detect unerupted, impacted, supernumerary or missing teeth
- To recognize periapical lesions, root resorption, dental size-shape abnormalities
- To estimate dental age
- To detect tooth eruptive patterns and true tooth-size, jaw-size discrepancies

22. Name the Landmarks and the Reference Planes in the Next Posterior-Anterior Cephalometric Radiograph

The most frequently hard tissue landmarks and reference planes (Fig. **8**) [21, 22] are:

a. ***Landmarks***
   - **m**: mandibular midpoint.
   - **ag**: antegonion. The highest point in the antegonial notch.
   - **ma**: mastoid. The lowest point of the mastoid process.
   - **um**: maxillary molar. The most prominent lateral point on the buccal surface of the first permanent maxillary molar.
   - **mx**: maxillare. The intersection of the maxillary alveolar process and the contour of the maxillozygomatic process of the maxilla.
   - **iif**: incisor inferior frontale. The midpoint of the mandibular incisors at the level of the incisal edges.
   - **isf**: incisor superior frontale. The midpoint of the maxillary incisors at the level of the incisal edges.
   - **lpa**: lateral piriform aperture. The point of the lateral aspect of the piriform aperture.
   - **za**: zygomatic arch. The point of the lateral aspect of the zygomatic arch.
   - **mzmf**: zygomaticofrontal medial suture point.

- **lzmf**:zygomaticofrontal lateral suture point.
- **lo**: latero-orbitale. The intersection of lateral orbital contour with the innominate line.
- **mo**: The point on the medial orbital margin.
- **om**: orbital midpoint. The projection of the line lo-lo of the top of the nasal septum at the base of the crista galli.
- **tns**: top nasal septum. The highest point on the superior aspect of the nasal septum.
- **ans**: anterior nasal spine.

c. ***References Planes***

- Symmetry:Dropping a line through crista galli perpendicular to the line connecting the zygomatic arches.
- Nasal cavity width: A line connecting the lateral piriform aperture **(lpa)**.
- Mandibular width: Measured from left to right antegonion (**ag**).
- Maxillary width: Inrelation to mandibular width by dropping two lines from the zygomaticofrontal medial suture **(mzmf)** to the antegonion point **(ag)**. The distances between these lines and the maxillare point (**mx**) define the relationship between the maxillary and mandibular width.
- Dental symmetry: The relationship between the incisor inferior frontale **(iif)** and the incisor superior frontale **(isf).**

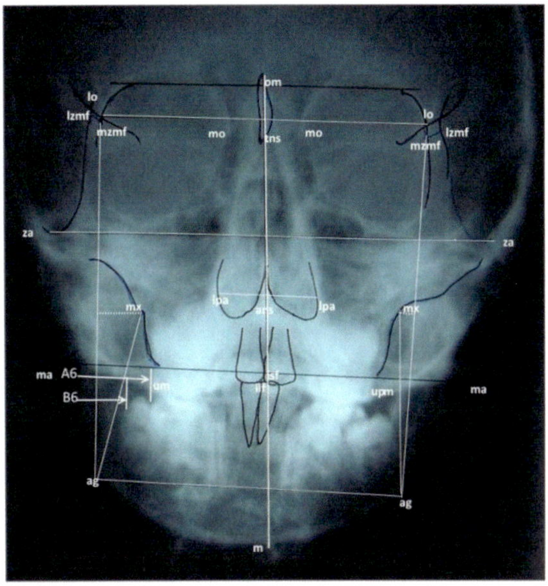

Fig. (8). Landmarks and the reference planes in the posterior-anterior cephalometric radiograph.

23. Name the Advantages and the Disadvantages of Cone-Beam Computed Tomography (CBCT) in Orthodontics

Table 1. Advantages and disadvantages of CBCT [3, 23, 24].

Advantages	Disadvantages
3-D visualization of the morphology of the face and cranium; quantifying discrepancies in cases of facial asymmetry (Fig. **9**)	Higher radiation dose compared to conventional radiograph.
High sensitivity for localization of impacted teeth.	Inability to represent curving form in three dimensions.
High precision for identification of root resorption (Fig. **10**)	Inability to capture soft tissue texture, which results in difficulties in the identification of landmarks that are dependant of surface colour.
High accuracy for visualization of bone geometry TMJ anatomy and upper airway dimensions.	Slowness of method, making distortion of scanned image likely.
Sharp visualization of buccal and lingual alveolar bone plates.	High cost.

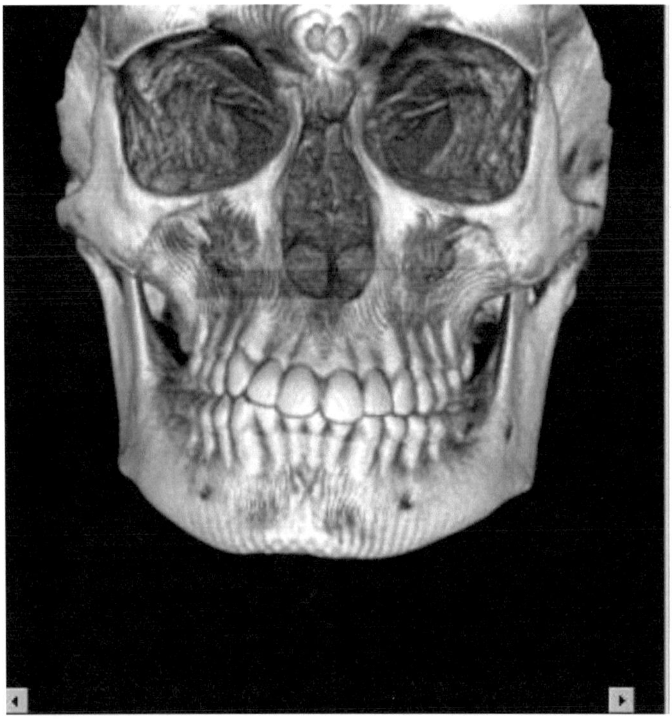

Fig. (9). Facial asymmetry.

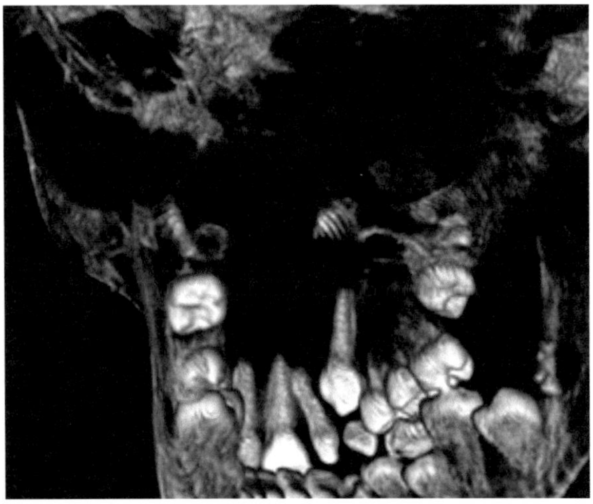

Fig. (10). Canine impaction and lateral incisor root position.

24. Provide the Effective Dose Expressed in Micro-Sieverts (msv) Produced by CBCT in Comparison with Multi-Slice CT and Conventional Radiographs

Table 2. Msv produced by different radiographs [3, 23, 24].

Examination	Effective Dose (msv)
CBCT of face and cranium (FOV > 15 cm)	52 to 1073
CBCT of face (FOV 10 - 15 cm)	61 to 603
CBCT of the jaws (FOV < 10 cm)	18 to 333
Multi-slice CT	426 to 1160
Panoramic radiograph	2 to 10
Cephalogram	2 to 10

25. Provide the Recommendations for CBCT use in Orthodontics

Table 3. CBCT recommendations in Orthodontics [3, 23, 24].

The younger the patient, the less should be the indications for asking a CBCT **examination (cleft patients). Preference is given to patients older than 16 years of age.**
CBCT scan proves advantageous for the diagnosis and treatment of severe craniofacial anomalies with malformation of the midface and mandible.
TMJ patients. CBCT scans provide clear imaging of articular fossa and condyles.
CBCT exams seem to permit the orthodontists to be more confident in diagnosing and treatment planning for impacted teeth and related root resorption.

(Table 3) contd.....

CBCT should be indicated to assess buccolingual thickness in the alveolar ridge of periodontal patients or under some circumstances in patients for whom skeletal anchorage devices will be considered.
Because of the low reliability and reproducibility of soft-tissue landmarks identification in CBCT scans, there is not enough evidence to support CBCT efficacy for orthognathic-surgery patients.

PART B. DENTAL CLASSIFICATION

1. a. What is Normal Occlusion?
b. What is Malocclusion?
c. What is the Aetiology of Malocclusion?

a. Normal occlusion is an occlusion within the accepted deviation of the ideal that does not constitute an aesthetic or functional problem.
b. Malocclusion is the anomaly which causes disfigurement or which impedes function and requires treatment if the disfigurement or functional defect is likely to be an obstacle to the patient's physical or emotional well-being.
c. Considerable genetic background exists in at least two aspects:
   i. Teeth size-morphology and
   ii. Growth pattern of both the maxilla and mandible. Genetic factors have long been regarded as significant in the aetiology of malocclusion since there are obvious familial tendencies in facial features (The Hapsburg jaw). Because the dentition is in equilibrium within its environment force system, malocclusions could be considered to be the result of a complex and interrelated pathway among a large number of hereditary and environmental factors.

2. Why Do We Need a Classification System for Malocclusion?

a. To divide the wide range into smaller groups.
b. To provide a verbal and mental picture unifying the communication.
c. To simplify the documentations.
d. To help to select treatment modality.

3. What is Normal Occlusion According to Angle Classification? What Are Class I, II, III Angle's Malocclusion?

Normal Occlusion [3]: Mesiobuccal cusp of the upper molar occludes in the buccal groove of the lower molar, all teeth arranged on a smoothly curving line of occlusion (Fig. **11**).

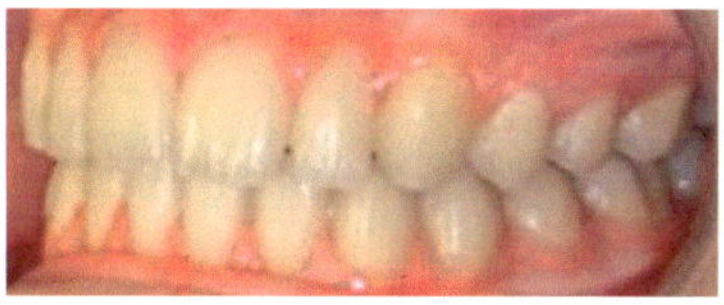

Fig. (11). Normal occlusion.

Class I Malocclusion [3]: Normal molar relationship, but line of occlusion incorrect because of rotations, ectopic or malposed teeth (Fig. **12**).

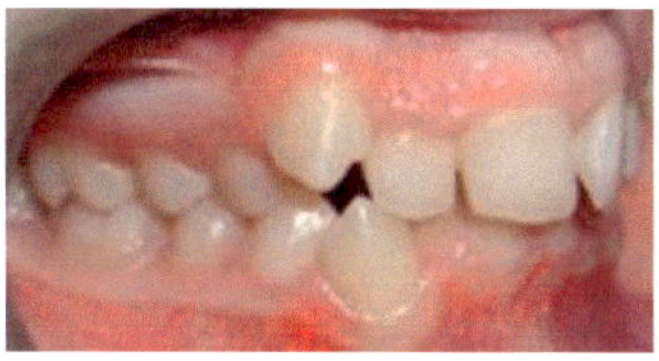

Fig. (12). Class I malocclusion.

Class II Malocclusion [3]: as having a distal relationship of the mandibular molar relative to the maxillary molar of more than one-half the width of the cusp. Angle characterised [25] two types of Class II malocclusions based on the inclination of the maxillary central incisors:

Class II/I Malocclusion (Fig. 13): It is characterized by labial inclined maxillary incisors, an increased overjet with deep or open bite. Class II division 1 subdivision malocclusion has a normal occlusal relation on one side and Class II occlusion on the other side.

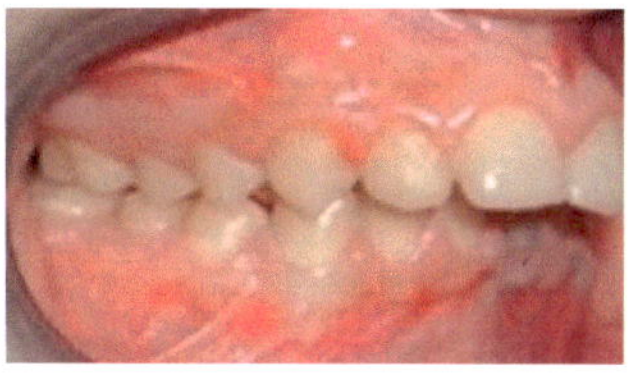

Fig. (13). Class II/I malocclusion.

Class II/II Malocclusion (Fig. 14): The buccal groove of the first mandibular molar occludes distal to the mesiobuccal cusp of the first maxillary molar. It is described as having an excessive lingual inclination of the maxillary central incisors accompanied by a deep overbite and minimal overjet.

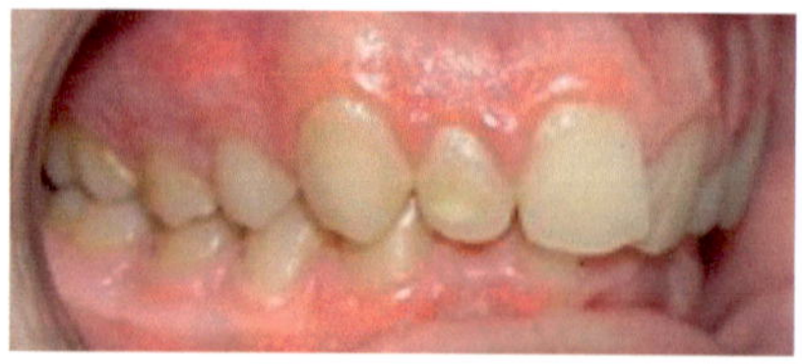

Fig. (14). Class II/II malocclusion.

Class III Malocclusion (Fig. 15): Refers to a condition where the mesio buccal cusp of the upper first molars occludes between the lower first and second molars. Crowding of the upper anterior teeth and lingual inclination of the lower anterior teeth compose the mosaic of Angle's classification. Class III malocclusion subdivision has a normal occlusal relation on one side of the arches and Class III occlusion on the other side.

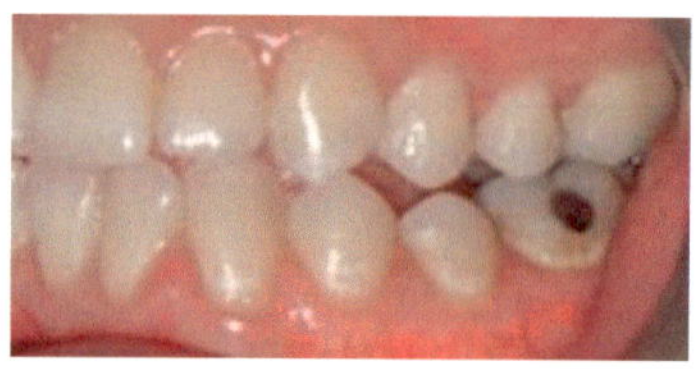

Fig. (15). Class III malocclusion.

4. Describe the Van-Deer-Linden Types of Class II/II Malocclusion

- Type A: Maxillary central incisors and laterals are retroclined (Fig. **16**).
- Type B: Maxillary lateral incisors are overlapping the retroclined maxillary central incisors (Fig. **17**).
- Type C: Maxillary central and lateral incisors are retroclined and overlapped by the maxillary canines (Fig. **18**) [26].

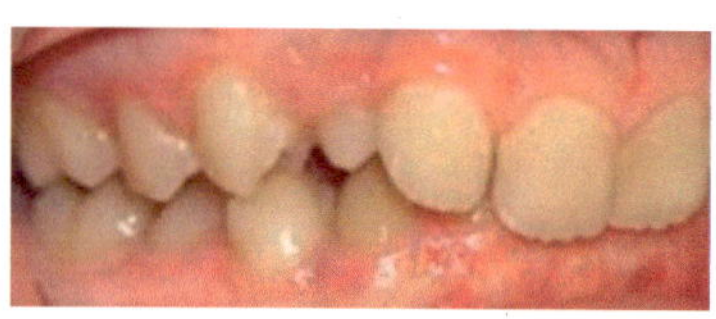

Fig. (16). Type A.

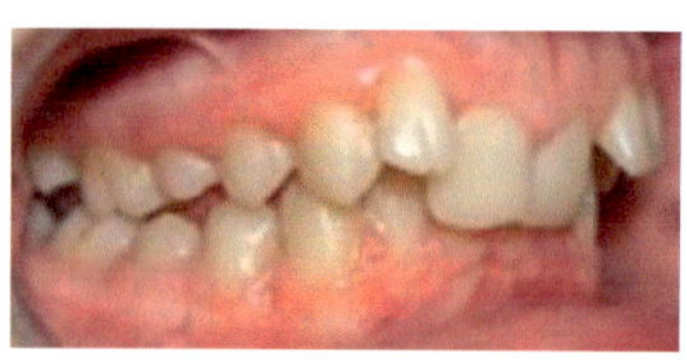

Fig. (17). Type B.

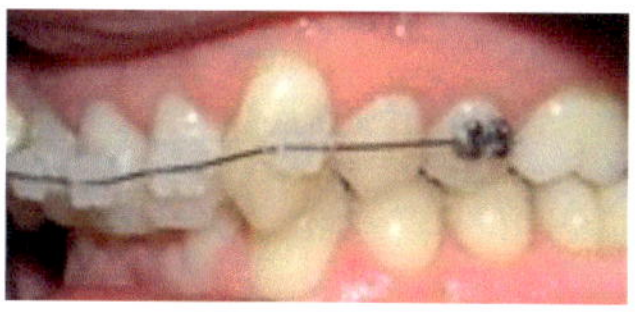

Fig. (18). Type C.

5. Why is Angle Classification not Enough to Describe the Class II, III Orthodontic Anomalies?

The class II, III malocclusion could be composed of skeletal, functional, and dental discrepancies, which may or may not be associated with each other. The classification by Angle is **restricted only to dental relationships** without considering the other factors. Although Angle's classification has been used for many years, his assumptions on the aetiology and diagnosis of the malocclusion lack definitive evidence.

6. Name Andrews' '*Six Keys to Normal Occlusion*' and the *Roth Philosophy* of Ideal Occlusion

'***Six Keys to Normal Occlusion***' [27].

a. **Molar Relationship:** The mesio-buccal cusp of the upper first permanent molar falls within the groove between the mesial and middle cusps of the lower first permanent molar. In addition, the distobuccal cusp of the upper first molar should contact the mesiobuccal cusp of the lower second molar.
b. **Crown Angulation (tip):** The angulation of the facial axis of the clinical crown (FACC) of every clinical crown should be positive. The gingival part of the long axis of each crown in the upper jaw should be positioned distally to the occlusal part of this axis.
c. **Crown Inclination (torque):** Refers to the labiolingual or buccolingual inclination of the crowns of the teeth. A positive reading is given if the gingival portion of the crown is lingual to the incisal portion. A negative reading is recorded when the gingival portion of the crown is labial to the incisal portion.
d. No rotations.
e. No spaces.
f. **Occlusal Plane:** The occlusal plane should be either flat or slightly curved.

Roth's philosophy of the 'ideal' occlusion is based on the dynamic features of occlusion during functional movement adding some keys to the previous six keys to normal occlusion by Andrew:

a. *Centric relationship* and *centric occlusion* should be coincident.
b. In protrusion, the incisors should disclude the posterior teeth, with the guidance being provided by the lower incisal edges along the palatal contour of the upper incisors.
c. In lateral excursions of the mandible, the canine should guide the working side whilst all other teeth on that side and the other side should be discluded.
d. When the teeth are in *centric occlusion*, there should be even bilateral contacts in the buccal segments.

7. What Are the IOTN, ICON and PAR Indices?

The *Index of Orthodontic Treatment Need* (IOTN) consists of two components – the *Dental Health Component* (DHC) and the *Aesthetic Component* (AC). The index value is determined by the presence and severity of anomalies belonging to one of the five categories: missing teeth, overjet, crossbite, displacement of anatomical contact points and overbite. The IOTN is particularly useful because, based on the severity of individual occlusal anomalies; it allows the patients to be classified into one of the five groups: no need for treatment, slight need for treatment, moderate/borderline need for treatment, need for treatment, and definite need for orthodontic treatment [28].

The *Index of Complexity, Outcome, and Need* (ICON) was proposed as a multipurpose occlusal index which could be used to assess orthodontic treatment need and complexity of orthodontic treatment, and can also be used to assess improvement from orthodontic treatment [29, 30].

PAR (*Peer Assessment Rating*) index was developed in recent years to evaluate the treatment results and it is considered as a simple, objective and reliable approach to evaluating the stability after orthodontic treatment. PAR considers five components of occlusion which are believed to be important outcomes of orthodontic treatment [30, 31].

Contact Point Displacements: Scores and their respective displacements to be used while assessing the alignment of anterior segment of the dentition (in the mixed dentition average widths are used to calculate space discrepancies).

Buccal Segment Relationship is recorded for both left and right sides in the three planes of space and summed for each buccal segment.

Overjet as well as anterior teeth in cross-bites are recorded together.

In **overbite** assessment, the worst positive or negative overlap of any of the four incisors are recorded.

Dental **midline** discrepancies were assessed, too.

CONCLUDING REMARKS

Although the majority of experienced orthodontists are confident in diagnosing without the use of a cephalometric radiograph, since its introduction, the lateral cephalometric radiograph has become a standard tool in the orthodontic community. Although the clinical assessment of the patients is of paramount importance, radiographic evaluation seems necessary, particularly for patients with profound skeletal imbalances. This radiograph provides skeletal size, position, proportion and symmetry of the individual, by which it is possible to assess skeletal disharmonies. Moreover, CBCT imaging is only justified if the expected additional information is therapeutically relevant compared with conventional orthodontic 2-D imaging.

REFERENCES

[1] Athanasiou AE. Orthodontic cephalometry. Maryland Heights, MI, USA: Mosby-Wolfe 1995.

[2] Burstone CJ, James RB, Legan H, Murphy GA, Norton LA. Cephalometrics for orthognathic surgery. J Oral Surg 1978; 36(4): 269-77.
[PMID: 273073]

[3] Proffit WR, Fields HM, Sarver DM, Eds. 2013. United States, St Louis, Missouri: Mosby. Contemporary Orthodontics.

[4] Riedel RA. Esthetics and its relation to orthodontic therapy. Angle Orthod 1950; 20(3): 168-78.
[PMID: 14790327]

[5] Downs WB. Analysis of the dentofacial profile. Angle Orthod 1956; 26: 191-212.

[6] McNamara JA Jr. A method of cephalometric evaluation. Am J Orthod 1984; 86(6): 449-69.
[http://dx.doi.org/10.1016/S0002-9416(84)90352-X] [PMID: 6594933]

[7] Ricketts RM, Roth RH, Chaconas SJ, Schulhof RJ, Engle GA. Orthodontic diagnosis and planning. USA: Rocky Mountain Data Systems 1982.

[8] Steiner CC. Cephalometrics for you and me. Am J Orthod 1953; 39: 729-55.
[http://dx.doi.org/10.1016/0002-9416(53)90082-7]

[9] Steiner CC. Cephalometrics in clinical practice. Angle Orthod 1959; 29: 8-29.

[10] Steiner CC. The use of cephalometrics as an aid to planning and accessing orthodontic treatment. Am J Orthod 1960; 46: 721-35.
[http://dx.doi.org/10.1016/0002-9416(60)90145-7]

[11] Adenwalla ST, Kronman JH, Attarzadeh F. Porion and condyle as cephalometric landmarks--an error study. Am J Orthod Dentofacial Orthop 1988; 94(5): 411-5.
[http://dx.doi.org/10.1016/0889-5406(88)90130-8] [PMID: 3189243]

[12] Chen YJ, Chen SK, Huang HW, Yao CC, Chang HF. Reliability of landmark identification in cephalometric radiography acquired by a storage phosphor imaging system. Dentomaxillofac Radiol 2004; 33(5): 301-6.
[http://dx.doi.org/10.1259/dmfr/85147715] [PMID: 15585806]

[13] Durão AR, Pittayapat P, Rockenbach MI, *et al.* Validity of 2D lateral cephalometry in orthodontics: a systematic review. Prog Orthod 2013; 14: 31.
[http://dx.doi.org/10.1186/2196-1042-14-31] [PMID: 24325757]

[14] Miloro M, Borba AM, Ribeiro-Junior O, Naclério-Homem MG, Jungner M. Is there consistency in cephalometric landmark identification amongst oral and maxillofacial surgeons? Int J Oral Maxillofac Surg 2014; 43(4): 445-53.
[http://dx.doi.org/10.1016/j.ijom.2013.08.007] [PMID: 24055177]

[15] da Silveira HL, Silveira HE. Reproducibility of cephalometric measurements made by three radiology clinics. Angle Orthod 2006; 76(3): 394-9.
[PMID: 16637717]

[16] Holdaway RA. A soft-tissue cephalometric analysis and its use in orthodontic treatment planning. Part I. Am J Orthod 1983; 84(1): 1-28.
[http://dx.doi.org/10.1016/0002-9416(83)90144-6] [PMID: 6575614]

[17] Holdaway RA. A soft-tissue cephalometric analysis and its use in orthodontic treatment planning. Part II. Am J Orthod 1984; 85(4): 279-93.
[http://dx.doi.org/10.1016/0002-9416(84)90185-4] [PMID: 6585146]

[18] Björk A. Prediction of mandibular growth rotation. Am J Orthod 1969; 55(6): 585-99.
[http://dx.doi.org/10.1016/0002-9416(69)90036-0] [PMID: 5253957]

[19] Jarabak JR, Fizzel JA. Technique and treatment with lightwire appliances. St Louis: CV Mosby 1972.

[20] Tweed CH. The Frankfort – mandibular incisor angle (FMIA) in orthodontic diagnosis, treatment planning and prognosis. Angle Orthod 1954; 24: 121-69.

[21] Ricketts RM, Grummons.D. Frontal cephalometrics: practical applications, Part I. World J Orthod 2003; 4: 297-316.

[22] Grummons DC, Kappeyne van de Coppello MA. A frontal asymmetry analysis. J Clin Orthod 1987; 21(7): 448-65.
[PMID: 3476493]

[23] American Academy of Oral and Maxillofacial Radiology. Clinical recommendations regarding use of cone beam computed tomography in orthodontics. [corrected]. Position statement by the American Academy of Oral and Maxillofacial Radiology. Oral Surg Oral Med Oral Pathol Oral Radiol 2013; 116(2): 238-57.
[http://dx.doi.org/10.1016/j.oooo.2013.06.002] [PMID: 23849378]

[24] Alqerban A, Jacobs R, Fieuws S, Nackaerts O, Willems G. Comparison of 6 cone-beam computed tomography systems for image quality and detection of simulated canine impaction-induced external root resorption in maxillary lateral incisors. Am J Orthod Dentofacial Orthop 2011; 140(3): e129-39.
[http://dx.doi.org/10.1016/j.ajodo.2011.03.021] [PMID: 21889061]

[25] Angle EH. Classification of malocclusion. Dental Cosmos 1899; 4: 248-64.

[26] Van der Linden . Development of the Human Dentition 2014.

[27] Andrews LF. The six keys to normal occlusion. Am J Orthod 1972; 62(3): 296-309.
[http://dx.doi.org/10.1016/S0002-9416(72)90268-0] [PMID: 4505873]

[28] Daniels C, Richmond S. The development of the index of complexity, outcome and need (ICON). J Orthod 2000; 27(2): 149-62.
[http://dx.doi.org/10.1093/ortho/27.2.149] [PMID: 10867071]

[29] Brook PH, Shaw WC. The development of an index of orthodontic treatment priority. Eur J Orthod 1989; 11(3): 309-20.
[http://dx.doi.org/10.1093/oxfordjournals.ejo.a035999] [PMID: 2792220]

[30] Richmond S, Shaw WC, Roberts CT, Andrews M. The PAR Index (Peer Assessment Rating): methods to determine outcome of orthodontic treatment in terms of improvement and standards. Eur J Orthod 1992; 14(3): 180-7.
[http://dx.doi.org/10.1093/ejo/14.3.180] [PMID: 1628684]

[31] Templeton KM, Powell R, Moore MB, Williams AC, Sandy JR. Are the peer assessment rating index and the index of treatment complexity, outcome, and need suitable measures for orthognathic outcomes? Eur J Orthod 2006; 28(5): 462-6.
[http://dx.doi.org/10.1093/ejo/cji120] [PMID: 16648208]

CHAPTER 4

Development of the Occlusion

Abstract: The mixed dentition period spans the period where both primary and permanent teeth are present. This period of dental development requires complex coordination between resorption of primary tooth roots, alveolar bone development and eruption of succedaneous permanent teeth. A thorough knowledge of dental arch dimensions changes, as a result of growth and development, is of paramount importance to the clinician. The purpose of this chapter with the question-answer format is to provide in depth the relationship between the tooth eruption pattern and dental arch changes during the transition from mixed to permanent dentition. In the second part of the chapter, through clinical examples and a problem-based approach, a thorough knowledge of the tooth eruption sequence, as well as tooth eruption abnormalities and arch space loss is provided.

Keywords: Dental arch length, Dental space deficiency, Late mesial shift, Leeway space, Mixed dentition, Tooth development.

INTRODUCTION

The process of occlusal development passes through three stages: the primary, mixed and permanent dentition. In the primary dentition, all the primary teeth erupt into the previously edentulous alveolar. In the early mixed dentition, the primary central and lateral incisors are replaced by the permanent central and lateral incisors, while the first permanent molars crupt distally to the second primary molars. In the late mixed dentition, the primary canines and the first and second primary molars are replaced by the permanent canines and premolars. The mixed dentition period seems to be the most critical time period to attain the proper occlusal relationship between the upper and lower dental arches.

PART A. TOOTH ERUPTION- DENTAL ARCH CHANGES

1. What is Tooth Eruption and What is Tooth Emergence?

Eruption is the movement of the teeth within and through the alveolar bone and the overlying mucosa, in order to appear in the oral cavity and contact the opposing teeth [1]. The eruption of the teeth has a circadian rhythm following the

George Litsas

pattern of growth hormone [2]. **The emergence** of a tooth is the first sign of its appearance in the oral cavity [1, 3, 4].

2. Describe the Stages of Tooth Eruption

There are three stages of eruption:

a. **Pre-Eruptive Stage:** before the crown is formed. This stage begins when the crown is complete and the root starts to form. Resorption of the alveolar bone and the roots of the primary dentition is necessary to allow pre-emergent eruption [2, 3].
b. **Pre-Functional Eruptive Stage:** begins at the initiation of root formation and ends when the teeth reach occlusal contact. The emergence of a tooth is the first sign of its appearance in the oral cavity. This usually occurs when the 2/3 of the final root length is established. Eruption speed is usually faster during the post–emergent eruption phase [2 - 4].
c. **Functional Eruptive Stage:** Eruption does not stop at this stage but continues to equal the vertical growth of the face [2 - 4].

3. Could You Provide a Timing of Primary Teeth Development?

a. Five months in utero, all crowns start calcification.
b. One year (11–12 months), all crowns complete formation.
c. Two and a half years, all primary teeth emerge.
d. Four years, all primary teeth complete root formation [5 - 7].

4. Describe the Timing of the Eruption of the Primary Teeth. What Are the Differences in the Sequence of Eruption between the Upper and Lower Primary Teeth?

Despite of the large individual variations regarding the timing of the primary tooth eruption, most children follow the "six/four" rule. Every six months, four primary teeth are erupted.

The "six/four" rule for primary tooth emergence

1. 6 months: 4 teeth (lower and upper centrals)
2. 12 months: 8 teeth (+ upper and lower laterals)
3. 18 months: 12 teeth (+ upper and lower 1st molars)
4. 24 months: 16 teeth (+ upper and lower canines)
5. 30 months: 20 teeth (+ lower & upper 2nd molars)

The sequence in the emergence of the primary dentition in the majority of the children *is the same* for both upper and lower arches [8, 13, 14].

5. i. What is the Eruption Sequence of Permanent Teeth? ii. Report the Criteria to Assess the Timing of Eruption

i. The most frequently observed sequence and time of the eruption of permanent teeth in both arches is as shown in (Table **1**). Eruption of the mandibular teeth usually precedes that of the corresponding maxillary teeth. Upper canines and lower second premolars are usually the last teeth to erupt anterior to the first molars and are often malpositioned in the dental arch [1, 7]. *Deviation from the typical sequence of eruption does not necessarily result in the malpositioning of teeth if space is reserved for all of the permanent teeth.*
ii. Criteria generally [2, 5, 8] used to assess the timing of the eruption of permanent teeth are:
   - ***Number of Teeth Present***: Conventionally, determination of the number of the teeth present in the mouth is made according to the chronological age of the patient. The values are compared with the normative charts. This method does not take into account the fact that individuals vary greatly in their schedules of maturation.
   - ***Tooth Maturation***: The most reliable method to estimate the timing of the eruption of the teeth for a given child is upon the maturational status of the teeth prior to eruption. Tooth eruption has been found to be more closely associated with the stage of root formation than with chronological age. A tooth should erupt once 2/3 of its root is formed.
   - ***Local Factors***: A significant role in the eruption of an individual tooth could be the malocclusion, early or delayed loss of primary tooth, lack of guidance by the adjacent tooth due to its premature loss, splinting (as when a space maintainer is attached to the crown) and inflammation.

6. How do you Assess Dental Maturity?

Dental maturity can be determined by the stage of tooth eruption or the stage of tooth formation. Tooth eruption is unreliable because many factors such as space available, ankylosis, and early or delayed exfoliation of primary teeth alter the eruption of the permanent successors. Various radiological methods have been proposed to estimate dental maturity based on the degree of calcification of the permanent teeth [6].

7. a. Summarise the Demirjian Method of Dental Age Assessment b. Give the Main Disadvantages of this Method

a. Demirjian *et al.* [6], using the first seven teeth of the left lower quadrant of French-Canadian children, developed a simplified scoring system for dental maturation assessment by giving the teeth a score from A to H. A digit maturity score was assigned for each of these teeth and was differentiated for boys and girls. Adding these scores results in an overall maturation score that can be converted to an estimated dental age using tables and curves developed separately for boys and girls.

b. There are two main disadvantages of this method:
   - Even though it is easy to use and is a highly reproducible method, the eight calcification stages that describe the developing tooth are based on discernible tooth formation changes rather than dividing tooth formation into equal time intervals. This means that the times taken for a tooth to develop from one stage to the next are not identical, affecting the accuracy of age estimation.
   - The secular trend in growth and development in the last decades and the ethnic disparity between French-Canadian children and the examining group.

Table 1. Sequence and time of the eruption of permanent teeth.

Jaw	Tooth	Time of emergence (years)	Root completed (years)	Emergence sequence
Max (upper)	1	7–8	10	4
	2	8	10–11	6
	3	11–13	14–15	12
	4	10–12	12–14	8
	5	10–12	13–14	10
	6	6–7	9–10	2
	7	11–13	15–16	14
	8	17–20	18–25	16
Mand (lower)	1	6–7	9	3
	2	7–8	9–10	5
	3	8–10	12–13	7
	4	10–12	12–14	9
	5	11–13	14–15	11
	6	6–7	9–10	1
	7	11–13	14–15	13
	8	17–20	18–25	15

8. a. What is Tooth Ankylosis? Which Teeth are Most Affected? b. What Are Hypodontia, Oligodontia and Hyperdontia?

a. *Tooth Ankylosis*, the fusion of bone and cementum, is a progressive anomaly of tooth eruption. Tooth ankylosis may be due to a disturbed metabolism.

Primary teeth become ankylosed far more frequently than permanent teeth (10/1), and lower teeth are ankylosed more (2/1) than upper teeth. *The first and second primary molars are the most commonly involved* teeth, with the second deciduous molars generally causing more damage [10]. A vertical occlusal deficiency (submerge) characterizes the ankylosed tooth as a result of the continuous eruption of the adjacent teeth (Fig. **1**). Frequently, tooth ankylosis is related to a congenital missing second permanent premolar. Clinically, the crown is located below the occlusal plane, while the eruption of adjacent teeth continues concomitantly with vertical alveolar bone growth. Such teeth are believed to be potential sites of malocclusion, with a risk of tipping of neighbouring teeth and loss of space. Extraction has therefore been the most widely recommended treatment [2, 4, 9].

b. *Hypodontia*: The most common developmental anomaly of human dentition in which one or two permanent teeth are congenitally missing. Excluding third molars, the prevalence of tooth agenesis is approximately 4.3 to 7.8% and the mandibular second premolars are the most commonly missing teeth, followed by the maxillary lateral incisors and maxillary second molars The prevalence of hypodontia in the primary dentition is very low (0.3%) [10].
c. *Oligodontia*: *More than six missing permanent teeth*. Often other organs of ectodermal origin are involved (ectodermal dysplasia) [11].
d. *Hyperdontia*: A supernumerary tooth in the permanent dentition called mesiodens is the most common type of hyperdontia. A mesiodens located in the maxillary central incisor region; the overall prevalence of mesiodentes is between 0.15% and 1.9%. It is a common finding in syndromes linked to hyperactivity of dental lamina such as Apert, Crouzon, Gardner and Down syndrome as well as to cleft palate patients. Sometimes, a supernumerary tooth could also be observed in the maxillary lateral incisor area without any other interesting findings [10, 11].

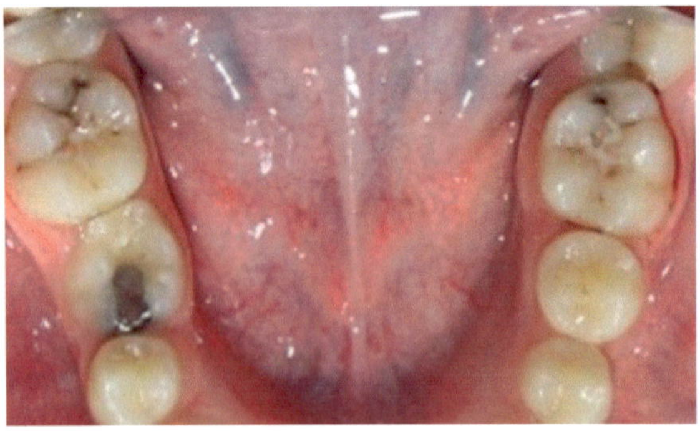

Fig. (1). Tooth ankylosis.

9. Provide the Definition of the Terms: i) Midline Diastema, ii) Ugly Duckling Stage and iii) Insisor Liability?

i. Midline diastema is the space between the permanent central incisors after their eruption. The midline space is normal [2, 3] at this age when:
  a. Is less than 2mm
  b. No supernumerary teeth or peg shape laterals
  c. No digit habits and
  d. No high labial frenum (Fig. **2**).

ii. If the laterals are flared or inclined distally, the diastema persists and this normal stage of development is referred to as"*ugly duckling*" (Fig. **3**). These spaces normally close spontaneously after the eruption of the upper permanent canines [2, 3].

iii. In the manibular arch, when the *lateral incisors erupt*, there is on average *1.6 mm less space* available for the four mandibular incisors than is required to perfectly align them. This difference between the amount of space needed and the available space is termed as "*incisor liability*" or "*physiological crowding*" [2].

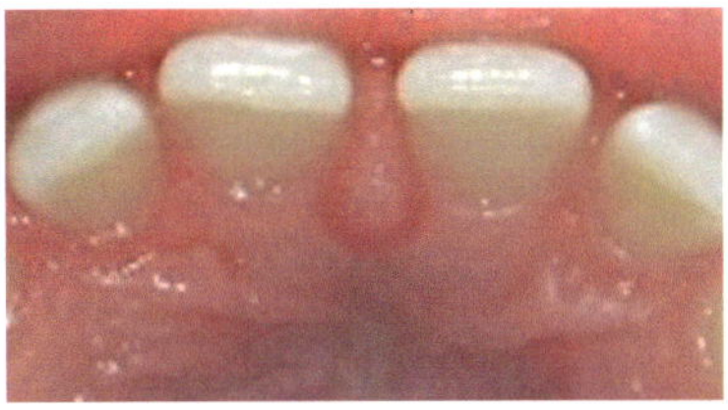

Fig. (2). Midline diastema because of a high labial frenum.

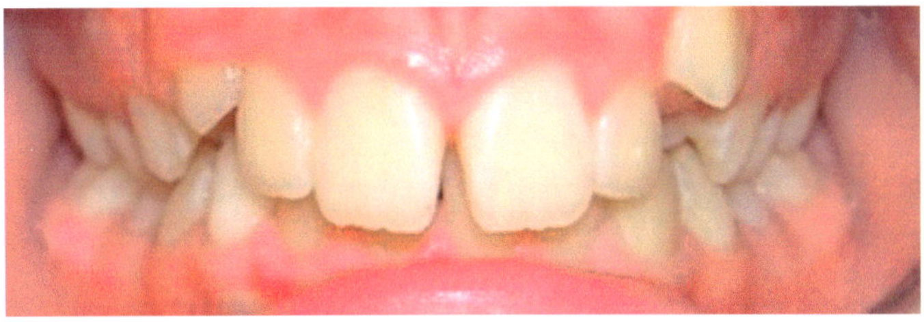

Fig. (3). "Ugly duckling" stage of development.

10. What are the Types of Primary Dentition, According to Baume? Describe the Characteristics of the Most Common Type

The types of primary dentition, according to Baume, are:

Type I: spaced dentition (70%), Type II: closed dentition

In Type I, primary dentition the incisors are spaced, positioned vertically in the alveolus, while the largest spaces, called primate spaces, are located distally to the lower canines and mesial to the upper canines. The overbite and the overjet are shallow and the distal edges of the upper and lower primary molars are flush. If there no spaces or even crowding in the primary dentition, crowding is inevitable in the permanent dentition [12, 13].

11. i) What is the Terminal Plane Relationship in the Following Figures? ii) Could You Predict the Molar Relationship in the Permanent Dentition?

i. It denotes the relationship between the distal surfaces of the upper and lower second primary molars in the primary dentition. It is a method of classifying the sagittal relationship between the maxillary and mandibular dentition prior to the eruption of the permanent teeth. The terminal plane determines the initial first permanent molar relationship, given that the first permanent molars are guided into occlusion by the second deciduous second molars. The classification of the terminal plane [2, 3] is flush terminal plane (Fig. **4**), mesial step (Fig. **5**), and distal step (Fig. **6**).
ii. The flush terminal plane will result in either Class I or Class II permanent molar relationship, depending on the amount: i) of the differential maxillary and mandibular growth and ii) the forward shift of first permanent molars after the exfoliation of the second primary ones. The mesial step it is quite possible to progress in Class III molar relationship in 20% of individuals if it is more than 2mm and if it is less than 2mm in Class I molar relationship in 80% of individuals. The distal step developed in Class II permanent molar relationship [2, 14 - 16].

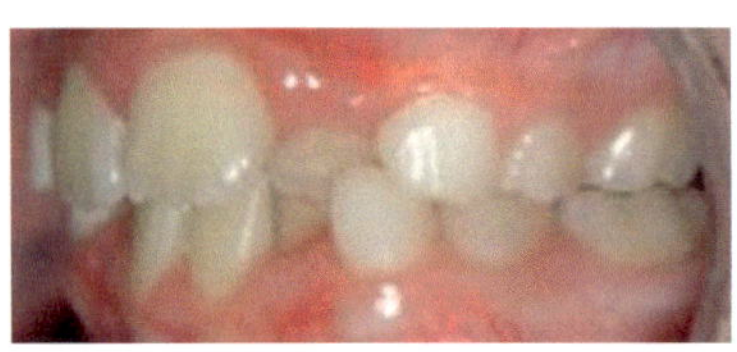

Fig. (4). Flush terminal plane.

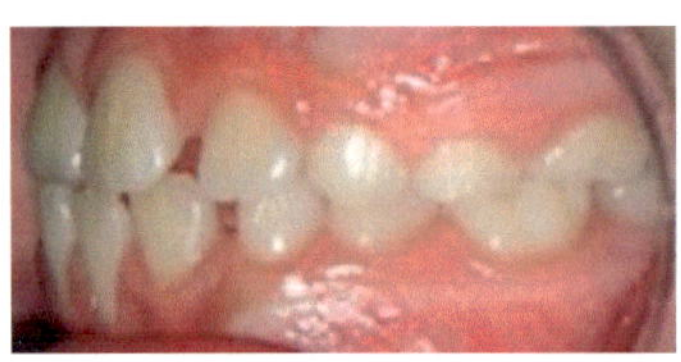

Fig. (5). Mesial step.

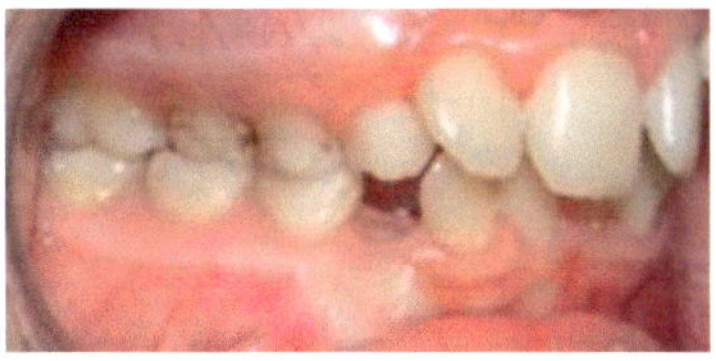

Fig. (6). Distal step.

12. i. What Do You See in the Next Figures? ii. Do You Know the Major Limitations of These Concepts?

i. The left figure (Fig. 7) represents the *"early mesial shift"*. According to the *early mesial shift* concept, in spaced primary dentition with a flush terminal plane relationship, the lower primary molars drift forward to the mandibular primate space during the eruption of the permanent first molars so that there can be a transition from a flush-terminal-plane to a mesial step during the early mixed dentition period [12, 13].
The right figure (Fig. **8**) represents the *"late mesial shift"*. The concept of the *late mesial shift* is thought to be a mechanism by which an End-to-End first molar relationship in the mixed dentition can change to a Class I molar occlusion in the permanent dentition. The larger "leeway space" in the mandible compared tothe maxillary permits the mesial movement of the molars necessary to acquire the normal adult occlusal relationship [12, 13].

ii. Both of them are supported by serial dental cast studies which could not provide information about the role of skeletal growth and tooth movement relative to basal bone in the development of the occlusion [12 - 15].
Early mesial shift: Cephalometric investigations have shown that the replacement of the mandibular primary incisors by their larger (5-6mm) permanent successors could result in a distal drifting of the mandibular primary canine into the mandibular primate space. The excessive mandibular growth seems to explain the mesial shift and the class I molar relationship [16 - 20].
Late mesial shift: According to cephalometric studies, even if the first permanent molar in the mandible seems to shift forward after the exfoliation of the second primary one, the same is true in the maxillary arch. Indeed, the principal factor in the occlusal adjustment of the buccal segments of the dental arches is the differential growth of the maxilla and the mandible [21, 22].

13. Classify the Stage of Dentition in the Next Figures

First transitional stage (6-8) yrs (Figs. **9**, **10**). During that stage the first permanent molars and the four permanent incisors erupt in both arches. The first stage is followed by a 2-year *intermediate period*.

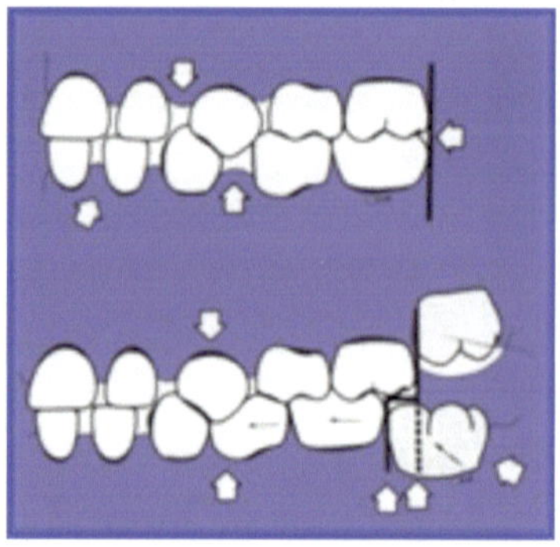

Fig. (7). Early mesial shift.

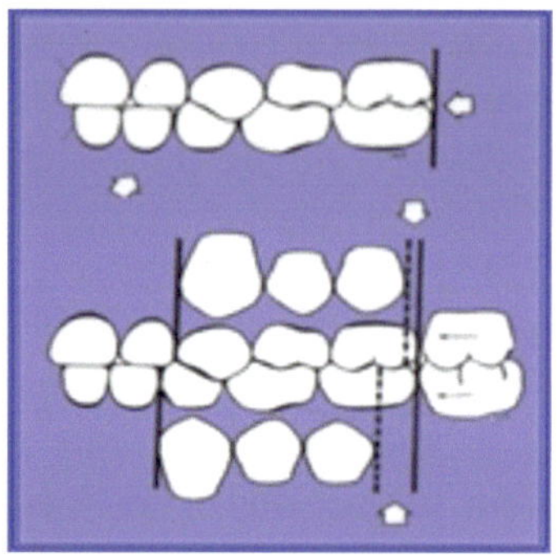

Fig. (8). Late mesial shift.

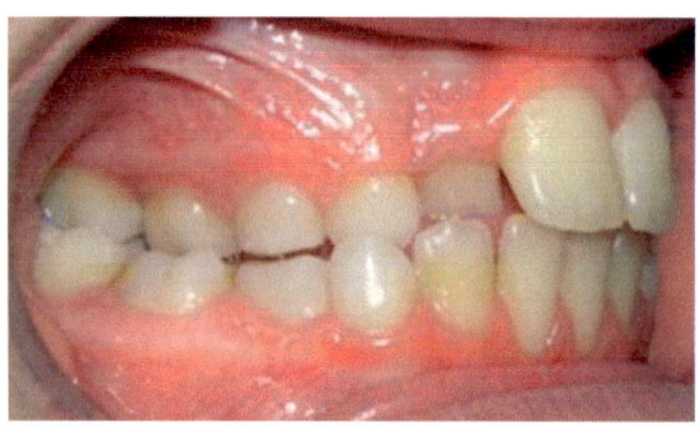

Fig. (9). First transitional stage.

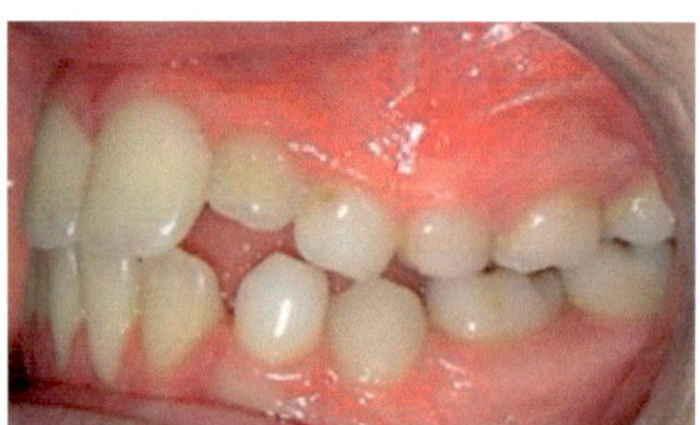

Fig. (10). First transitional stage.

Second transitional stage (10-12) yrs (Figs. **11** & **12**). During that stage the premolars and the canines erupt [2, 21, 22].

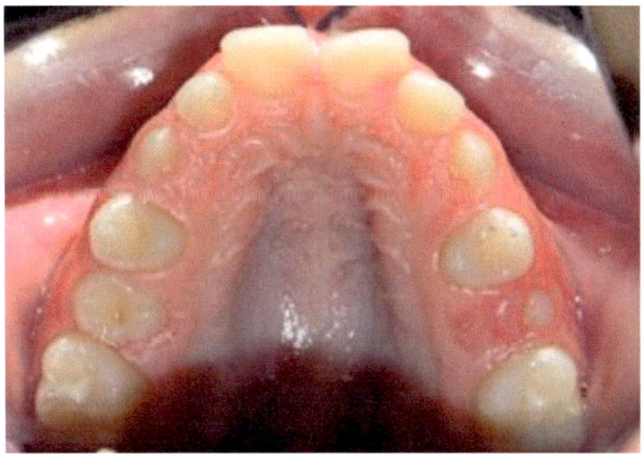

Fig. (11). Second transitional stage.

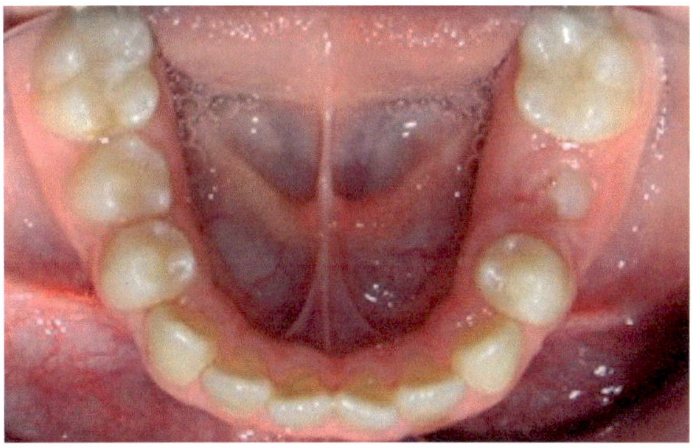

Fig. (12). Second transitional stage.

14. i. What is Leeway Space? ii. What Does it Represent Clinically? Describe the Differences (mm) between the Upper and the Lower Dental Arches

i. The size difference between the primary canines and primary molars and the corresponding permanent teeth is called *"Leeway Space"*. It is approximately *2.5mm per side in the mandible and about 1.5mm per side in the maxilla.* Leeway space is required to permit the mesial movement of the molars necessary to acquire the normal adult occlusal relationship [2 - 4, 21, 22].

ii. It represents the mesio-distal difference between the second primary molar and the second premolar (E-space) because the mesio-distal diameter of the primary canine and the first primary molar (13.64 mm) is approximately equal to the mesio-distal diameter (13.85 mm) of the permanent canine and first premolar [21, 22].

15. Which Parameters Determine How the Leeway Space is Utilised?

- The first permanent molar occlusion during the mixed dentition period.
- The sequence of exfoliation and eruption of the maxillary and mandibular primary posterior teeth.
- The pattern of skeletal growth [16 - 22].

16. i. Define the Distance *"d"*. ii. What Changes Occur in this Distance from Full Primary to Full Permanent Dentition for Both Arches?

i. *Dental Arch length.* Is the distance from the midpoint of most labial points of the central incisors to the line connecting the mesial points of first permanent molars (Fig. **13**).

ii. *Upper dental arch length*: In the first transitional period increases because of the more labial eruption of the upper permanent incisors (0.5mm during the eruption of the centrals and 1mm during the eruption of the laterals).
In the second transitional period decreases about 1.5mm per side because of replacement of the primary molars and canine by premolars and permanent canines. The upper dental arch length is slightly longer between the full primary and permanent dentition [23].

iii. *Lower dental arch length*: No significant change occurs or increases slightly during the first transitional period because the lower permanent incisors erupted almost into the same position of the primary ones.
There is a considerable decrease 2.6-3.3mm in the second transitional period arch because of the mesial migration of the first permanent molars during the replacement of the primary molars by the premolars. The lower dental arch length decreases about 2-3mm between the full primary and permanent dentition. In addition, decreases approximately 3mm between 15 and 26 years old [24, 25].

17. Describe the Maxillary and Mandibular Arch Length Changes up to 45 yrs of Age in the Following Diagrams

Maxilla (Fig. **14**): 3 to 13 yrs the arch length *increases significantly* for both sexes [4] (4.00 mm in males and 2.4 mm in females).

After that the maxillary arch *decreases significantly* until the age of 45 yrs [4] (5.7 mm for males and 4.6 mm for females).

Mandible (Fig. **15**): The mandibular arch length *increases significantly* until the age of 8 yrs (1.9 mm in males and 2.00 mm in females), and then *decreases* *significant* during the next 5 yrs (13 yrs). Between 13 and 45 yrs *decreases significantly;* 7.4 mm in males and 8.3 mm in females [23].

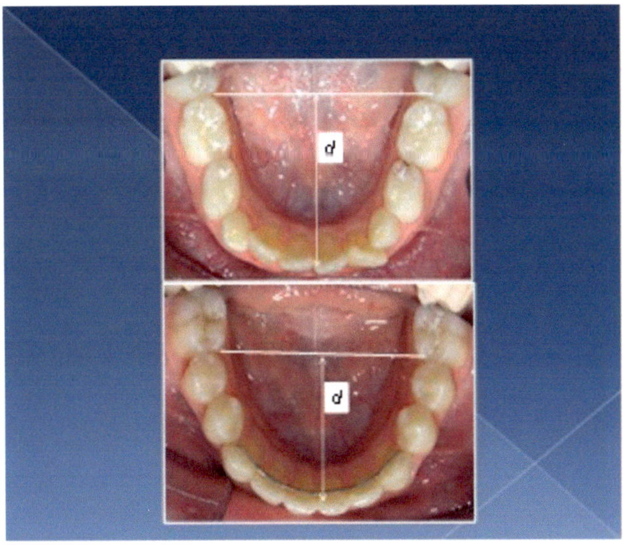

Fig. (13). Dental arch length.

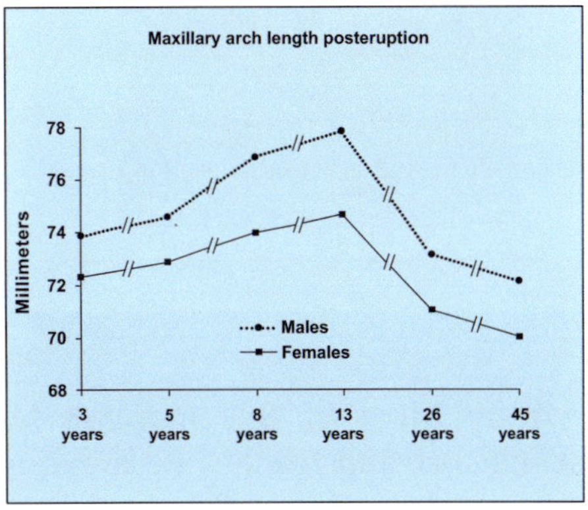

Fig. (14). Maxillary arch length.

18. Define the Distance "α". What Changes Occur in this Distance from Primary to Full Permanent Dentition?

Intercuspid width. It is determined by measuring the distance between the crown tips of the cuspids (Fig. **16**).

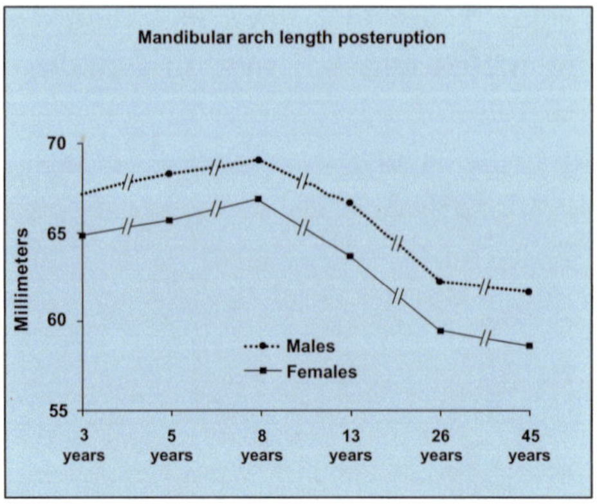

Fig. (15). Mandibular arch length.

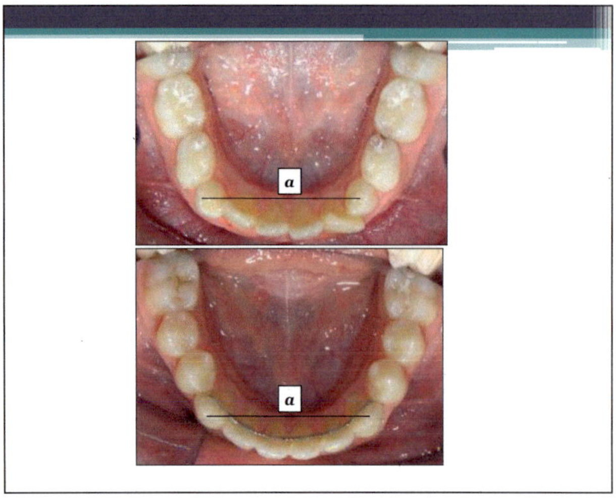

Fig. (16). Intercuspid width.

Mandibular intercuspid width. Most of this increase takes place during the eruption of the permanent incisors and reaches its maximum size at the time of exfoliation of the primary cuspids. When the permanent cuspids have fully erupted, the intercuspid diameter remains stable or decreases slightly. Thereafter, it decreases slightly, beginning at the age of 11 or 12 years until the age of 18 years [20 - 25].

In total, from 2 to 18 years, the intercuspid width increases by 3 mm in males and 2.5 mm in females.

Maxillary intercuspid width. Increases about 3 mm between 6 and 9 years of age during the eruption of incisors. After the eruption of the lateral incisors, there is dimensional stability until the primary cuspids are exfoliated. An additional 2.5 mm increases when the permanent canines erupt. At that time, it is found to be greater. A small decrease of this dimension is observed until the age of 18 years [20 - 25].

In total from 6 to 16 years, the intercuspid width increases by 5 mm in males and 4 mm in females.

19. Can You Describe the Cuspid Width Changes in the Following Diagram in Accordance with the Study of Moorrees?

Maxilla: The inter-canine width (Fig. **17**) increases after the age of 6, at the point at which the permanent lateral incisors erupt. At that time, the primary cuspids move distally and laterally, and an increase occurs until the permanent cuspids are erupted [2, 3, 5].

Mandible: The inter-canine width *stays* similar up until age 6, and then significantly increases around the age of 6 with the eruption of the permanent incisors. The mandibular inter-canine width does not show significant changes from age 8-10 yrs, whereas it decreases slightly after 12 yrs [2, 3, 5].

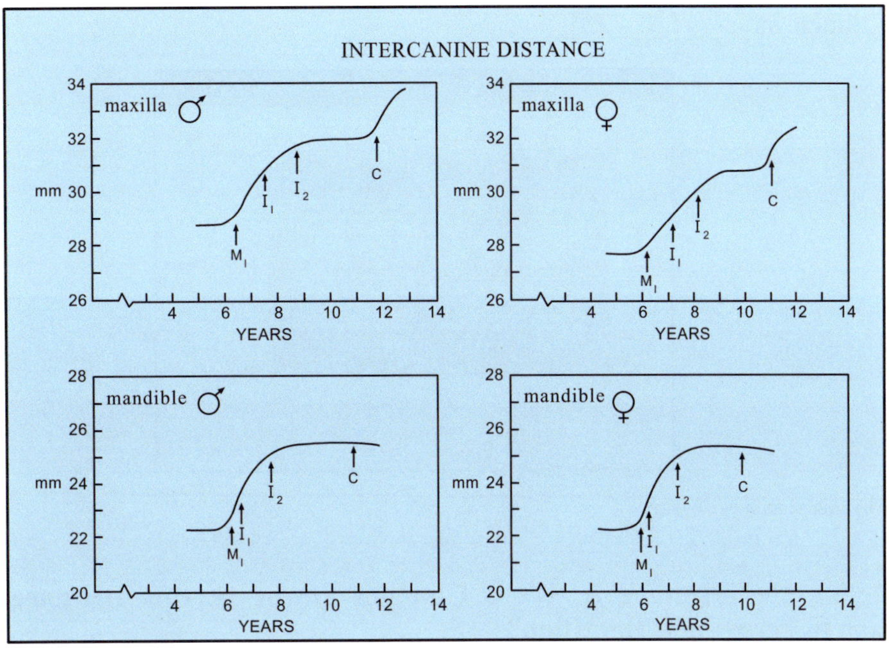

Fig. (17). Inter-canine distance.

20. Define the Line in the Following Picture. What Changes Occur in this Dimension from Primary to Permanent Dentition?

Dental Arch Perimeter. It is measured by connecting the interproximal contact points of the posterior teeth and the incisal edges of incisor teeth into a smooth curve (Fig. **18**). The anterior segment of both dental arches, from cuspid to the midline of central incisors, increases during the eruption of the incisors and reaches its maximum size after the exfoliation of the primary cuspid. In the posterior segment (cuspid to distal of second bicuspid or second primary molar), there is a reduction in the maxillary, as well as in the mandibular arch, due to the leeway space [20 - 25].

Maxilla: increases approximately 4 to 5 mm from 6 to 11 years of age and decreases 3 to 4 mm between 11 and 16 years of age.

Mandible: increases approximately 2.5mm during the first transitional period and decreases significantly during the second transitional period due to:

- Late growth changes in the mandible.
- Since the mandibular incisors are enclosed by maxillary incisors, the increase in size and forward growth of the mandible will result in the uprighting of the mandibular incisors [20 - 25].

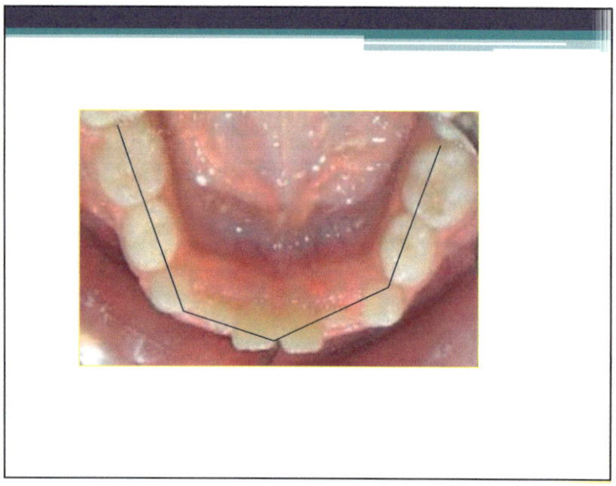

Fig. (18). Dental arch perimeter.

21. Define the Distance *b*. What Changes Occur in this Distance from Primary to Permanent Dentition?

Intermolar width: It is obtained by measuring the distance between the mesiolingual cusps of the first permanent molars (Fig. **19**). In the mandible there is no real increase from 6 to 11 years of age because of the molars' convergent eruption path. Maxillary inter-molar molar width increases steadily from 6 to 12 years of age about 5mm for both sexes due to the remodelling of the alveolus, transverse jaw growth as well as because the permanent first molars occupy a position farther distally and bucally on the diverging segments of the arch [20 - 25].

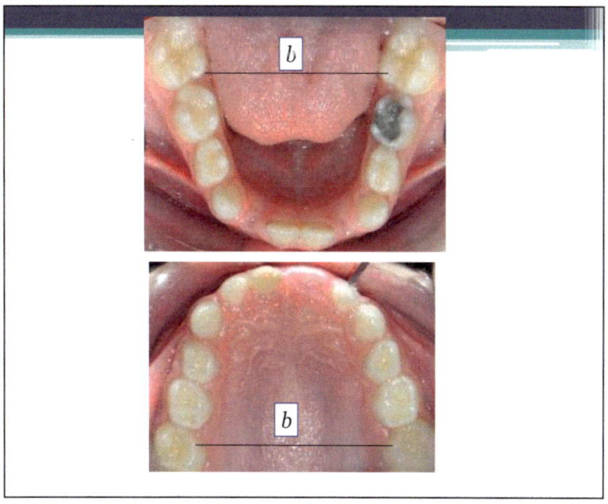

Fig. (19). Inter-molar width.

22. Describe the Average Transverse Arch Changes by Sillman

a. From birth to 4 years much of the transverse jaw growth is achieved (Fig. **20**).
b. From 4 to 8 years of age growth increments are less pronounced.
c. From 8 to 12 yrs the maxilla have a larger rate of change than the mandible.
d. Decrease in transverse dimension observed from ages 16 to 20 years [26].

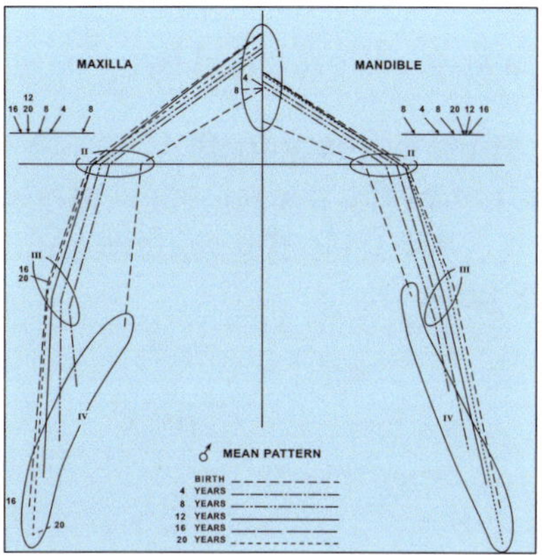

Fig. (20). Transverse arch changes by Sillman.

PART B. CLINICAL EXAMPLES

1. a. At What Stage of Dental Development is this Child?
b. Describe the Mandibular Incisors' Path of Eruption.
c. Describe the Maxillary Incisors' Path of Eruption.

a. Early mixed dentition period.

b. **Mandible**: The central incisors have erupted. The space for mandibular lateral incisor eruption is sufficient (Figs. **21**, **22**). Their roots converge towards the midline. The mandibular lateral incisors erupt after the mandibular and maxillary centrals. The lateral incisors have emerged in an adequate space (Fig. **23**). As the permanent lateral incisors erupt, they resorb the lingual aspect of the primary lateral incisor roots. The occlusal path of eruption is oblique and labial relative to the primary ones. Problems of eruption may be occurring because the lateral incisors are proportionately larger than the permanent central incisors and tend to be positioned lingual; thus, they are dependent on the available space.
If the available space is not sufficient, the erupting lateral incisors tend to push the primary canines into the primate space or, if there is no primate space, may erupt lingual or cause root resorption and premature exfoliation of the primary canines.

c. **Maxilla**: The left central incisor has emerged (Fig. **23**) in a divergent direction (normal at this age). Primate space deficiency in the maxillary arch has been observed. The maxillary central incisors (Fig. **24**) are erupted more labial and obliquely compared to the mandibular centrals and their crowns are tilted distally (normal at this age), causing a midline diastema.

2. During the Eruption of the Upper and Lower Incisors, an Additional Space of about 7-8.00 mm and 5-6.00 mm is Required. How is it Solved?

In the maxillary arch the extra space is provided by:

a. The **interdental spacing** of the primary teeth,
b. The greater **labial inclination** of the permanent centrals,
c. The **primate space,** which is mesial to the canines and
d. The **transverse maxillary** growth.

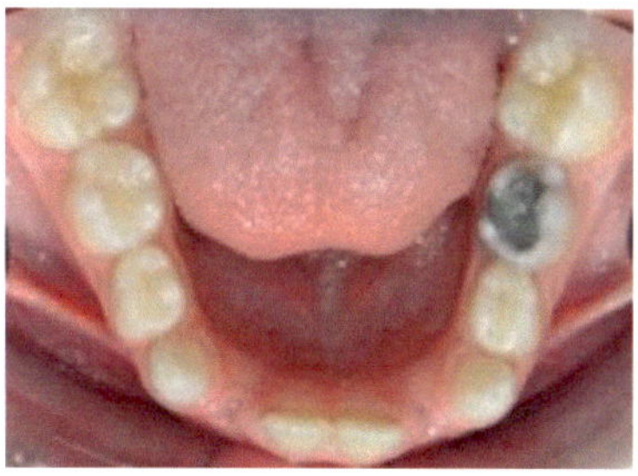

Fig. (21). Mandibular occlusal view.

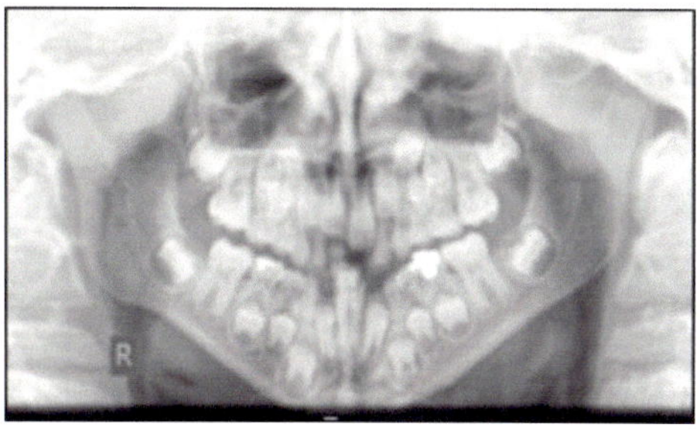

Fig. (22). Panoramic X-Ray.

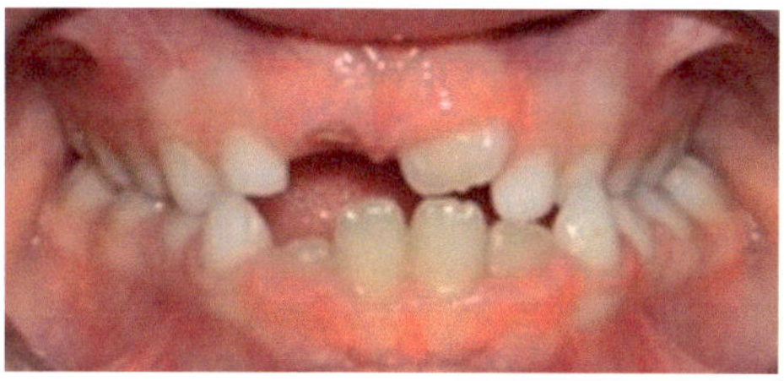

Fig. (23). Anterior occlusal view.

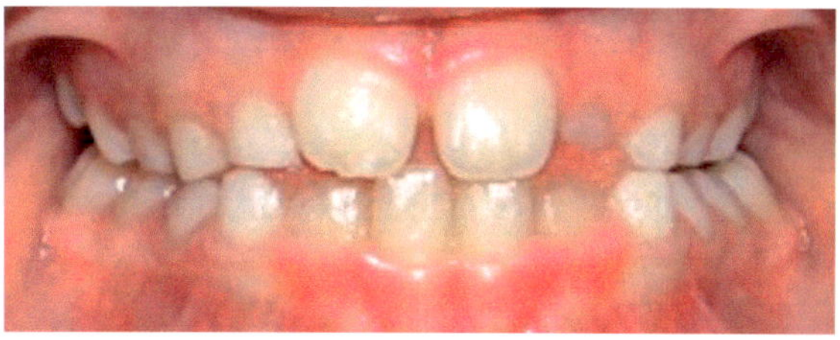

Fig. (24). Anterior occlusal view.

In the mandibular arch the incisors neither erupt to a wider dental arch circumference nor can transverse growth take place. The extra space could be provided by:

a. The **interdental spacing** of the primary teeth, and
b. The **repositioning of the canines** into the primate space because of the "pushing effect" during the eruption of the lateral incisors.

3. a. At What Stage of Dental Development is this Child?
b. What Do You See Here that is Unusual?
c. What Are the Possible Causes of this Malocclusion?

a. Early mixed dentition period.
b. Unerupted-impacted permanent central incisor (Fig. **25**).
c. A supernumerary tooth called mesiodens is the most likely cause of the unerupted permanent incisor (Fig. **26**). A mesiodens located in the maxillary central incisor region; the overall prevalence of mesiodentes is between 0.15% and 1.9%. Mesiodentes frequently interfere with the eruption and alignment of the maxillary incisors.

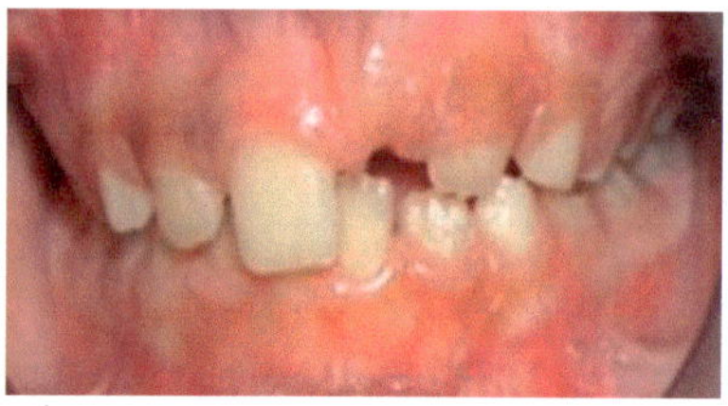

Fig. (25). Anterior occlusal view.

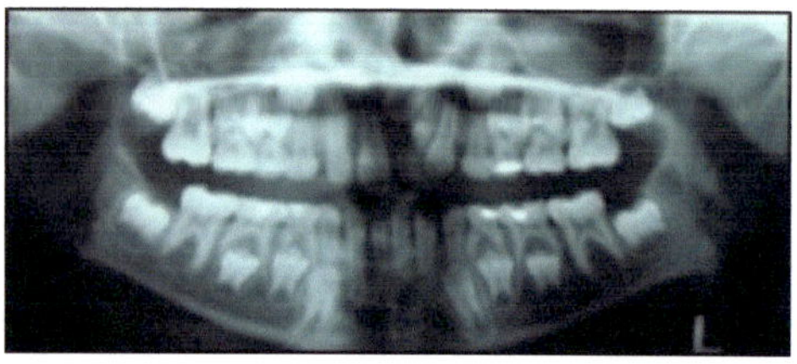

Fig. (26). Panoramic X-Ray.

4. a. At What Stage of Dental Development is this Child?
b. What Do You See in the Following Patient?
c. What Are the Possible Causes of this Malocclusion? How Do You Treat this Orthodontic Problem?

a. Permanent dentition.
b. Unerupted permanent central incisors and dental crowding (Fig. **27**).
c. Multiple supernumerary teeth in the maxillary central incisor region (Fig. **28**). They may cause ectopic eruption, impaction, rotation or labial displacement of

one or both permanent incisors, removal of supernumerary tooth and extensive orthodontic treatment.

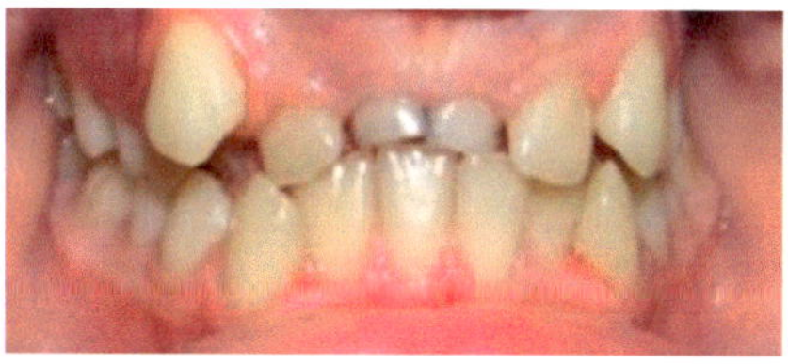

Fig. (27). Anterior occlusal view.

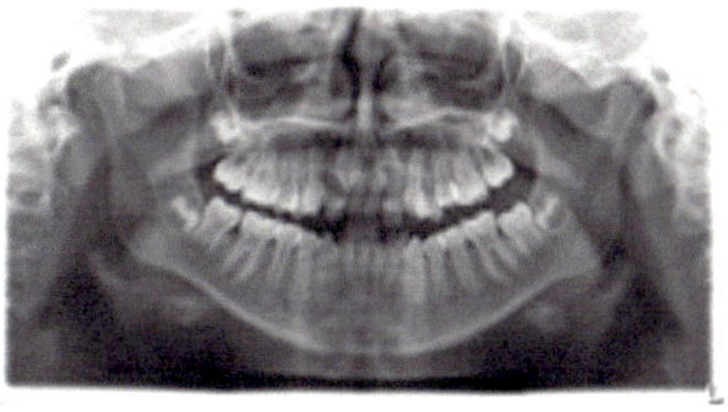

Fig. (28). Panoramic X-Ray.

5. This Patient Has a Class I Skeletal Relationship and Good Facial Balance.
a. At What Stage of Dental Development is this Child? What Do You See Here?
b. What Are the Possible Dental Causes of this Anterior Malocclusion?
c. When and Why Do You Manage this?

a. Early mixed dentition period (Fig. **29**). Anterior cross-bite of the two upper central incisors with the three lower incisors (Fig. **30**).
b. Anterior dental cross-bites originate from the abnormal axial inclination of the maxillary anterior teeth. Various etiological factors have been reported for the palatal pathway eruption of the maxillary incisors such as:
   - Trauma to the primary maxillary incisors resulting in lingual displacement of the permanent tooth buds
   - Presence of supernumerary anterior teeth or odontomas
   - An over-retained deciduous tooth or root and
   - Delayed exfoliation of the primary incisors

   If the permanent incisors are erupting in an edge-to-edge relationship, the patient most probablytends to bring the mandible forward, avoiding the traumatic occlusion, but worsening the malocclusion.
c. Correction of this malocclusion by removable orthodontic appliances should be done as soon as possible to prevent the gingival recession of the lower incisors to correct the axial inclination of both the upper and lower incisors and

to create space and guidance for the upper laterals to erupt. Various orthodontic appliances could be used such as a removable appliance with a fun-type screw and posterior bite blocks.

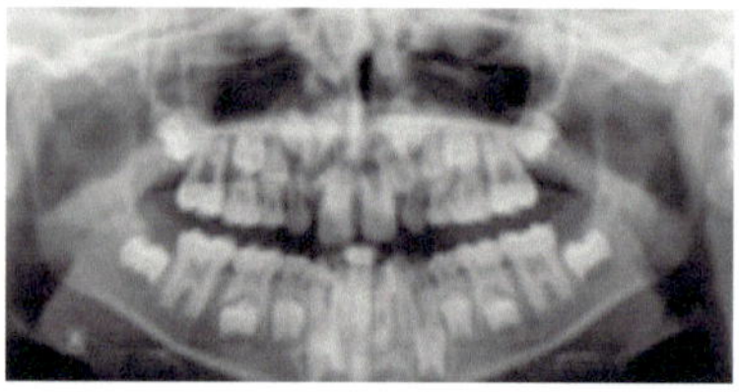

Fig. (29). Panoramic X-Ray.

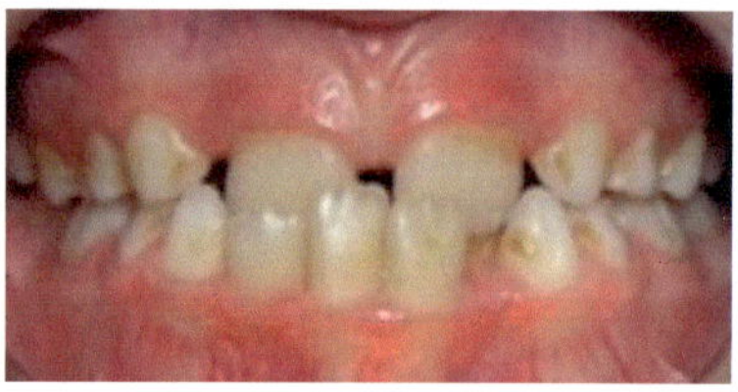

Fig. (30). Anterior occlusal view.

6. What Do You See Here? How do You Manage this Problem?

a. Intra-oral pictures radiograph illustrating supernumerary right permanent lateral incisor and crowding (Figs. **31**, **32**).
b. Supernumerary teeth extraction and extensive orthodontic treatment is required.

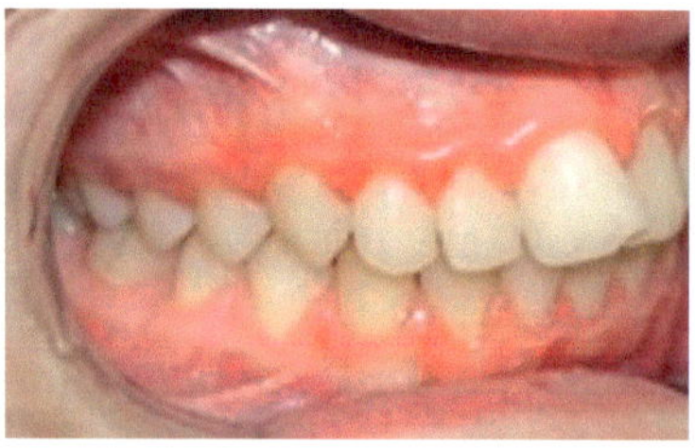

Fig. (31). Right occlusal view.

7. What Do You See Here?

Mandible: The permanent central incisors are congenitally missing (Figs. **33**, **34**) and the permanent lateral incisors upon their eruption shifted towards the midline, occupying part of their space. The lateral incisors provided proper guidance for the eruption of the cuspids occupying their position.

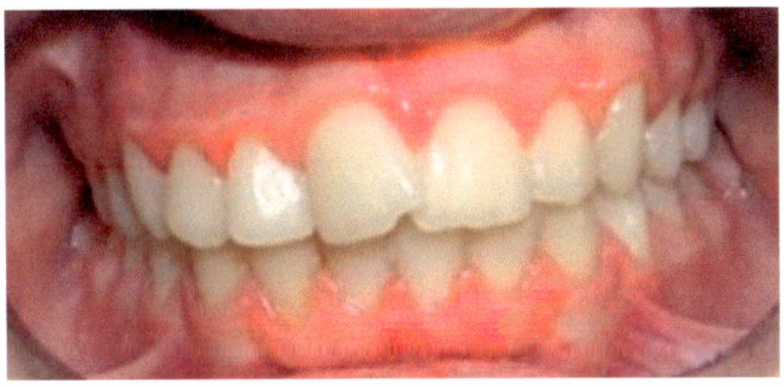

Fig. (32). Frontal occlusal view.

Maxilla: Congenitally missing the right lateral incisor. The right maxillary canine upon its eruption occupiedthe lateral's position.

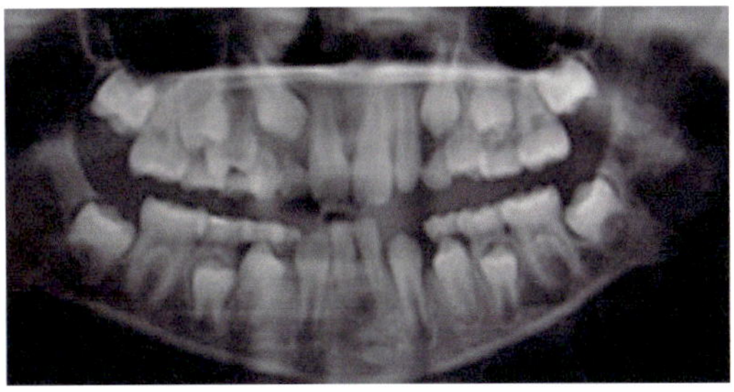

Fig. (33). Panoramic X-Ray.

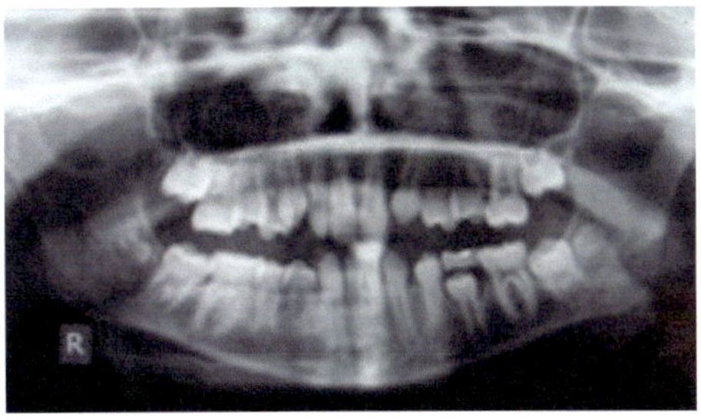

Fig. (34). Panoramic X-Ray.

8. a. What Do You See Here in the Maxillary Anterior Arch?
b. What Are the Possible Causes of the Upper Lateral Position?
c. Describe the Position of the Upper Cuspids.

a. Abnormal palatal path of eruption for both the lateral incisors and an abnormal buccal-mesial path of eruption for the canines (Figs. **35**, **36**).
b. The position of the lateral incisors could be affected:
   - By the abnormal root position of the primary lateral incisors,
   - By the inherent straight insteadof labial path of eruption or
   - Lack of space during the early mixed dentition period causes them to erupt

into a palatal position.

c. The position of the permanent cuspids into the dental arch is determined most of the times by the position of the lateral incisors. In this patient, the permanent cuspids are not guided into their proper positions and have erupted buccally and mesially.

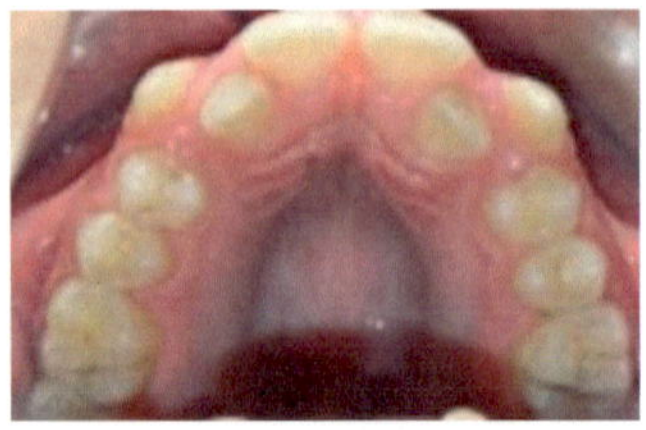

Fig. (35). Upper occlusal view.

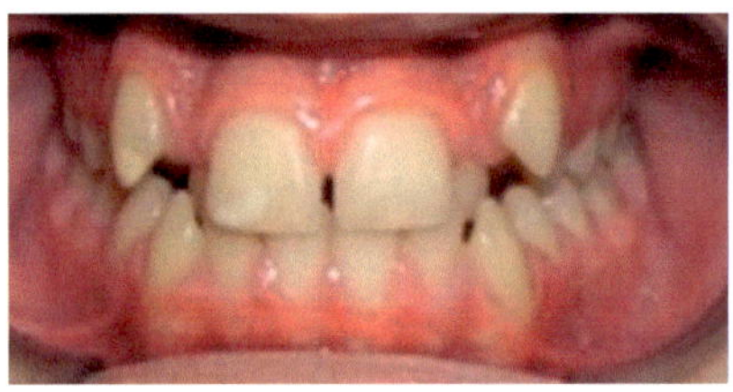

Fig. (36). Frontal occlusal view.

9. a. Define the Malocclusion.
b. What Are the Possible Causes of the Upper Lateral Position?
c. Describe the Position of the Upper Cuspids.

a. Class II/II malocclusion (Figs. **37**, **38**).
b. Possible cause of the labial position of the lateral incisors is the reversed infra-bony position relative to the permanent incisors during their development.
c. The position of the permanent cuspids is not affected because the distal aspect of the permanent lateral incisors is able to guide them correctly.

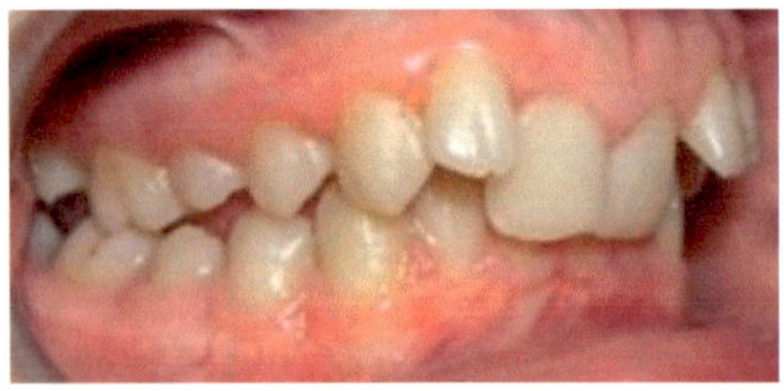

Fig. (37). Right occlusal view.

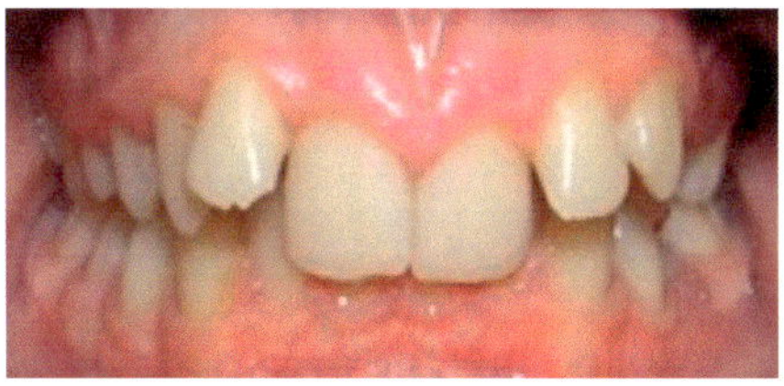

Fig. (38). Frontal occlusal view.

10. a. At What Stage of Dental Development is this Child? b. In Which Chronological Ages Do the Following Radiographs Belong? c. Describe the Canines' Path of Eruption.

a. Early mixed dentition period.
b. Panoramic radiograph at the age of 8 yrs (Fig. **39**).
   Panoramic radiograph at the age of 9 yrs (Fig. **40**).
c. The mandibular canines begin their infrabony movement mesially and lingually along the distal side of the roots of the permanent lateral incisors. The maxillary permanent canines are sited vertically at the distal side of the apical part of the maxillary lateral incisors (Fig. **39**).

Normal path of eruption for the permanent canines. Note the proper positions of both the maxillary and the mandibular permanent cuspids at the distal sides of the lateral incisors (Fig. **40**).

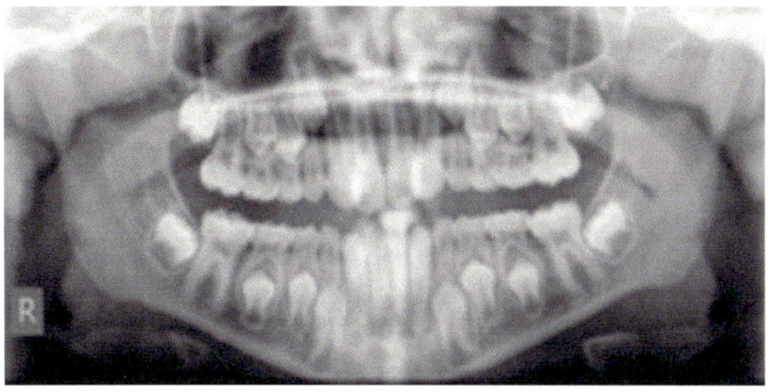

Fig. (39). Panoramic X-Ray.

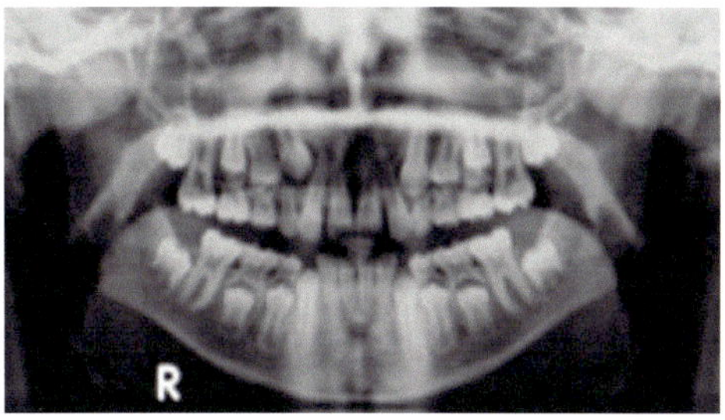

Fig. (40). Panoramic X-Ray.

11. Describe the Mandibular Canines' Pattern of Eruption

The position of the permanent canines depends on the position of the permanent lateral incisors (Fig. **41**). Lingually positioned lateral incisors result inlabially erupted permanent canines. Space analysis and extensive orthodontic treatment is required.

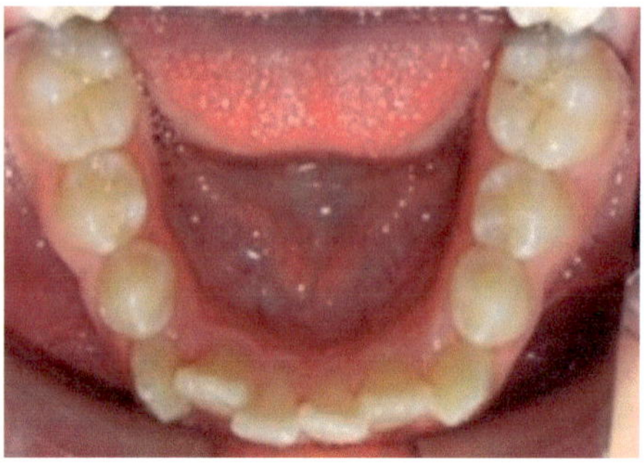

Fig. (41). Lower occlusal view.

The permanent cuspids lose their path of eruption due to lingually positioned laterals and erupted mesial (Fig. **42**). The present position of the lateral occurs because of their failure to obtain a labial path of eruption (*e.g.* retained primary laterals). Space analysis and extensive orthodontic treatment is required.

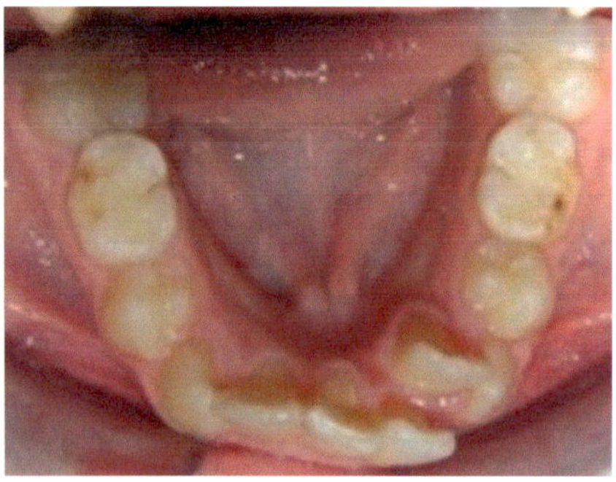

Fig. (42). Lower occlusal view.

Buccal maxillary canine displacement: The major etiological cause of buccal maxillary canine displacement **is the space deficiency** (Figs. **43** & **44**). The maxillary cuspid follows a more difficult path of eruption than any other tooth. It is high in the maxilla, with its crown directed mesially and somewhat lingually. It moves towards the occlusal plane, gradually uprighting itself until it seems to strike the distal aspect of the root of the lateral incisor. It then seems to be deflected to a more vertical and mesial position.

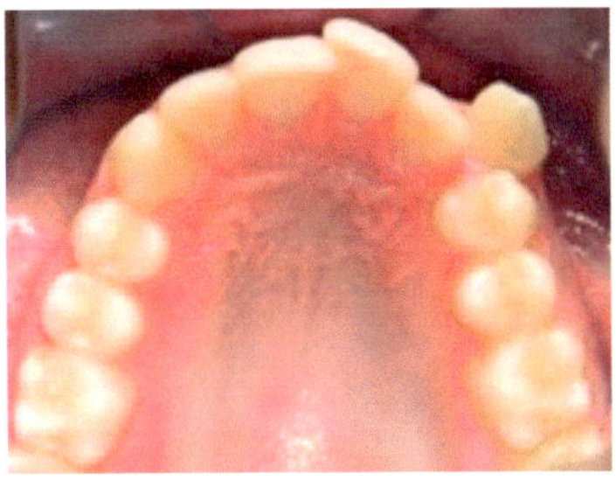

Fig. (43). Upper occlusal view.

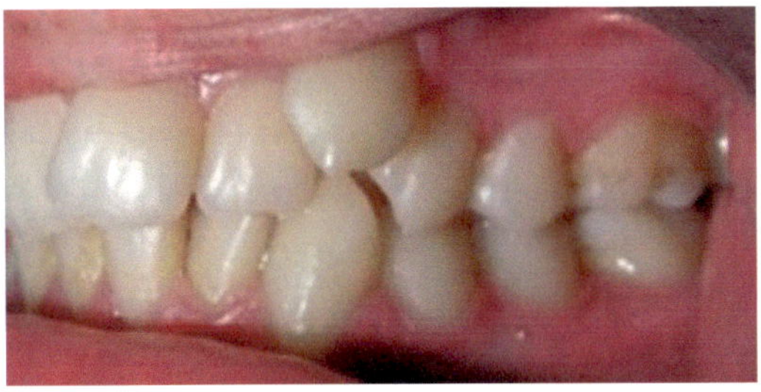

Fig. (44). Left occlusal view.

Palatal Canine Displacement (PDC): The anomalous infraosseous position of the canine before the expected time of eruption (Fig. **45**). Most of the time, palatal displacement of the maxillary canine results in impaction *(see following chapter)*.

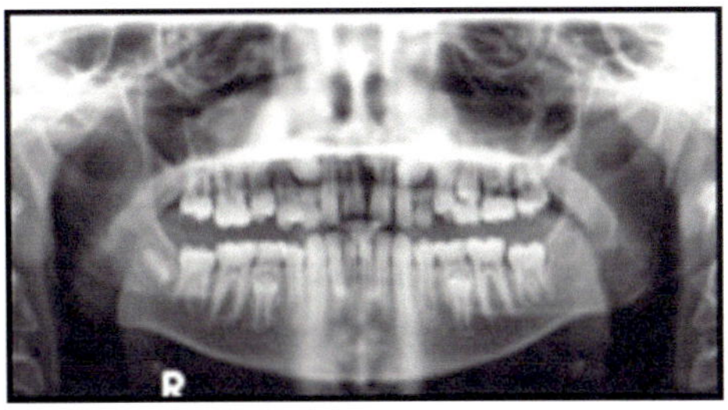

Fig. (45). Panoramic X-Ray.

Palatal Canine Impaction: The anomalous infraosseous position of the tooth after the expected time of eruption (Fig. **46**).

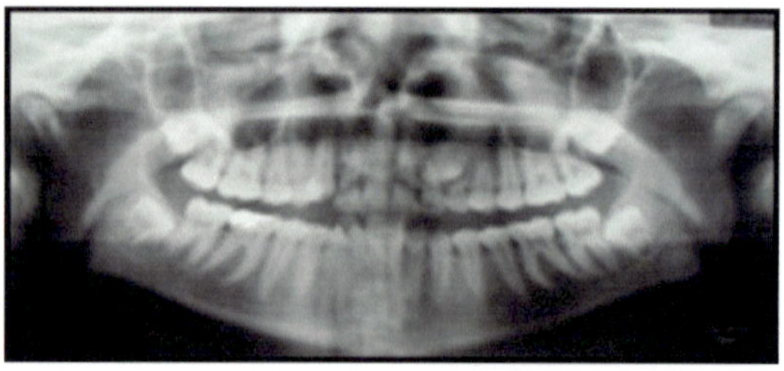

Fig. (46). Panoramic X-Ray.

12. Describe the Eruption Pathway of the Bicuspids in the Following Figures

The eruption of mandibular second premolars is of special interest (Fig. **47**). As the second premolar erupts, it resorbs the distal root of the second primary molar erupting close to the mesial surface of the first permanent molar. It is the safest eruption path regarding the minimum loss of space during the replacement procedure.

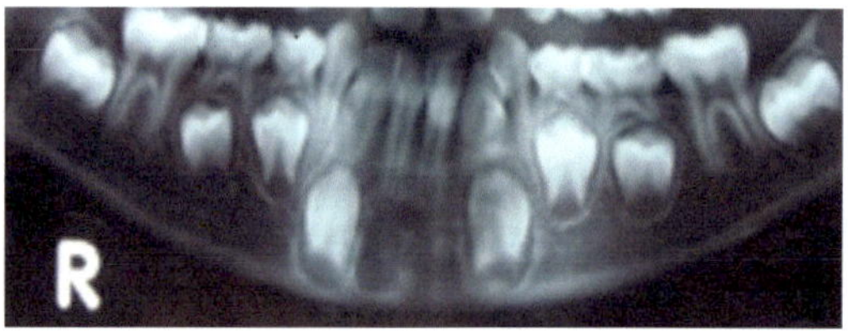

Fig. (47). Lower arch X-Ray.

Radiograph depicting the least desirable path of eruption for the mandibular second bicuspids (Fig. **48**). The tooth erupted mesially and resorbed the mesial root of its predecessors. On the right side, the first premolar is experiencing interference in its eruption by the mesial root of the second primary molar, whereas the second premolar seems to be blocked by the first one.

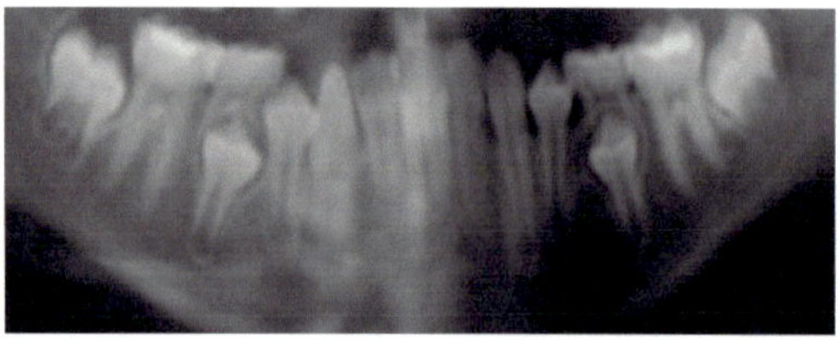

Fig. (48). Lower arch X-Ray.

Early loss of the mandibular left second primary molar *(after the eruption of the first permanent molar)* can cause the mesial inclination of the first permanent molars, distal eruption of the first bicuspidand impaction of the second bicuspid

(Figs. **49** & **50**). However, considerable loss in arch length can occur if the first permanent molars erupt without the second primary molar as an eruptive guide. Space loss more than 8 mm in a maxilla and up to 4 to 6 mm in a mandible has been reported.

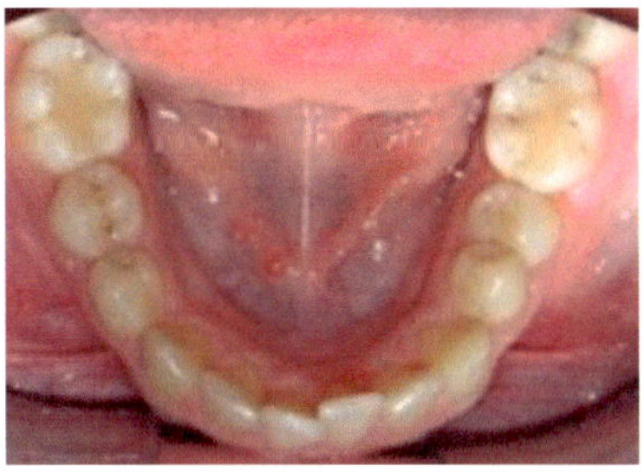

Fig. (49). Lower occlusal view.

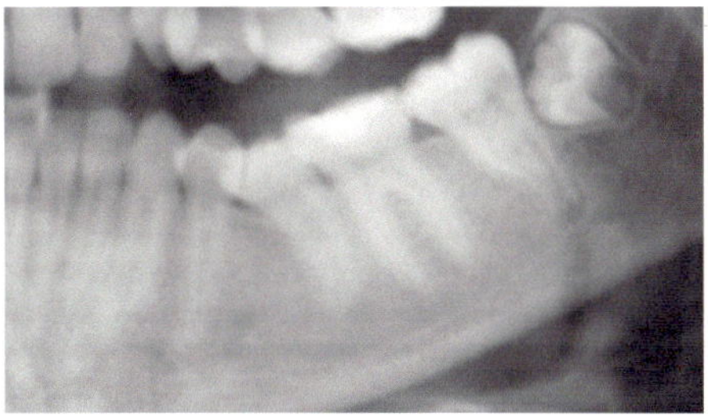

Fig. (50). Left mandible X-Ray.

The first primary molars have been lost prematurely; leeway space has been lost; reversed sequence of eruption for the premolars; the first premolar has been blocked by the permanent canine and the second premolar (Figs. **51** & **52**).

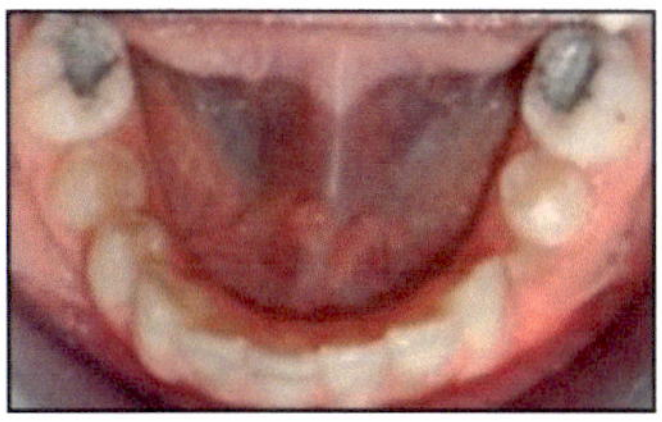

Fig. (51). Lower occlusal view.

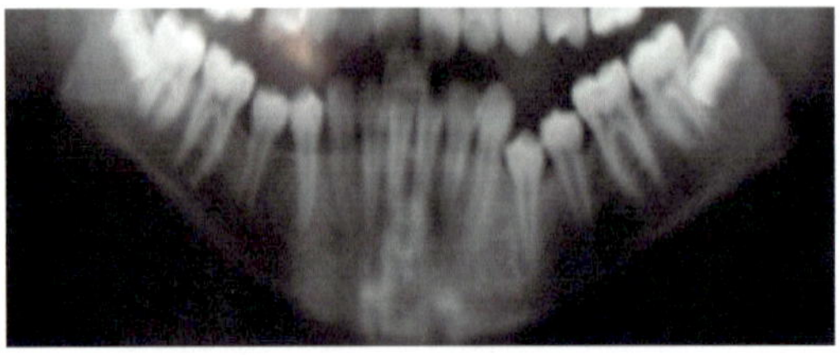

Fig. (52). Lower arch X-Ray.

Unilateral premature exfoliation of the maxillary right second primary molar (Fig. **53**). Mesial crown movement and rotation of the maxillary right permanent molar around the palatal root and distal tipping of the first primary molar. The second maxillary bicuspid has become impacted.

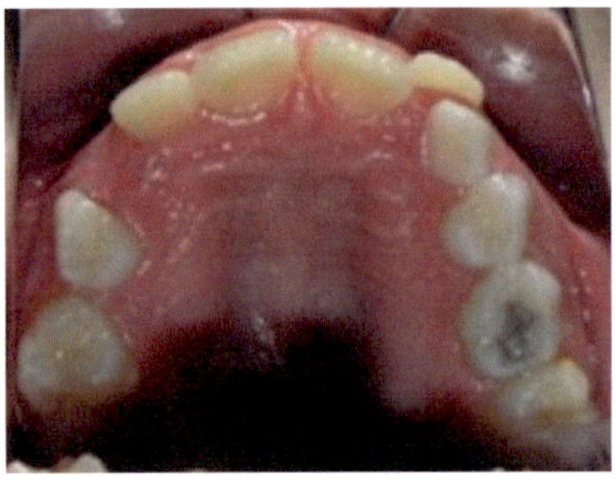

Fig. (53). Upper arch view.

Bilateral premature loss of the maxillary second primary molars. Mesial crown movement and rotation around the palatal root of the first maxillary permanent molars, distal tipping of the first bicuspids and second maxillary bicuspid impaction (Fig. **54**).

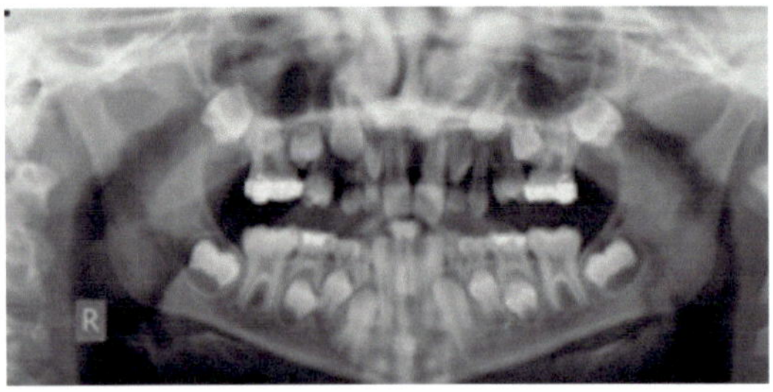

Fig. (54). Panoramic X-Ray.

Early Loss of the Maxillary First Primary Molar. The primary cuspid shifts distally the first year after the premature exfoliation; the primary second maxillary molar could move mesially (depending on the age and the duration of tooth loss) and the erupting first bicuspid could erupt mesially because of the mesially shifted second primary molar (Fig. **55**).

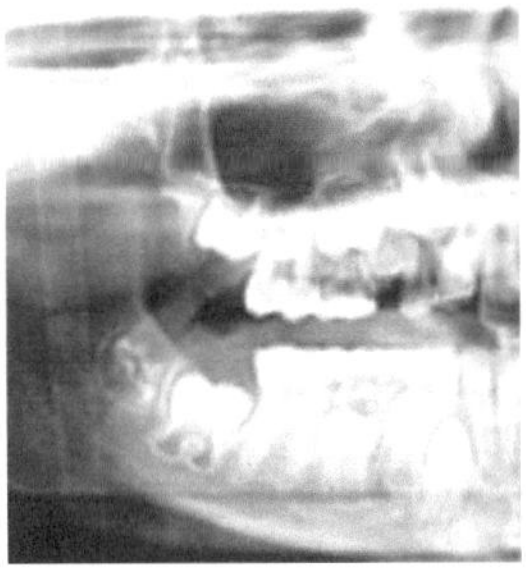

Fig. (55). Left arch X-ray.

CONCLUDING REMARKS

Occlusion development begins with the formation of the primary dentition, continuing to the mixed dentition and finally concludes with the formation of the permanent dentition. Much of the adjustment from mixed dentition to permanent dentition in normal growth patients relies on the proper utilisation of the leeway space.

REFERENCES

[1] Nolla CM. Development of the permanent teeth. J Dent Child 1960; 27: 254.

[2] Proffit W. Contemporary Orthodontics. 4th ed., St. Louis: Mosby 2007.

[3] Moyers RE. Handbook of Orthodontics. 3rd ed., Chicago: Year Book Medical Publishers 1973.

[4] Moyers RE, Van der Linden FP, Riolo ML, *et al.* Standards of Human Occlusal Development Monograph 5 Craniofacial Growth Series. Ann Harbor, MI: Center of Human Development, the University of Michigan 1976.

[5] Moorrees CF, Grøn AM, Lebret LM, Yen PK, Fröhlich FJ. Growth studies of the dentition: a review. Am J Orthod 1969; 55(6): 600-16. [http://dx.doi.org/10.1016/0002-9416(69)90037-2] [PMID: 4890736]

[6] Demirjian A, Goldstein H, Tanner JM. A new system of dental age assessment. Hum Biol 1973; 45(2): 211-27. [PMID: 4714564]

[7] Garn SM, Smith BH. Developmental communalities in tooth emergence timing. J Dent Res 1980; 59(7): 1178. [http://dx.doi.org/10.1177/00220345800590072501] [PMID: 6929821]

[8] Nanda S. The development basis of occlusion and malocclusion. Chicago: Quintessence Publishing Co. 1982.

[9] Dugoni SA. Comprehensive treatment during mixed dentition period. Am J Orthod Dentofacial Orthop 1998; 113: 75-84.

[http://dx.doi.org/10.1016/S0889-5406(98)70278-1] [PMID: 9457021]

[10] Brook AH, Jernvall J, Smith RN, Hughes TE, Townsend GC. The dentition: the outcomes of morphogenesis leading to variations of tooth number, size and shape. Aust Dent J 2014; 59 (Suppl. 1): 131-42.
[http://dx.doi.org/10.1111/adj.12160] [PMID: 24646162]

[11] Arte S, Nieminen P, Apajalahti S, Haavikko K, Thesleff I, Pirinen S. Characteristics of incisor-premolar hypodontia in families. J Dent Res 2001; 80(5): 1445-50.
[http://dx.doi.org/10.1177/00220345010800051201] [PMID: 11437217]

[12] Baume LJ. Physiological tooth migration and its significance for the development of occlusion; the biogenesis of accessional dentition. J Dent Res 1950; 29(3): 331-7.
[http://dx.doi.org/10.1177/00220345500290031301] [PMID: 15428568]

[13] Baume LJ. Physiological tooth migration and its significance for the development of occlusion; the biogenesis of the successional dentition. J Dent Res 1950; 29(3): 338-48.
[http://dx.doi.org/10.1177/00220345500290031401] [PMID: 15428569]

[14] Paulsen HU. Changes in sagittal molar occlusion during growth. Tandlaegebladet 1971; 75(12): 1258-67.
[PMID: 5290992]

[15] Clinch LM. An analysis of serial models between three and eight years of age. Dent Rec (London) 1951; 71(4): 61-72.
[PMID: 24540970]

[16] Brin I, Kelley MB, Ackerman JL, Green PA. Molar occlusion and mandibular rotation: a longitudinal study. Am J Orthod 1982; 81(5): 397-403.
[http://dx.doi.org/10.1016/0002-9416(82)90077-X] [PMID: 6960726]

[17] Kim YE, Nanda RS, Sinha PK. Transition of molar relationships in different skeletal growth patterns. Am J Orthod Dentofacial Orthop 2002; 121(3): 280-90.
[http://dx.doi.org/10.1067/mod.2002.119978] [PMID: 11941342]

[18] Kerr WJ. A longitudinal cephalometric study of dento-facial growth from 5 to 15 years. Br J Orthod 1979; 6(3): 115-21.
[http://dx.doi.org/10.1179/bjo.6.3.115] [PMID: 297456]

[19] Lundström A, McWilliam JS. Dento-alveolar compensation for antero-posterior variations between the upper and lower apical bases. Eur J Orthod 1984; 6(2): 116-22.
[http://dx.doi.org/10.1093/ejo/6.2.116] [PMID: 6587968]

[20] Nanda RS, Merrill RM. Cephalometric assessment of sagittal relationship between maxilla and mandible. Am J Orthod Dentofacial Orthop 1994; 105(4): 328-44.
[http://dx.doi.org/10.1016/S0889-5406(94)70127-X] [PMID: 8154458]

[21] Bishara SE, Hoppens BJ, Jakobsen JR, Kohout FJ. Changes in the molar relationship between the deciduous and permanent dentitions: a longitudinal study. Am J Orthod Dentofacial Orthop 1988; 93(1): 19-28.
[http://dx.doi.org/10.1016/0889-5406(88)90189-8] [PMID: 3422119]

[22] Bishara SE, Treder JE, Jakobsen JR. Facial and dental changes in adulthood. Am J Orthod Dentofacial Orthop 1994; 106(2): 175-86.
[http://dx.doi.org/10.1016/S0889-5406(94)70036-2] [PMID: 8059754]

[23] Bishara SE, Jakobsen JR, Treder J, Nowak A. Arch length changes from 6 weeks to 45 years. Angle Orthod 1998; 68(1): 69-74.
[PMID: 9503137]

[24] DeKock WH. Dental arch depth and width studied longitudinally from 12 years of age to adulthood. Am J Orthod 1972; 62(1): 56-66.
[http://dx.doi.org/10.1016/0002-9416(72)90125-X] [PMID: 4503706]

[25] Burdi AR, Moyers RE. Development of the dentition and occlusion. Handbook of orthodontics. 4th ed., Chicago: Year Book Medical Publishers 1988.

[26] Sillman JH. Dimensional changes of the dental arches: Longitudinal study from birth to 25 years. Am J Orthod 1964; 50(11): 824-42. [http://dx.doi.org/10.1016/0002-9416(64)90040-5]

CHAPTER 5

Interceptive Treatment

Abstract: Early diagnosis and successful treatment of developing malocclusions can have both short-term and long-term benefits while achieving the goals of occlusal harmony and function and dentofacial aesthetics. Guidance of eruption and the development of permanent dentition is an integral component of comprehensive oral health care for all paediatric orthodontic patients. Such guidance should contribute to the development of a permanent dentition that is in a stable, functional, and aesthetically acceptable occlusion and normal subsequent dentofacial development. The purpose of this chapter with the question-answer format is to provide the principles for proper occlusal guidance, prevention of developing malocclusions and proper interceptive orthodontic treatment during the mixed dentition period. In the second part of the chapter, a series of clinical examples and the paediatric orthodontic intervention treatment are provided.

INTRODUCTION

Space management of the developing occlusion is an important part of interceptive and preventive dental care. Space maintenance involves using an appliance to passively hold teeth in position in order to allow for the eruption of permanent successors into occlusion deal arch form, which is dependent on the presence and correct alignment of every erupted tooth in the mouth. The premature loss of a tooth or tooth structure, if not compensated for, may result in a loss of arch circumference, crowding and/or malocclusion due to the shifting and/or drifting of adjacent teeth. In the mixed dentition period, one mechanism for alignment is to preserve the leeway space. Most clinicians expect that interceptive orthodontics could correct malocclusion, avoiding permanent tooth extractions at the later stage of treatment.

PART A. SPACE MANAGEMENT IN THE MIXED DENTITION

1. What is Space Management and What is Dental Crowding?

Space maintenance involves using an appliance to passively hold teeth in position in order to allow for the eruption of permanent successors into occlusion. Dental crowding is the difference between the space needed in the dental arch and the space available in that arch. A common form is tooth size arch length discrepancy.

George Litsas

Negative space available results in crowding and positive space available results in spacing between the teeth [1, 2]. Crowding is one of the most prevalent malocclusions and the most common reasons patients seek orthodontic treatment [3].

2. Why Do You need to Study Models in the Mixed Dentition Period?

You should evaluate the models in the mixed dentition period [4, 5] in order to:

a. Evaluate the dental arch form
b. Evaluate the dental anatomy
c. Check the intercuspation
d. Make dental arch space analysis

3. Describe the Moyers, Tanaka and Johnston Mixed Dentition Analysis. List the Reasons for Using the Mandibular Incisors as Reference Teeth. Provide the Main Advantages and Disadvantages of these Methods.

a. **Moyers analysis** (Fig. **1**) uses the sum of the widths of the lower incisors and the prediction charts to obtain the estimated value of the unerupted teeth [4]. This method has good accuracy and makes allowance for different levels of probability. No radiographs are required.
b. **Tanaka and Johnston's** method (Fig. **2**) used a regression equation to predict the sizes of the unerupted canines and premolars [5]. The equation takes 1/2 of the sum of the mesio-distal widths of the permanent central and lateral mandibular incisors plus 11 mm for the maxillary and plus 10.5 mm for the mandibular teeth. This equation predicts the width of the unerupted premolars and canines at the seventy-fifth percentile level. This method has good accuracy; neither radiographs nor tables are required.
c. The reasons for using the mandibular incisors [2, 3] as reference teeth are:
   1. The first teeth in the sequence of eruption
   2. They have less variability in shape and size
   3. They can be measured easily and accurately
d. The main **advantages** of both analyses are the ease and speed of using by direct measurement of teeth in the oral cavity without any radiographic exposure to young children [9].

The main **disadvantages are** that they neither take into account the axial inclination of the mandibular anterior teeth, the effects of the curve of Spee, ethnic group biases or facial profile, all of which can affect the amount of crowding and space required in the analyses. Studies comparing these methods with their respective populations have observed either overestimation or underestimation [6, 7].

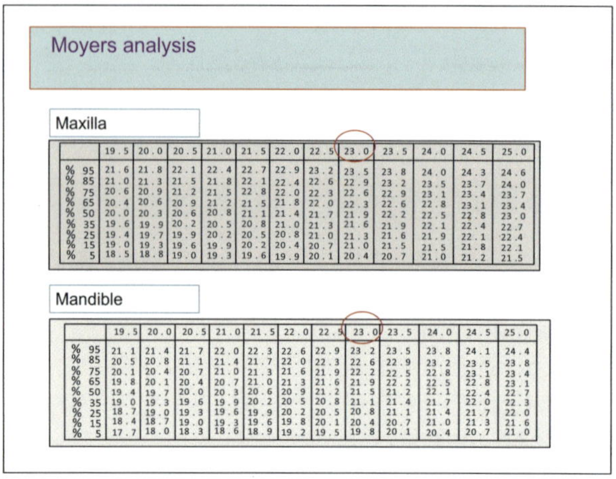

Moyers analysis

Maxilla

	19.5	20.0	20.5	21.0	21.5	22.0	22.5	23.0	23.5	24.0	24.5	25.0
% 95	21.6	21.8	22.1	22.4	22.7	22.9	23.2	23.5	23.8	24.0	24.3	24.6
% 85	21.0	21.3	21.5	21.8	22.1	22.4	22.6	22.9	23.2	23.5	23.7	24.0
% 75	20.6	20.9	21.2	21.5	22.8	22.0	22.3	22.6	22.9	23.1	23.4	23.7
% 65	20.4	20.6	20.9	21.2	21.5	21.8	22.0	22.3	22.6	22.8	23.1	23.4
% 50	20.0	20.3	20.6	20.8	21.1	21.4	21.7	21.9	22.2	22.5	22.8	23.0
% 35	19.6	19.9	20.2	20.5	20.8	21.0	21.3	21.6	21.9	22.1	22.4	22.7
% 25	19.4	19.7	19.9	20.2	20.5	20.8	21.0	21.3	21.6	21.9	22.1	22.4
% 15	19.0	19.3	19.6	19.9	20.2	20.4	20.7	21.0	21.5	21.5	21.8	22.1
% 5	18.5	18.8	19.0	19.3	19.6	19.9	20.1	20.4	20.7	21.0	21.2	21.5

Mandible

	19.5	20.0	20.5	21.0	21.5	22.0	22.5	23.0	23.5	24.0	24.5	25.0
% 95	21.1	21.4	21.7	22.0	22.3	22.6	22.9	23.2	23.5	23.8	24.1	24.4
% 85	20.5	20.8	21.1	21.4	21.7	22.0	22.3	22.6	22.9	23.2	23.5	23.8
% 75	20.1	20.4	20.7	21.0	21.3	21.6	21.9	22.2	22.5	22.8	23.1	23.4
% 65	19.8	20.1	20.4	20.7	21.0	21.3	21.6	21.9	22.2	22.5	22.8	23.1
% 50	19.4	19.7	20.0	20.3	20.6	20.9	21.2	21.5	21.2	22.1	22.4	22.7
% 35	19.0	19.3	19.6	19.9	20.2	20.5	20.8	21.1	21.4	21.7	22.0	22.3
% 25	18.7	19.0	19.3	19.6	19.9	20.2	20.5	20.8	21.1	21.4	21.7	22.0
% 15	18.4	18.7	19.0	19.3	19.6	19.8	20.1	20.4	20.7	21.0	21.3	21.6
% 5	17.7	18.0	18.3	18.6	18.9	19.2	19.5	19.8	20.1	20.4	20.7	21.0

Fig. (1). Moyers analysis.

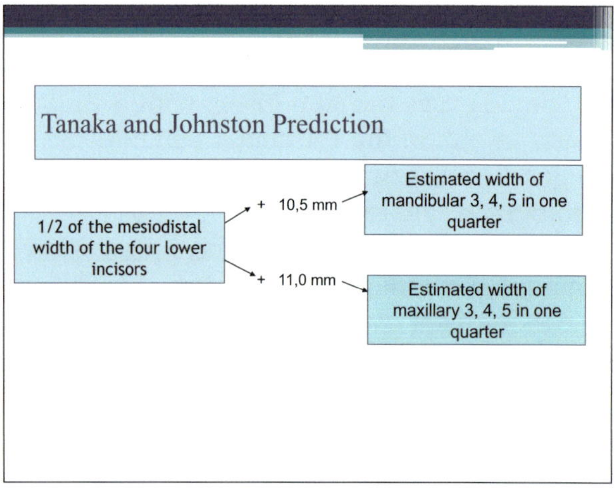

Fig. (2). Tanaka and Johnston method.

4. a. Which Factors Determine Whether the Space Loss Needs to be Maintained or not?

Which Could be the Possible Orthodontic Treatment in the Mixed Dentition if the Space Analysis in a Normal Growth Patient Revealed that the Required Space is: i) < 3.00mm, ii) 4.00mm-8.00mm and iii) > 8.00mm?

a. **Root development**: The less the root of the permanent succedaneous tooth has developed, the stronger the recommendation for space management procedures.
b. **Overlying alveolar bone**: The more the amount of the overlying bone, the stronger the recommendation for space maintenance.
c. **Type of tooth** lost [8 - 10].

i. **< 3mm: Localised space loss**. Interproximal stripping [6, 9, 13] of:
   - Mesial-distal surfaces of primary canines (Fig. **3**)
   - Mesial surfaces of first, second primary molars (Figs. **4-6**)

ii. **4-8mm: Space regaining- Extraction borderline cases**. Orthodontic intervention could be considered the E space reservation, maxillary expansion and maxillary permanent molar distalization procedures [8 - 11].

iii. **>8 mm: Serial extraction**. It could be defined as the extraction of permanent teeth in a planned sequence and guiding all permanent teeth to a good occlusion in order to prevent a gross malocclusion. The practice of serial dental extraction protocol aims at correcting definitive crowding, of a genetic aetiology [12, 13].

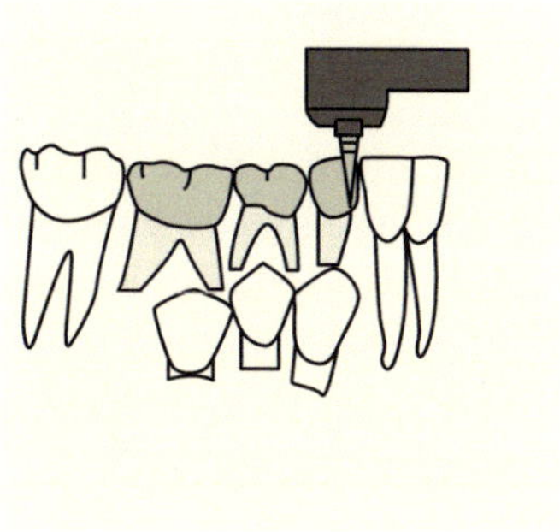

Fig. (3). Interproximal stripping.

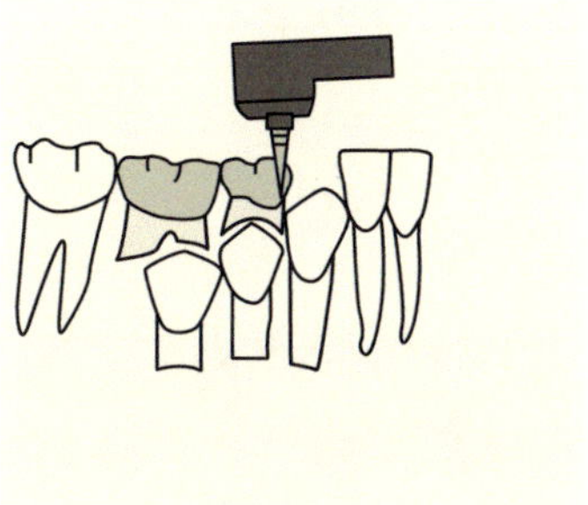

Fig. (4). Interproximal stripping.

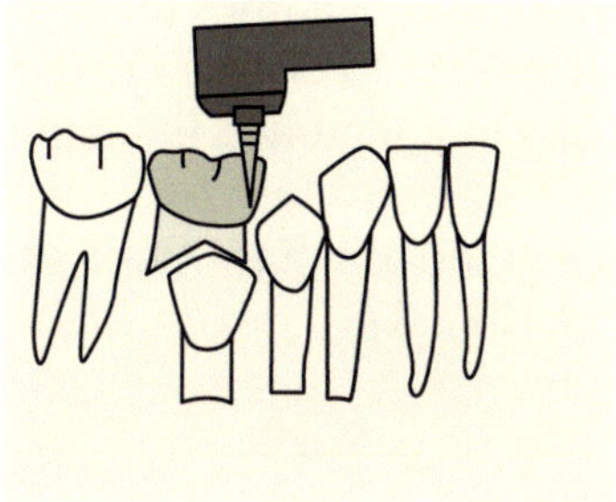

Fig. (5). Interproximal stripping.

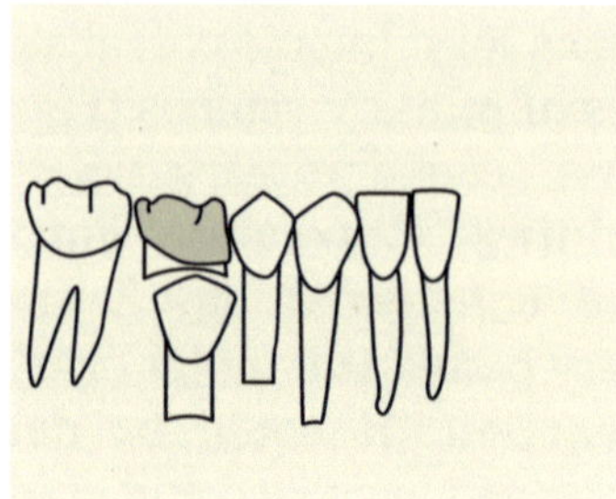

Fig. (6). Interproximal stripping.

5. a. What is Serial Extraction Treatment Protocol? List the Indications and Contraindications for Serial Extraction Protocol Treatment Protocol?

a. Serial extraction is a form of interceptive treatment which aims to relieve crowding at an early stage so that the permanent teeth can erupt into good alignment, reducing or avoiding the need for extensive orthodontic treatment at later stages [12].
b. The patient **indications** [3, 4, 13] for this protocol are:
    i. True tooth size – jaw size discrepancy
    ii. Orthognathic or bimaxillary protrusive profile
    iii. Normal or high angle vertical pattern
    iv. Class I or mesial step dental relationship
    v. Minimal overjet and overbite

The patient **contraindications** [3, 4, 13] for this protocol are:

a. Low angle
b. Class II or Class III skeletal relationship and
c. Class I bimaxillary retrusive profile

6. Describe the Serial Extraction Treatment Protocol

- Removal of upper and lower primary canines to align the permanent incisors.
- Removal of the first primary molars to encourage the eruption of first premolars
- Removal of the first premolars to encourage the eruption and distal movement of permanent canines (Fig. **7**)
- Removal of second primary molars and fixed appliance therapy after the eruption of second premolars (Fig. **8**)

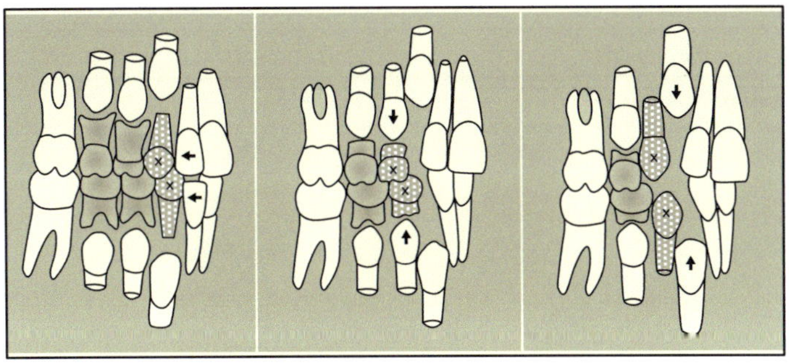

Fig. (7). Serial extraction, removal of the first premolars.

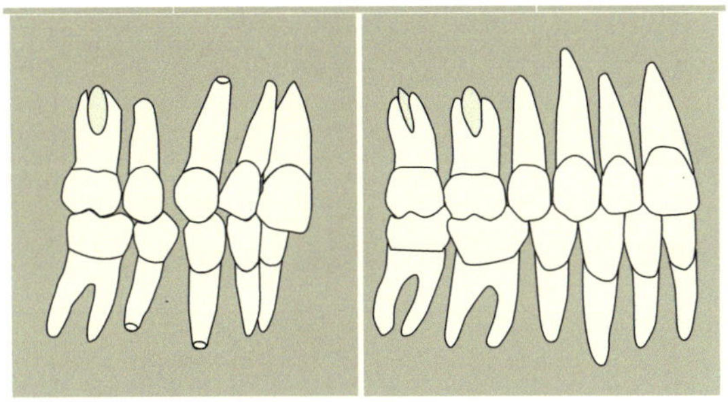

Fig. (8). Serial extraction, removal of second primary molars.

7. Give Some Clinical Reasons in the Early Mixed Dentition Period that Could Identify Potential Severe Crowding in Permanent Dentition (Table 1).

The **clinical "signs"** in mixed dentition that could identify potential severe crowding in permanent dentition [7, 9, 10] could be:

a. The permanent mandibular lateral incisor resorbing primary canine root, causing their exfoliation (Fig. **9**)
b. The mesial ectopic eruption of upper first permanent molars resorbing primary second molar roots, causing early exfoliation (Fig. **10**)
c. The hereditary crowding (tooth – jaw size discrepancy Fig. **11**).

8. List Some Skeletal Conditions in the Mixed Dentition that Would Make You Favour Bicuspid Extraction in the Permanent Dentition

Table 1. Skeletal conditions in the mixed dentition that encourage bicuspid extraction in the permanent dentition [13 - 15].

a. **Dolichofacial growth pattern with marked incisor protrusion**
b. **Protrusive upper lip with acute nasiolabial angle**

(Table 1) contd.....

c. **Skeletal open-bite**
d. **Bimaxillary protrusion**

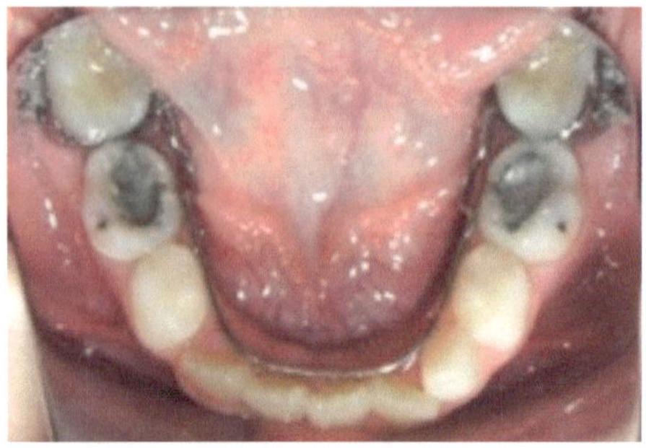

Fig. (9). Premature loss of right primary canine.

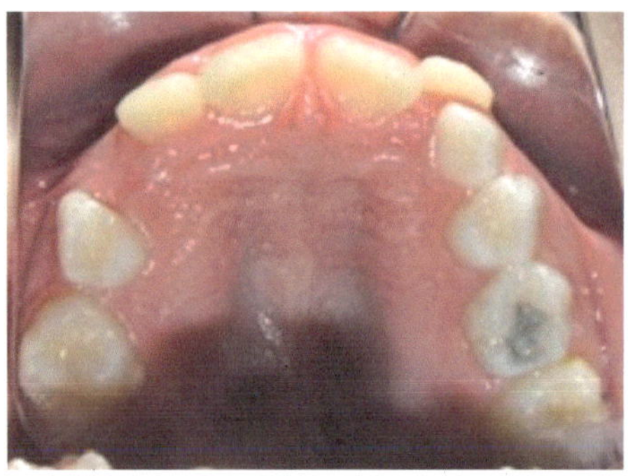

Fig. (10). Premature loss of 2nd primary molar.

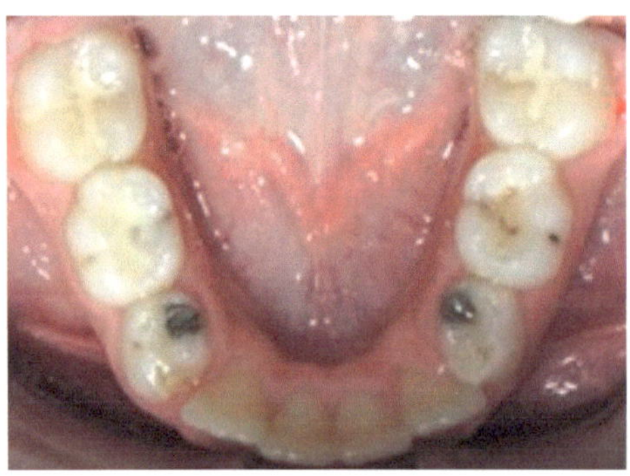

Fig. (11). Premature loss of primary canines because of hereditary crowding.

9. Which Tooth Eruption Sequence Variances Have an Arch Space Loss Possibility?

Eruption of mandibular second molars ahead of mandibular second premolars as well as the eruption of maxillary canines ahead of the first premolars. Moreover, left-right asymmetries in timing of eruption of permanent teeth can create local space loss [16].

10. Could You Describe the Most Likely Consequences After the Premature Exfoliation of the Second, First Primary Molars and Mandibular Primary Canines? (Tables 2-4).

2nd Primary Molars

Table 2. Possible consequencesafter premature exfoliation of the second primary molars [17 - 19].

Maxilla	Mandible
1) **Mesial crown-root movement as well as mesial rotation of the first permanent molars around the palatal root**	1) Mesial tipping of the first permanent molars
2) **Distal eruption of the first bicuspid**	2) Distal eruption of the first bicuspid
3) **Impaction of the second bicuspid**	3) Impaction of the second bicuspid

1st Primary Molars

Table 3. Possible consequences after premature exfoliation of the first primary molars [6, 11, 13].

Maxilla	Mandible
1) **The primary cuspid shifts distally (1st year after the premature exfoliation)**	1) Distal movement of the primary cuspid towards the extraction space
2) **The primary second maxillary molar could shift mesially** (***depending on the age and the duration of tooth loss***). **The erupting 1st bicuspid could erupt mesially because of the mesial shifted second primary molar.**	2) Mesial movement of the second primary and the first permanent molar
3) Space loss and possible impaction for the maxillary canine	

Generally speaking, there is more space loss associated with the loss of a second primary molar than with a first primary molar.

1st Primary Canines

Table 4. Possible consequences after premature exfoliation of the mandibular primary canines [3, 4, 20 - 22]

a. Lingual-distal positioning of the permanent incisors
b. Decreased arch length and deepening the bite

(Table 4) contd.....

c. Midline shift if the premature exfoliation is unilateral

11. List the Requirements of an Ideal Space Maintainer Appliance

An ideal space maintainer appliance [23, 24] should:

- *Encourage eruption of adjacent and succedaneous teeth*
- *Prevent over-eruption of antagonists*
- *Be compatible with masticatory function and soft tissues*
- *Avoid torque forces on abutment teeth*
- *Resist distortion*
- *Allow for adjustment or minor repair*

12. Could You Describe the Space Management Procedure After the Premature Exfoliation of the Primary Incisors, Mandibular Canines, First and Second Primary Molars?

- *Primary incisors*: No space maintainer procedures are required.
- *Mandibular canine*: Lower Lingual Arch (LLA Fig. **12**).
- *First primary molar*: Band and loop on the second primary molar or the first permanent molar (Fig. **13**).
- *Mandibular second primary molar*: Lower Lingual Arch (LLA) on the first permanent molar or "distal shoe" on the first primary molar, if it is lost before the eruption of the first permanent molar.
- *Maxillary second primary molar*: Nance Orthodontic appliance or Transpalatal arch (TPA) (Fig. **14**).

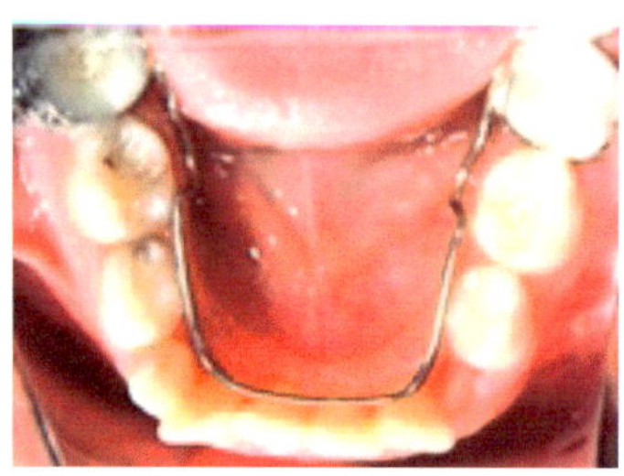

Fig. (12). Lower Lingual Arch (LLA).

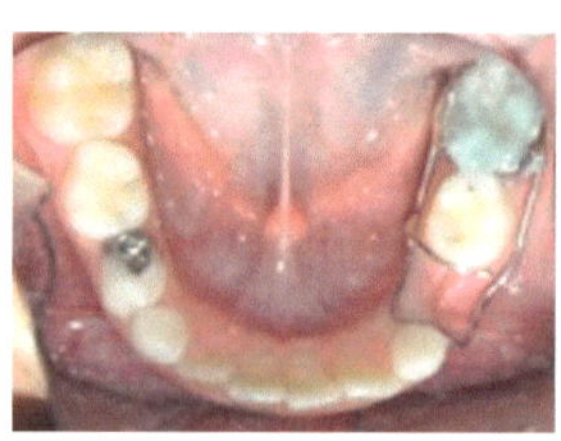

Fig. (13). Band and loop.

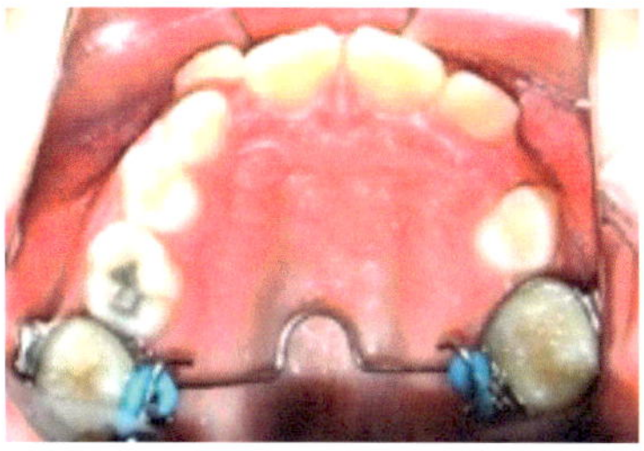

Fig. (14). Transpalatal arch (TPA)

13. What is the Band and Loop Space Maintainer Appliance?

The band and loop space maintainer appliance consists of a band which is placed on the abutment tooth and a loop soldered to the band to span the edentulous space. The loop should be wide buccal-lingual to allow for the eruption of the succedaneous tooth as well as to adapt 0.5 mm from the gingival tissue and to contact the adjacent tooth at the contact point [25].

14. a. What are the Main Advantages as well as the Disadvantages of Using the Lower Lingual Arch (LLA)?
b. Do you Know the Effectiveness of this Appliance?

a. In interceptive orthodontics, the use of a lower lingual arch **LLA** is a widely accepted procedure. A LLA (0.9 mm SS) is considered an ideal space maintainer appliance in the mixed dentition because of the following **advantages** [26 - 28] (Table **5**):

Table 5. Advantages of lower lingual arch.

easy construction and insertion
low cost
minimal breakage problems
normal oral hygiene needs
no child cooperation concerns

However, some **disadvantages** [28] have also been reported.

- Lower lingual arch appliance could provoke forward movement and proclination of lower incisors.
- Preventing the late mesial shift through preservation of the E-space, eruption of the mandibular second molars could also be affected if the **intermolar angulation is greater than 24 degrees.**

• Possible decalcification of the banded teeth.

b. The **effectiveness of the** LLA device has a wide range of variability ranging from an average decrease of **–0.44 (+/-1.35 mm) +2.9 mm** arch length gain, depending on different growth patterns. The changes in incisor and molar positions during the treatment with lingual arches were influenced by facial growth [26].

15. a. List the Indications of the Lower Lingual Arch (LLA)as a Space Maintainer Appliance
b. In Which Cases Should You Avoid Placing a LLA Appliance?

a. It is used to prevent the lingual collapse and the distal drifting of the lower incisors in cases of bilateral (Fig. **15**) or unilateral (Fig. **16**) premature loss of the mandibular primary canine in order
   - It is used to maintain the space after the premature loss of the 2nd mandibular primary molar. Early loss of the primary second molars has the greatest effect on dental arch length and results **in 2-4 mm** of space closure per quadrant in both arches.
   - It can also be used to resolve anterior mandibular crowding by preserving the leeway space in mixed dentition cases. A lingual holding arch placed during the mixed dentition will restrict the mesial migration and tipping and should even cause a slight increase of the total arch length by preventing the mandibular incisors from tipping lingually.
   - It can also be used in the case of the unilateral or bilateral loss of multiple mandibular primary teeth.

b. The LLA should not be placed [4],
   - Before the eruption of the permanent incisors because:1) Primary incisors do not offer sufficient anchorage and 2) the frequent lingual eruption path of the permanent incisors.
   - Class III growth pattern or Class II- high angle skeletal pattern (ANB >5 degrees).
   - Severe lower arch crowding that needs extensive orthodontic treatment.

16. a. Describe the Space Management Appliances in the Maxilla
b. Report the Indications of Using these Appliances as Space Maintainer Appliances

a. Whereas the lingual arch is commonly used for the lower arch, the Nance appliance (Fig. **17**) and the transpalatal arch (TPA) (Fig. **18**) are the appliances used for the upper arch. These appliances use a large wire to connect banded teeth on both sides of the arch that are distal to the extraction site. The difference between the two is that the Nance appliance incorporates an acrylic button that rests directly on the palatal rugae.It is an effective space maintainer, but soft tissue irritation can be a problem. The accumulation of bacteria and food debris will often result in palatal inflammation and, in many cases, pain [8].

The transpalatal arch is connected to molar bands and runs across the palatal vault, avoiding contact with the soft tissue. It is constructed from a 0.036-inch (0.9 mm) stainless steel wire. It could be soldered directly to molar bands or the prefabricated arch forms available in different length could be used. The TPA offers the option of expansion, rotation, contraction, and torque of the molars due to an omega loop in the centre of the vault.*It should be passive when inserted into the mouth. If the appliance is not passive, unexpected vertical and transverse movements of the permanent molars may occur* [29 - 31].

b. A transpalatal arch is best indicated when one side of the arch is intact and several primary teeth are missing on the other side. In this case, the rigid attachment to the intact side usually provides enough stability for space maintenance. However, when second primary molars have been lost bilaterally, a Nance appliance is preferred [30].

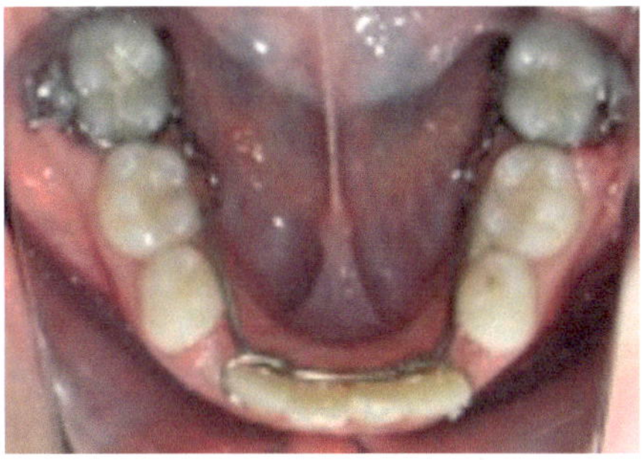

Fig. (15). Early loss of both primary canines.

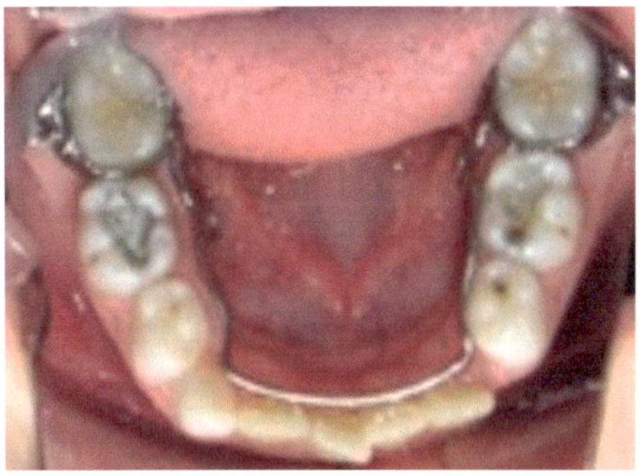

Fig. (16). Early loss of left primary canine.

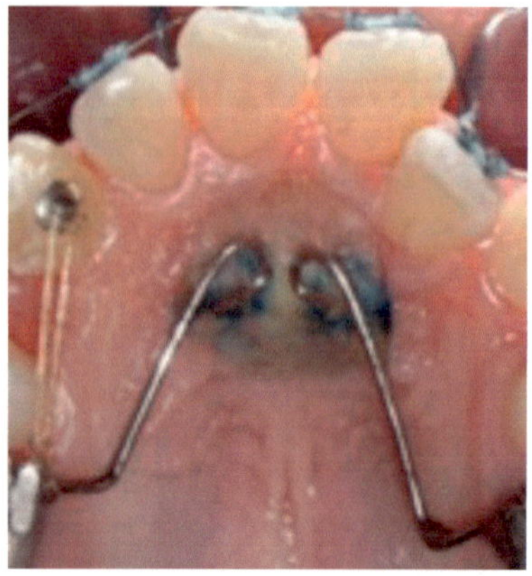

Fig. (17). Nance appliance.

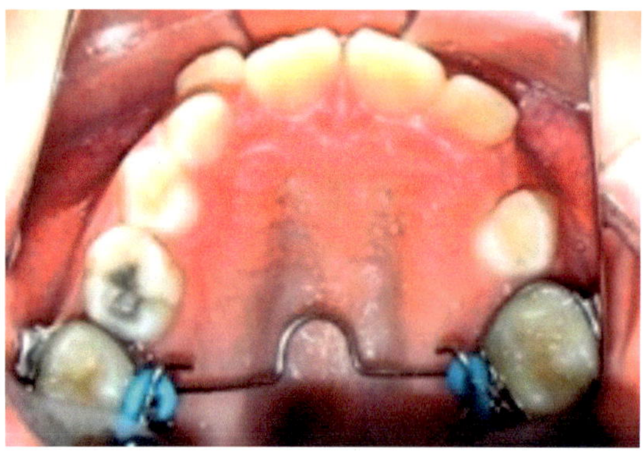

Fig. (18). Transpalatal arch (TPA).

17. a. List the Indications for a Transpalatal Arch (TPA) in the Mixed Dentition Period.
b. Describe the Proper Position of the Upper First Permanent Molar Ideal Rotational Position. How Much Arch Length Can be Gained by Correcting the Upper First Molar Rotations?

a. The indications for a Transpalatal arch (TPA) in the mixed dentition period are to:
   - Establish and maintain arch widths;
   - Derotate unilaterally or bilaterally rotated molars
   - Control their vertical position (*tongue pressure on the appliance's loop*)
   - Correct unilateral cross-bites for maxillary expansion and
   - Create buccal root torque of upper 1st molars

b. Distobuccal cusp and mesio-lingual cusps of the first molars should line up with the contralateral canine. If the molars are mesially rotated (as is almost always the case in class II malocclusions), correcting the rotations by TPA helps to establish class I molar relation 1-2 mm / side (Fig. **19**).

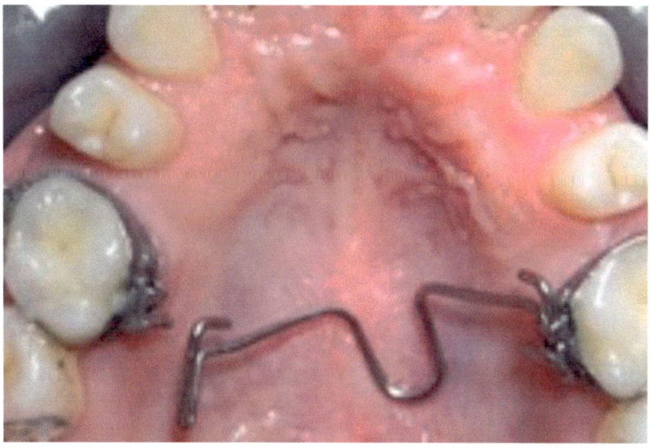

Fig. (19). Derotation of 1st permanent molars by TPA.

18. Do You Know How the Bolton Discrepancy is Calculated?

It is commonly accepted that the sizes of the maxillary and the mandibular teeth must be proportionate to accomplish excellent occlusal interdigitations with ideal overjet and overbite [1]. The Bolton analysis has been shown to be a reliable diagnostic tool for assessing tooth size discrepancy and subsequently aiding in the treatment planning of dental malocclusions.For an exact tubercule-fossa relationship there has to be a defined ratio (*91.2 for 12 teeth, 77.2 for 6 teeth*) between the widths of mesiodistal sizes of lower teeth to that of upper teeth [2].

When this ratio is out of regularity, the *Bolton Discrepancy* exists.

Bolton Ratio for 12 Teeth

M-D size sum of mandibular 12 teeth / M-D size sum of maxillary 12 teeth

> 91.2 → Mandibular excess
< 91.2→ Maxillary excess

Bolton Ratio for 6 Teeth

M-D size sum of mandibular 6 teeth / M-D sizesum of maxillary 6 teeth

> 77.2 →Mandibular excess
< 77.2 →Maxillary excess

PART B. CLINICAL EXAMPLES

A. Describe the Dental Space Loss as Well as the Proper Interceptive Orthodontic Treatment in the Next Patients

Patient 1

Maxilla: Space loss because of the premature exfoliation of the right second primary molars and mesial movement/ rotation of the first right permanent molar around the palatal root (Figs. **20** & **21**).

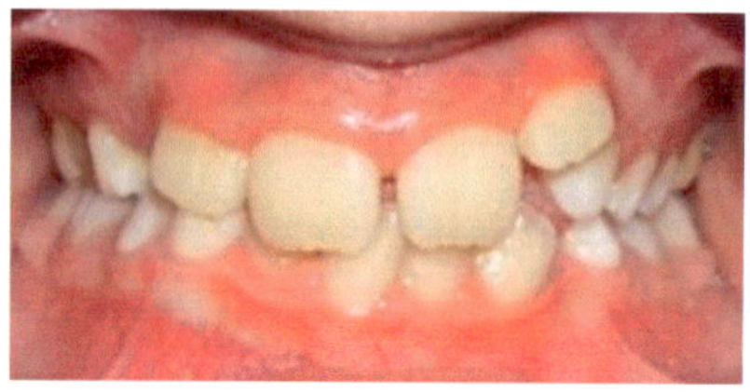

Fig. (20). Frontal occlusal view.

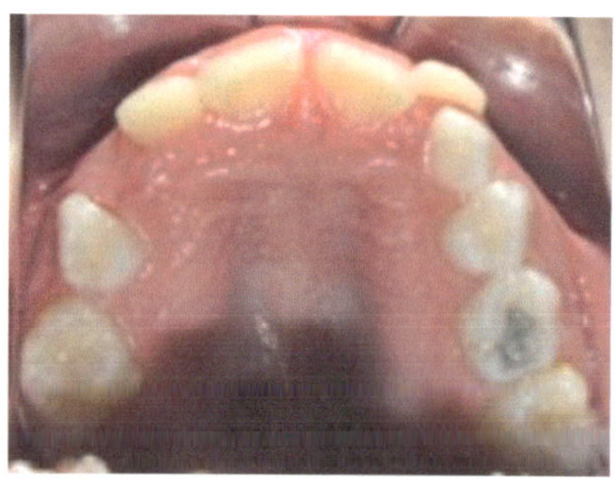

Fig. (21). Maxillary occlusal arch view.

Treatment: A transpalatal arch (TPA) could be inserted to recapture the lost space by derotating and tipping distally the first permanent molar (Fig. **22**).

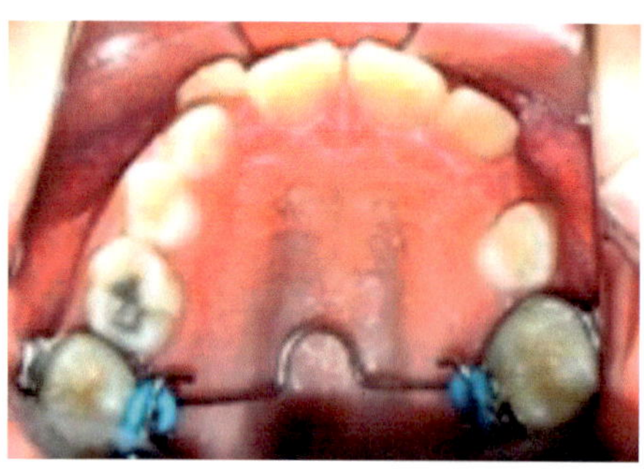

Fig. (22). Insertion of Transpalatal arch.

Mandible: Premature loss of the left mandibular primary canine (Fig. **23**). The permanent mandibular incisors shift to the left, changing the vertical axes as well as decreasing the arch length and disrupting the eruption of the left permanent cuspid.

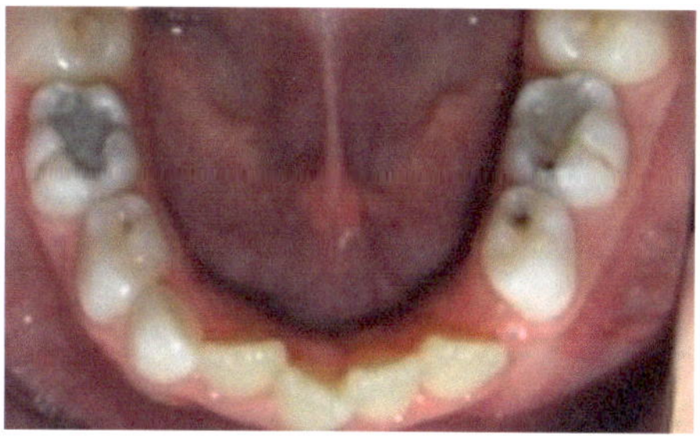

Fig. (23). Mandibular occlusal arch view.

Treatment: Extraction of the contralateral primary canine is indicated to allow the incisors to move freely and a fixed Lower Lingual Arch (LLA) was inserted to avoid more arch length loss (Fig. **24**). The LLA should be passive to prevent the labial tipping of the lower incisors and buccal expansion of the molars. However, we should notice that most of the time, the midline and the vertical axes of the mandibular incisors are not self-corrected and an extensive fixed orthodontic treatment is required.

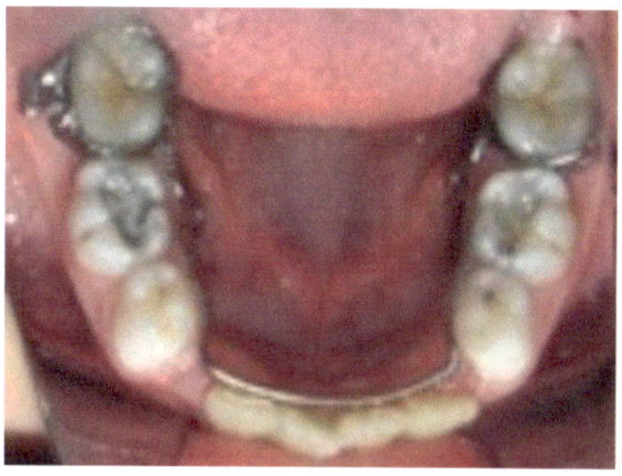

Fig. (24). Insertion of Lower Lingual Arch.

Patient 2

Mandibular Right Side: The mandibular right primary canine was extracted by mistake in order to align the four incisors (Fig. **25**). Only the right lateral permanent incisor shifted towards the extraction site.

Treatment: Extraction of the contralateral primary canine is indicated and a fixed Lower Lingual Arch was inserted (Figs. **26 & 27**).

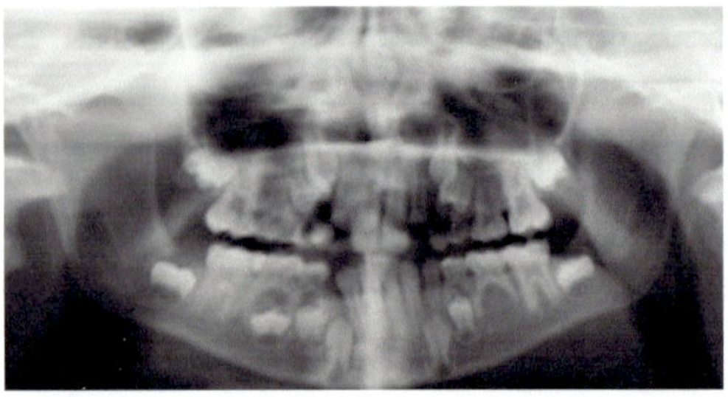

Fig. (25). Panoramic X-Ray.

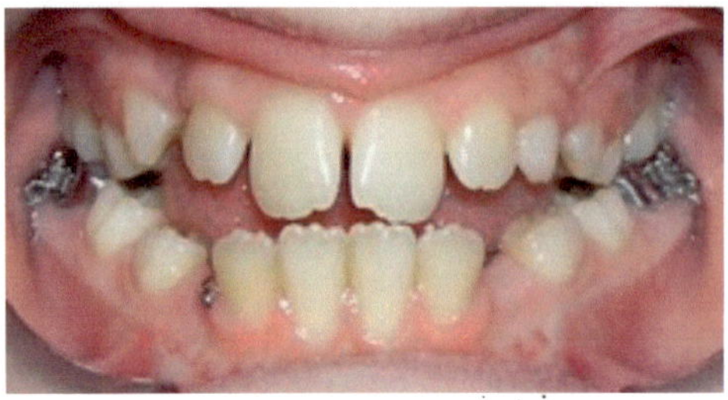

Fig. (26). Anterior occlusal view.

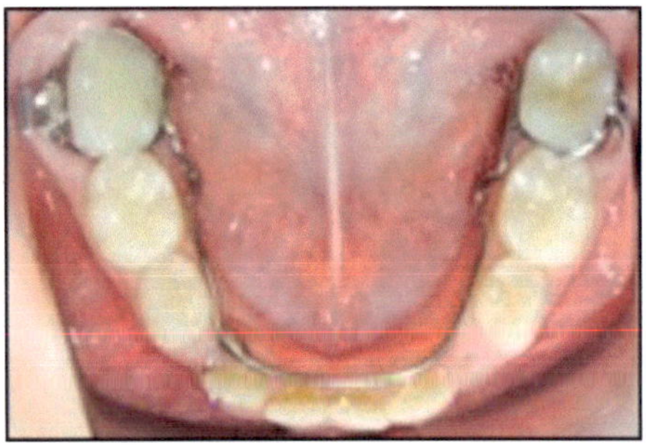

Fig. (27). Mandibular occlusal arch view.

Patient 3

Mandibular Right Side: The mandibular right primary cuspid has been lost prematurely. However, unlike the previous patient, all the permanent mandibular incisors shifted to the right (Figs. **28-30**), changing the vertical axes of these teeth as well as disrupting the eruption of the right permanent cuspid.

Treatment: Fixed orthodontic space regaining appliance (modified Crozat) was inserted to regain the space loss and a fixed Lower Lingual Arch (LLA) was inserted after the regaining procedure (Figs. **31** & **32**).

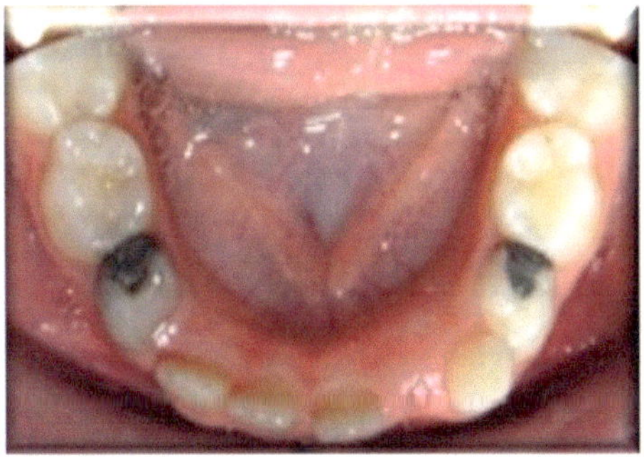

Fig. (28). Mandibular arch view.

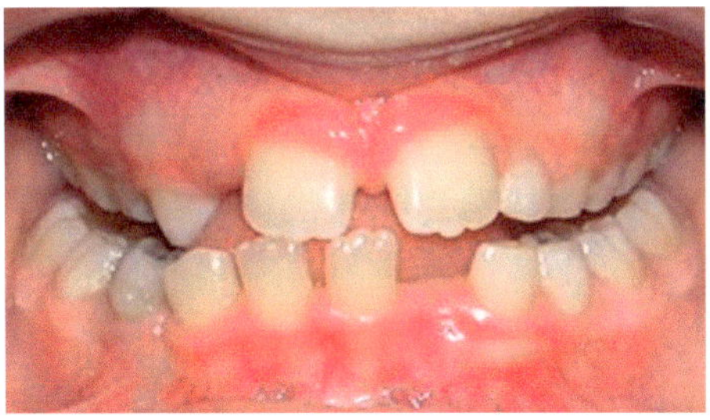

Fig. (29). Anterior occlusal view.

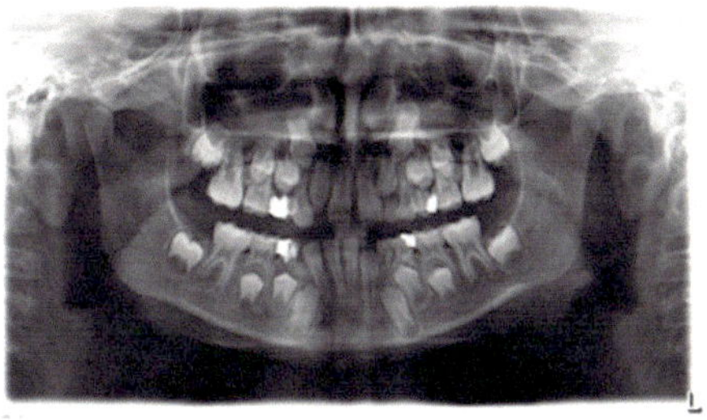

Fig. (30). Panoramic X-Ray.

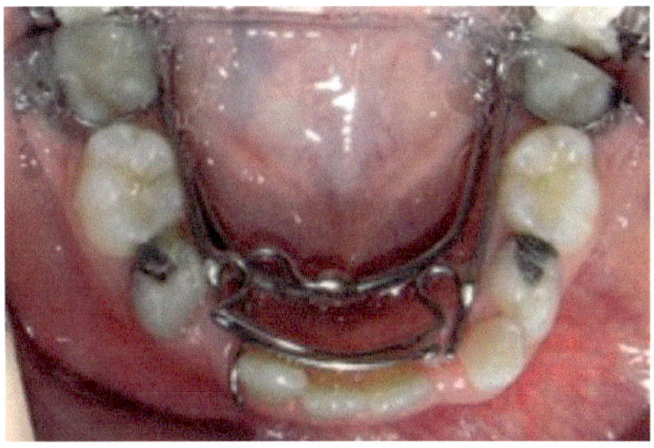

Fig. (31). Crozat appliance.

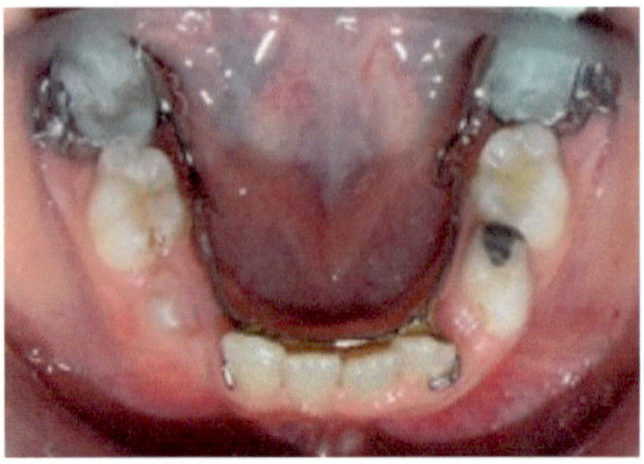

Fig. (32). Lower lingual arch.

Patient 4

Maxilla: The maxillary primary canines have been removed (by mistake) in order to find space for the lateral incisors' eruption and alignment (Figs. **33** & **34**).

Treatment: The lost space should be regained by repositioning the drifted lateral incisors (Fig. **35**). After the space discrepancy has been recaptured space maintenance is necessary until the succedaneous teeth have erupted.

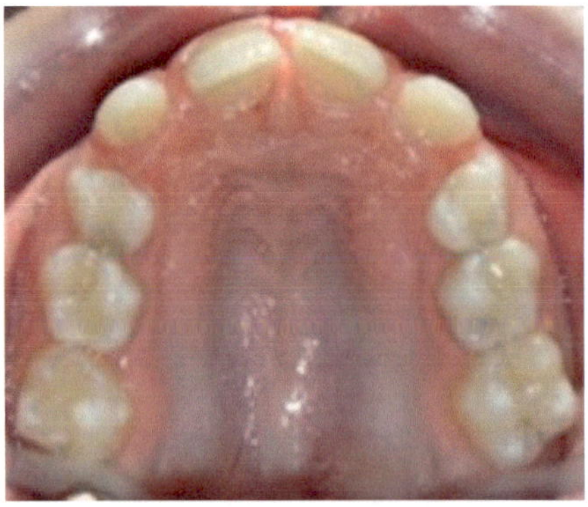

Fig. (33). Maxillary occlusal view.

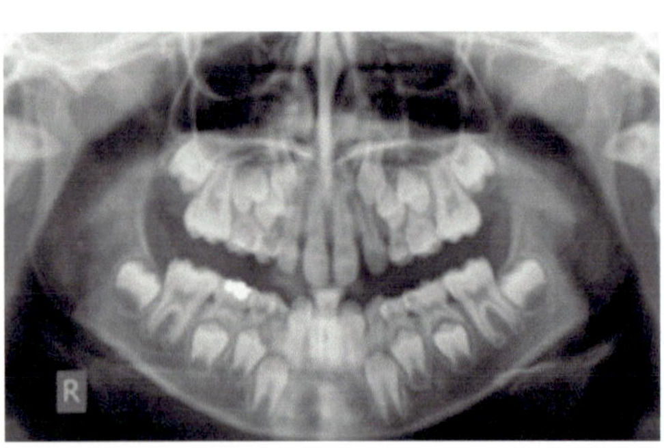

Fig. (34). Panoramic X-ray.

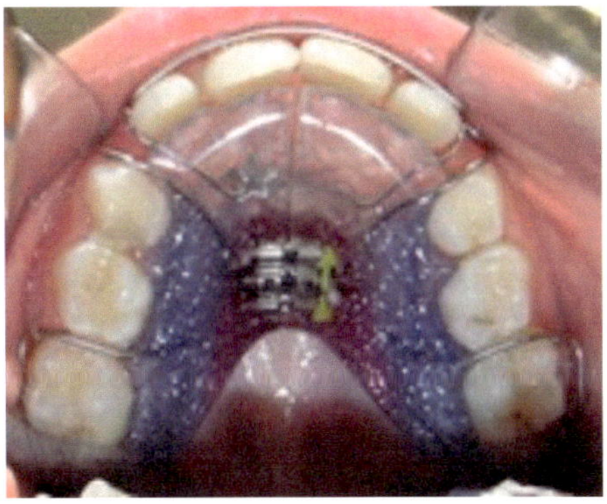

Fig. (35). Space regaining appliance.

Patient 5

Left Side: The eruption of the first premolar will be accelerated because of the early loss of the first permanent molar (Fig. **36**).

Treatment: Band and loop space maintainer is required (Figs. **37** & **38**).

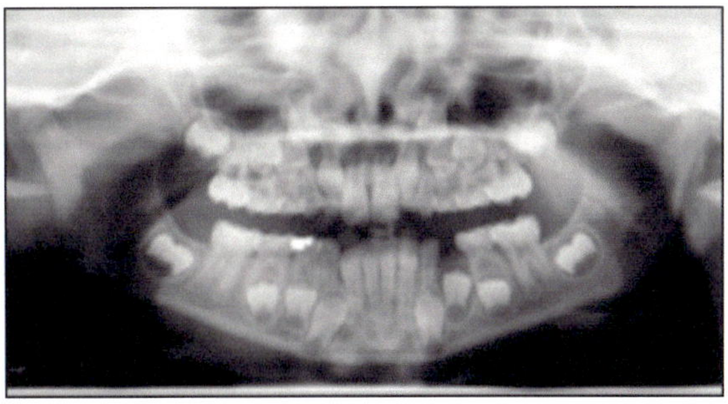

Fig. (36). Panoramic X-Ray.

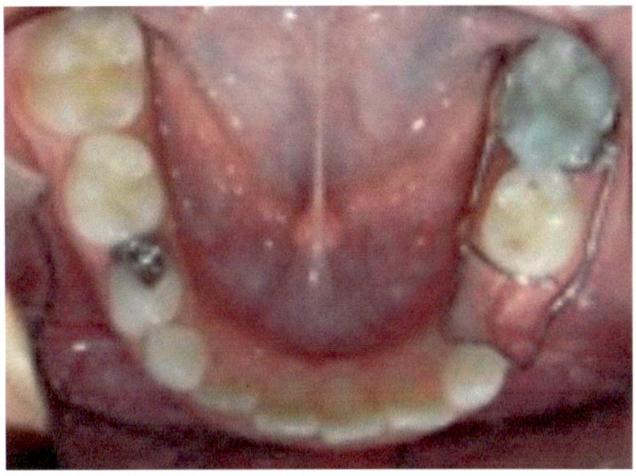

Fig. (37). Band and loop space maintainer.

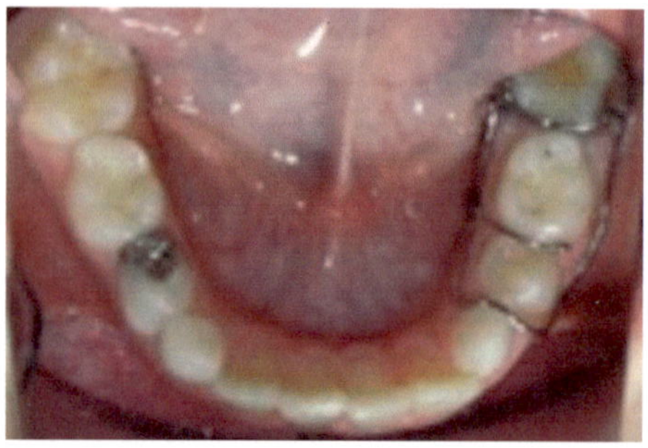

Fig. (38). Second premolar eruption.

Patient 6

Bilateral loss of the mandibular primary cuspids (Figs. **39** & **40**). The possible scenario is that the permanent lateral incisors resorb the roots of the primary cuspids during their eruption, resulting inthe premature primary cuspid exfoliation.

Treatment: This is a strong clinical indication for mandibular arch length deficiency. Definite orthodontic treatment plan (serial extraction treatment protocol) should be done at this point. A Lower lingual arch (LLA) could be inserted in order to maintain arch length by preventing the lingual collapse of the lower incisors. It is made of 0.9 mm SS, which is superior to that made of 1.25 mm SS in terms of arch length preservation.

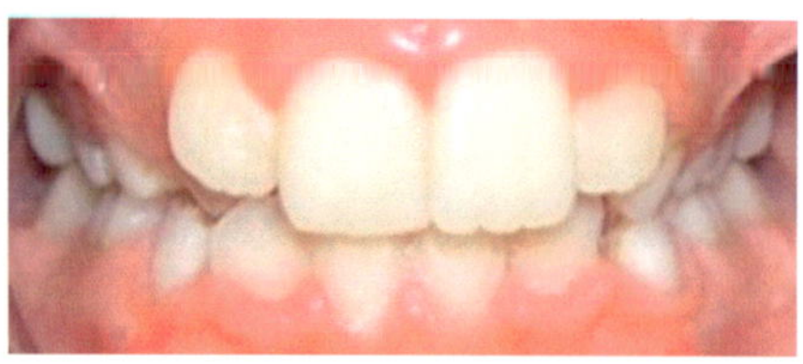

Fig. (39). Anterior occlusal view.

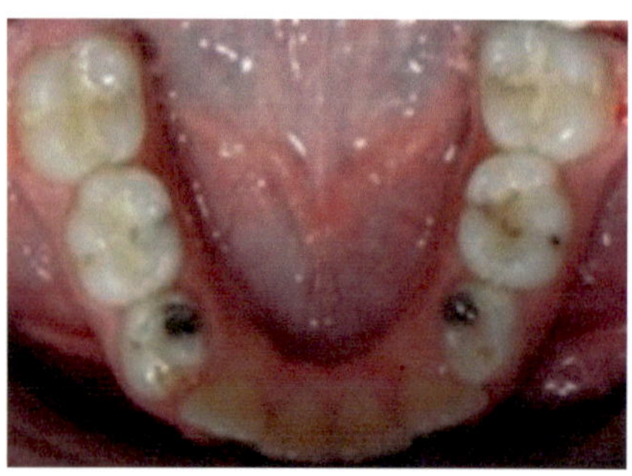

Fig. (40). Mandibular occlusal view.

Patient 7

Supposing that the following patient has 5.5mm crowding, skeletal and dental Class I Angle classification and good facial balance (Figs. **41** & **42**). How do you solve the crowding?

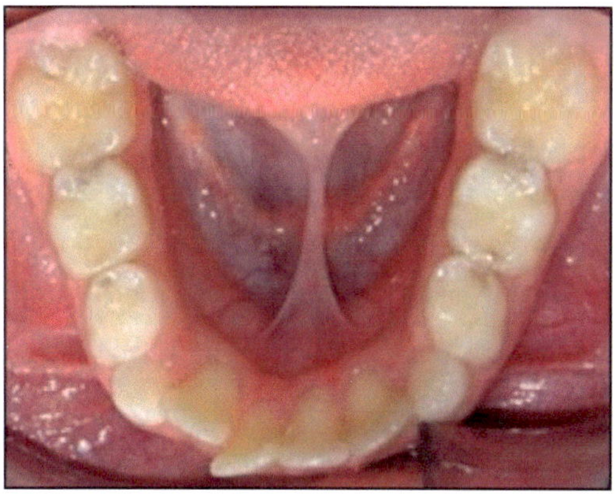

Fig. (41). Mandibular occlusal view.

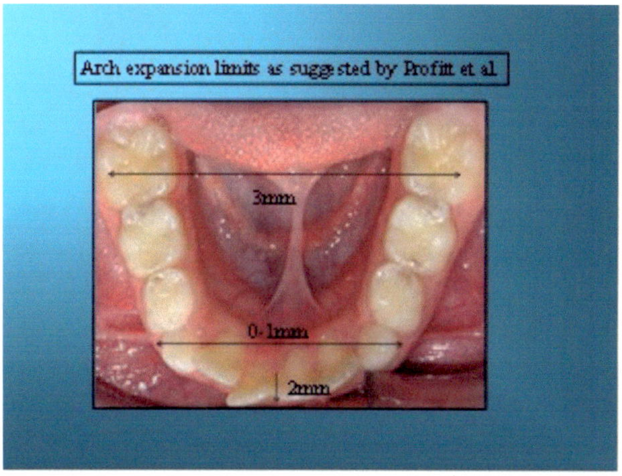

Fig. (42). Mandibular expansion limits

Treatment:

Space-creation	*Arch-perimeter Gain*
Intercanine width stable	*0.0 mm*
Intermolar width expansion 3mm	*0.9 mm*
Incisor advancement 2mm	*2.2 mm*

Contd.....

Space-creation	*Arch-perimeter Gain*
Inter-proximal stripping 0.5mm per contact from distal of #32 to distal #42 (five contacts)	*2.5 mm*
TOTAL	*5.6mm*

Patient 8

Right Side: The second primary molar has been prematurely lost; the second premolar is impacted because the first permanent molar has tipped mesial and the first premolar has shifted distally (Figs. **43-45**). Orthodontic space regaining procedures are mandatory.

Left Side: The second premolar is congenitally missing. The second premolar is congenitally missing.

Treatment: Extraction of the second primary teeth and mesial molar retraction by orthodontic means was applied (Figs. **46 & 47**).

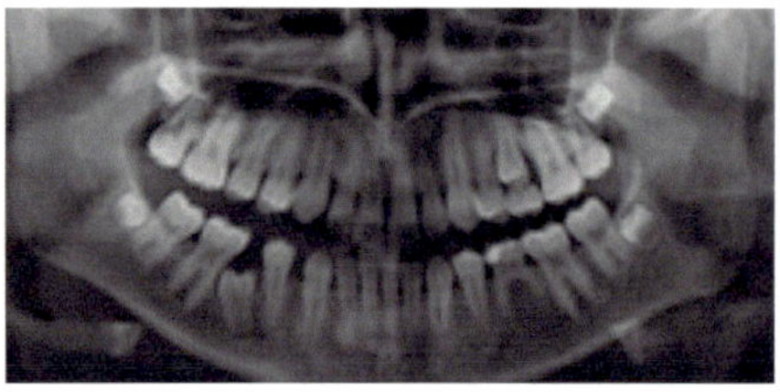

Fig. (43). Panoramic X-Ray.

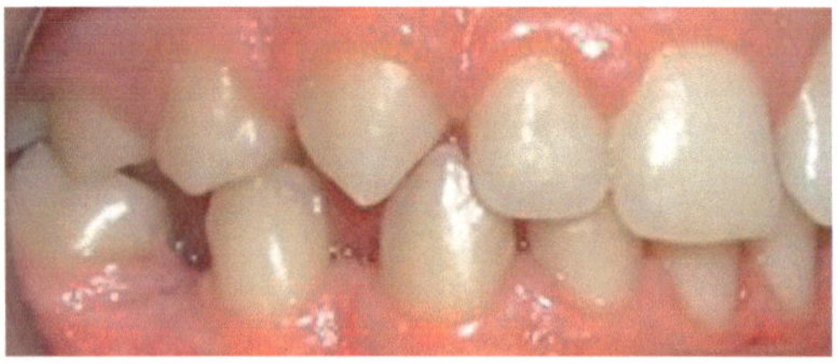

Fig. (44). Right occlusal view.

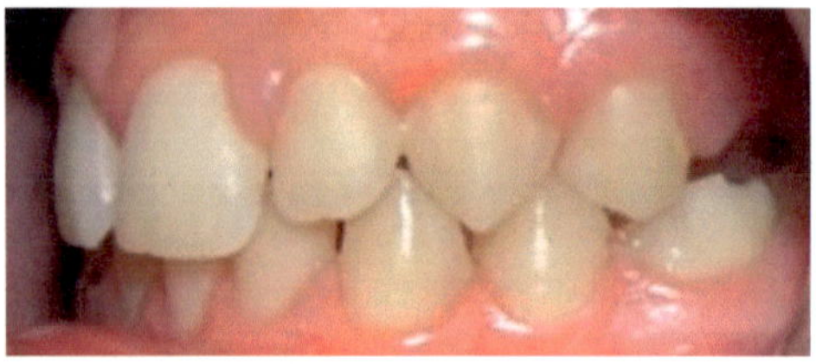

Fig. (45). Left occlusal view.

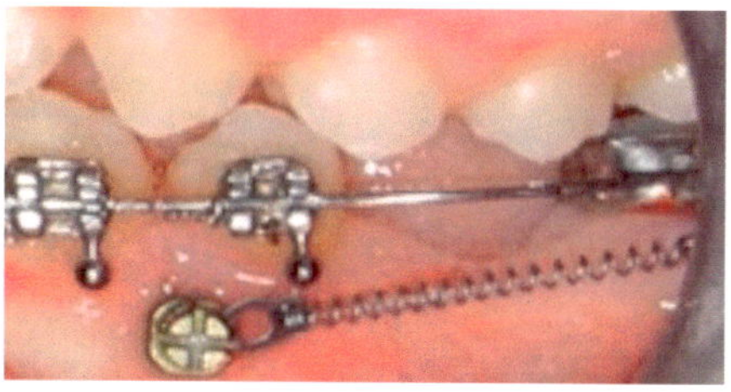

Fig. (46). Molar Mesialization.

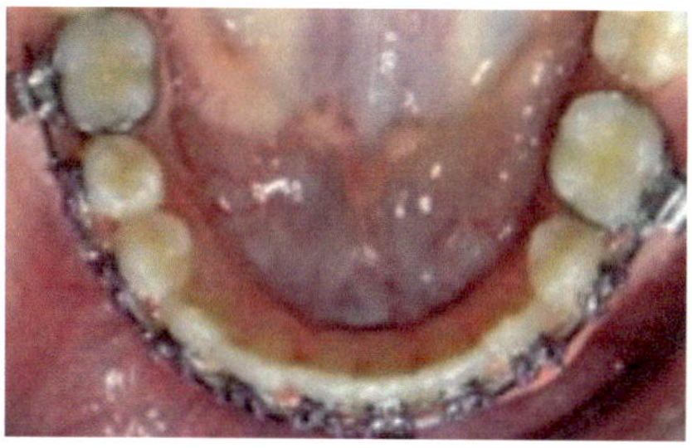

Fig. (47). Mandibular occlusal view.

Patient 9

Left Side: The left second premolar erupted mesially (unusual path) and resorbed the mesial root of the primary second molar. This eruptive path will not self-correct,even after the extraction of the second primary molar (Fig. **48**).

Right Side: Radiograph depicting the least desirable path of eruption for the mandibular second bicuspids. The teeth erupted mesially and resorbed the mesial root of their predecessors. The first premolar is experiencing interference in its eruption by the mesial surface of the second primary molar.

An extensive orthodontic treatment that includes surgical exposure and orthodontic traction of the impacted teeth is required (Figs. **49** & **50**).

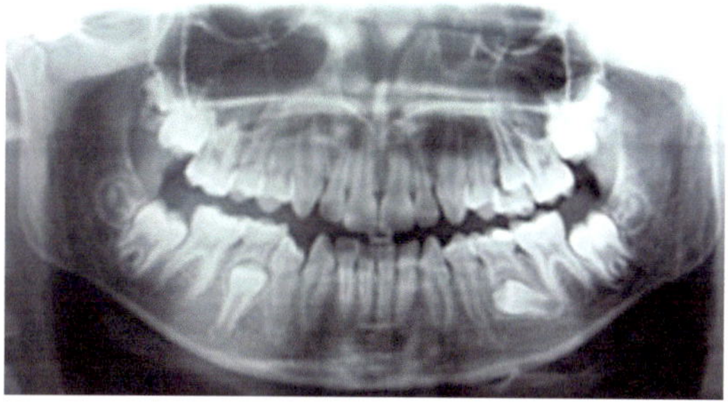

Fig. (48). Initial Panoramic X-Ray.

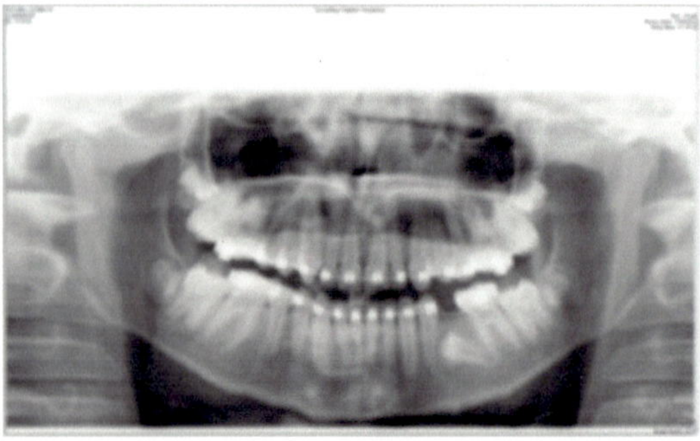

Fig. (49). Panoramic X-ray before surgical exposure and orthodontic traction of the impacted teeth.

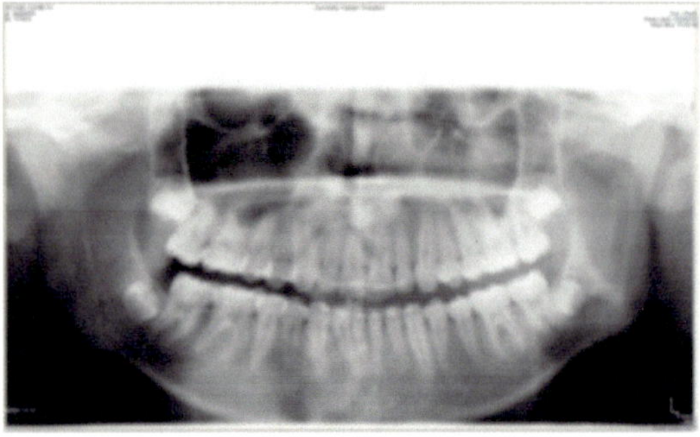

Fig. (50). Panoramic X-ray at the end of the treatment.

Patient 10

Right Side: The second premolar has erupted normally without losing the required guidance of the correctly positioned first permanent molar (Fig. **51**).

Left Side: The maxillary second primary molar has been lost prematurely. The break in the continuity of the dental arch allowed the first premolar to rotate and shift distally and the first molar to rotate mesially around the palatal root (Fig. **51**). On the side where the primary molar has been lost, the permanent second premolar was mechanically blocked.

Treatment: Orthodontic intervention is required to regain the space by de-rotating both the first molar and premolar. Some molar distalization has taken place too. One of the conventional intra-oral appliances for space regaining in the maxillary arch in patients with good soft tissue profile, without incisor overjet and with horizontal growth pattern, is done by using the Pendulum appliance. The Pendulum consists of the Nance palatal component and bilateral helical spring made out of titanium molybdenum alloy, which delivers a continuous 200 to 250 gms force against the maxillary first molars. The use of this beta titanium wire is to provide constant distal force near to the centre of the resistance of the molar, thus reducing the moment of force (Fig. **52**). A Transpalatal arch (TPA) is required to maintain the position of the first molars (Fig. **53**).

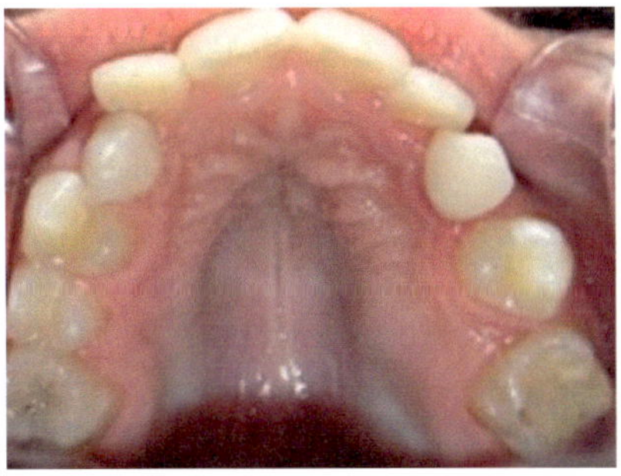

Fig. (51). Maxillary occlusal view.

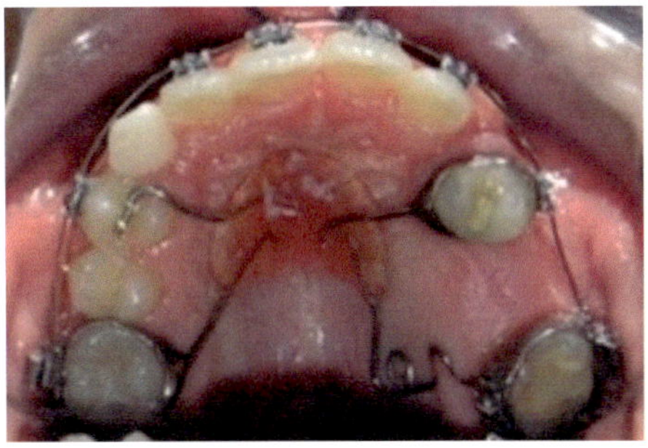

Fig. (52). Space regaining.

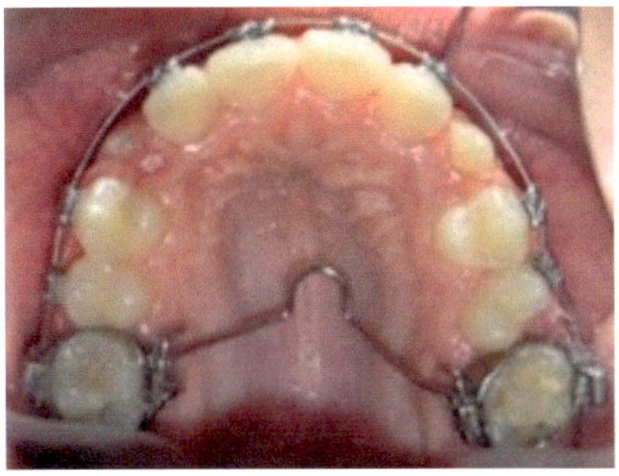

Fig. (53). TPA to stabilize the space.

Patient 11

This patient is another example of poor occlusal management during the mixed dentition period.

Maxilla: In both sides, the maxillary second primary molar has been lost prematurely and the permanent second premolar was mechanically blocked (Fig. **54**).

Treatment: Orthodontic intervention is required to regain the space by de-rotating the first molars and premolars at both sides. A Pendulum appliance was inserted, adding a midline screw in order to achieve some palatal expansion (Fig. **55**). Extensive orthodontic treatment is required.

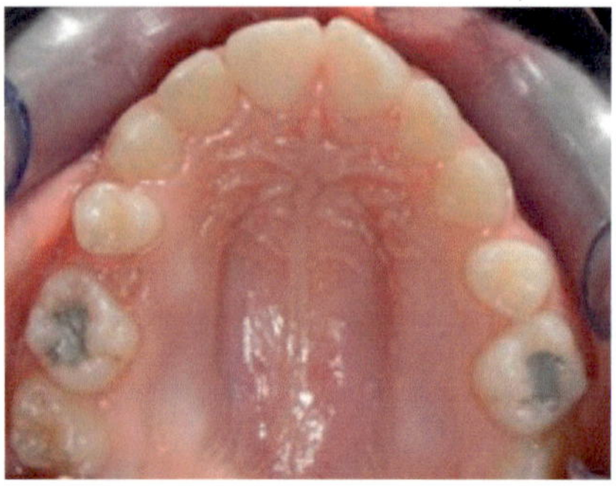

Fig. (54). Maxillary occlusal view.

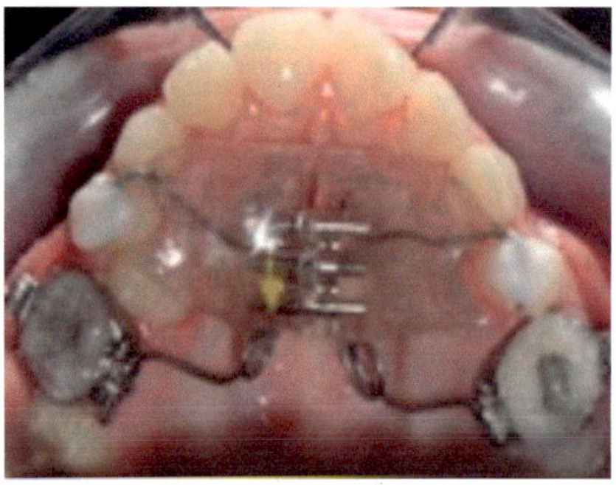

Fig. (55). Space regaining procedures.

CONCLUDING REMARKS

Thorough knowledge of tooth eruption sequence, their anomalies as well as the dental arch development during the mixed dentition period contribute to the development of a permanent dentition that is in a stable and functional acceptable occlusion and normal subsequent dentofacial development.

REFERENCES

[1] Bolton WA. Disharmony in tooth size and its relation to the analysis and treatment of malocclusion. Angle Orthod 1958; 28: 113-30.

[2] Bernabé E, Villanueva KM, Flores-Mir C. Tooth width ratios in crowded and noncrowded dentitions. Angle Orthod 2004; 74(6): 765-8.
[PMID: 15673138]

[3] Proffit W. Contemporary Orthodontics. 4th ed., St. Louis: Mosby 2007.

[4] Moyers RE. Handbook of Orthodontics. 3rd ed., Chicago: Year Book Medical Publishers 1973.

[5] Tanaka MM, Johnston LE. The prediction of the size of unerupted canines and premolars in a

contemporary orthodontic population. J Am Dent Assoc 1974; 88(4): 798-801. [http://dx.doi.org/10.14219/jada.archive.1974.0158]

[6] Sampson WJ, Richards LC. Prediction of mandibular incisor and canine crowding changes in the mixed dentition. Am J Orthod 1985; 88(1): 47-63. [http://dx.doi.org/10.1016/0002-9416(85)90106-X] [PMID: 3860012]

[7] Sayin MO, Türkkahraman H. Factors contributing to mandibular anterior crowding in the early mixed dentition. Angle Orthod 2004; 74(6): 754-8. [PMID: 15673136]

[8] Nance HN. The limitations of orthodontic treatment; mixed dentition diagnosis and treatment. Am J Orthod 1947; 33(4): 177-223. [PMID: 20291149]

[9] Dugoni SA. Comprehensive treatment during mixed dentition period. Am J Orthod Dentofacial Orthop 1998; 113: 75-84. [http://dx.doi.org/10.1016/S0889-5406(98)70278-1] [PMID: 9457021]

[10] Gianelly AA. Leeway space and the resolution of crowding in the mixed dentition. Semin Orthod 1995; 1(3): 188-94. [http://dx.doi.org/10.1016/S1073-8746(95)80022-0] [PMID: 9002915]

[11] Proffit WR. The timing of early treatment: an overview. Am J Orthod Dentofacial Orthop 2006; 129(4) (Suppl.): S47-9. [http://dx.doi.org/10.1016/j.ajodo.2005.09.014] [PMID: 16644417]

[12] Dewel BF. Serial extraction, second premolars, and diagnostic precautions. Am J Orthod 1978; 73(5): 575-7. [http://dx.doi.org/10.1016/0002-9416(78)90247-6] [PMID: 277071]

[13] Yoshihara T, Matsumoto Y, Suzuki J, Sato N, Oguchi H. Effect of serial extraction alone on crowding: relationships between tooth width, arch length, and crowding. Am J Orthod Dentofacial Orthop 1999; 116(6): 691-6. [http://dx.doi.org/10.1016/S0889-5406(99)70206-4] [PMID: 10587605]

[14] Woodside DG. The significance of late developmental crowding to early treatment planning for incisor crowding. Am J Orthod Dentofacial Orthop 2000; 117(5): 559-61. [http://dx.doi.org/10.1016/S0889-5406(00)70199-5] [PMID: 10799114]

[15] American Academy of Pediatric Dentistry. Policy on ethical responsibility to treat or refer. Pediatr Dent 2013; 35(special issue): 106. [PMID: 23635976]

[16] Nyström M, Peck L. The period between exfoliation of primary teeth and the emergence of permanent successors. Eur J Orthod 1989; 11(1): 47-51. [http://dx.doi.org/10.1093/oxfordjournals.ejo.a035964] [PMID: 2714392]

[17] McNamara JA, Brudon WL. Dentitional development.Orthodontics and Dentofacial Orthopedics. Ann Arbor, Mich: Needham Press, Inc 2001.

[18] Howe RP, McNamara JA Jr, O'Connor KA. An examination of dental crowding and its relationship to tooth size and arch dimension. Am J Orthod 1983; 83(5): 363-73. [http://dx.doi.org/10.1016/0002-9416(83)90320-2] [PMID: 6573844]

[19] Brin I, Camasuvi S, Dali N, Aizenbud D. Comparison of second molar eruption patterns in patients with skeletal Class II and skeletal Class I malocclusions. Am J Orthod Dentofacial Orthop 2006; 130(6): 746-51. [http://dx.doi.org/10.1016/j.ajodo.2005.02.027] [PMID: 17169737]

[20] Burson C. A study of individual variation in mandibular bicanine dimenstion during growth. Am J Orthod 1952; 38: 848-65. [http://dx.doi.org/10.1016/0002-9416(52)90040-7]

[21] Puri N, Pradhan KL, Chandna A, Sehgal V, Gupta R. Biometric study of tooth size in normal, crowded, and spaced permanent dentitions. Am J Orthod Dentofacial Orthop 2007; 132(3): 279.e7-279.e14.
[http://dx.doi.org/10.1016/j.ajodo.2007.01.018] [PMID: 17826594]

[22] Brennan MM, Gianelly AA. The use of the lingual arch in the mixed dentition to resolve incisor crowding. Am J Orthod Dentofacial Orthop 2000; 117(1): 81-5.
[http://dx.doi.org/10.1016/S0889-5406(00)70252-6] [PMID: 10629524]

[23] Qudeimat MA, Fayle SA. The longevity of space maintainers: a retrospective study. Pediatr Dent 1998; 20(4): 267-72.
[PMID: 9783298]

[24] Rajab LD. Clinical performance and survival of space maintainers: evaluation over a period of 5 years. ASDC J Dent Child 2002; 69(2): 156-160, 124.
[PMID: 12515058]

[25] Bell RA, Dean JA, McDonald RE, Avery DR. Management of the developing occlusion. McDonald and Avery's Dentistry for the Child and Adolescent. 9th ed., Maryland Heights, Mo: Mosby Elsevier 2011.
[http://dx.doi.org/10.1016/B978-0-323-05724-0.50031-X]

[26] Owais AI, Rousan ME, Badran SA, Abu Alhaija ES. Effectiveness of a lower lingual arch as a space holding device. Eur J Orthod 2011; 33(1): 37-42.
[http://dx.doi.org/10.1093/ejo/cjq022] [PMID: 20660503]

[27] Rebellato J, Lindauer SJ, Rubenstein LK, Isaacson RJ, Davidovitch M, Vroom K. Lower arch perimeter preservation using the lingual arch. Am J Orthod Dentofacial Orthop 1997; 112(4): 449-56.
[http://dx.doi.org/10.1016/S0889-5406(97)70054-4] [PMID: 9345158]

[28] Viglianisi A. Effects of lingual arch used as space maintainer on mandibular arch dimension: A systematic Review c. Am J Orthod Dentofacial Orthop 2010; 138(4): 382 e 1-4.
[http://dx.doi.org/10.1016/j.ajodo.2010.02.026]

[29] Rebellato J. Two-couple orthodontic appliance systems: transpalatal arches. Semin Orthod 1995; 1(1): 44-54.
[http://dx.doi.org/10.1016/S1073-8746(95)80088-3] [PMID: 8935043]

[30] Stivaros N, Lowe C, Dandy N, Doherty B, Mandall NA. A randomized clinical trial to compare the Goshgarian and Nance palatal arch. Eur J Orthod 2010; 32(2): 171-6.
[http://dx.doi.org/10.1093/ejo/cjp075] [PMID: 19959609]

[31] Zablocki HL, McNamara JA Jr, Franchi L, Baccetti T. Effect of the transpalatal arch during extraction treatment. Am J Orthod Dentofacial Orthop 2008; 133(6): 852-60.
[http://dx.doi.org/10.1016/j.ajodo.2006.07.031] [PMID: 18538249]

CHAPTER 6

Maxillary Expansion in Mixed Dentition

Abstract: Posterior crossbite is one of the most prevalent malocclusions in the mixed dentition period; it does not have a spontaneous correction and should be treated as early as possible, after an accurate diagnosis. Maxillary expansion is considered an effective and reliable method for increasing transverse dimension in patients with unilateral or bilateral posterior crossbites. Moreover, it seems that this not only enlarges the constricted maxillae, but also creates additional spaces in the dental arches to resolve borderline dental crowding in some patients. This chapter addresses the aetiology, diagnosis and treatment of maxillary transverse discrepancy in the mixed dentition period.

Keywords: Hyrax appliance, Maxillary expansion, Posterior cross-bite, Quad-helix appliance.

INTRODUCTION

An orthopaedic maxillary expansion treatment has been used for more than a century but has been popularised since the mid-1960s. Even if the primary goal of maxillary expansion treatment is to correct the posterior cross-bite by widening the constricted maxilla, it can also provide additional spaces in mixed dentition dental arches to increase dental arch dimensions, decrease the nasal resistance and broaden the smile. There are two treatment alternatives of the maxilla expansion in mixed dentition period, which are evaluated on the basis of the frequency of the activations, magnitude of the applied force and duration of the treatment. These ME) and slow maxillary expansion.

1. a. Give the Basic Clinical Characteristics of Maxillary Transverse Deficiency.
b. Give Some Etiological Factors of Maxillary Transverse Deficiency.
c. Which is the Most Common Form of Maxillary Transverse Deficiency in the Mixed Dentition Period?
d. What Range of Transverse Measurements between Upper First Molars is Considered Normal for Mixed Dentition and Permanent Dentition?

George Litsas

a. Maxillary transverse deficiency may be one of the most pervasive skeletal problems in the craniofacial region. These are the three basic clinical characteristics of the transverse maxillary deficiency:
   - Unilateral or bilateral cross-bites
   - Possible dental crowding due to transverse space deficiency
   - Buccal flared maxillary posterior teeth [1 - 3].

b. *Skeletal factors.* Maxillary growth deficiency (e.g. cleft-lip and palate, mouth breathing, prolonged finger sucking-tongue thrust, Class III).
   Dental factors. Prolong retention of primary teeth or ectopic eruption of first permanent molars, tooth-size arch-length discrepancies, abnormalities in tooth morphology and eruption sequence.
   Functional reasons. Lateral jaw shift as the teeth shift from centric relation (CR) to centric occlusion (CO) because of occlusal interferences. Patients with normal occlusion in the primary dentition were shown to develop a lateral cross-bite in 3.1% by the time the permanent dentition was reached [3].

c. The most common form of posterior crossbite in the mixed dentition period (Fig. **1**) is a unilateral presentation with a functional shift of the mandible toward the crossbite side. Proper attention should be given because what appears to be a unilateral crossbite in maximum interdigitation **is a bilateral crossbite with a functional lateral jaw shift** as the teeth shift from centric relation (CR) to centric occlusion (CO) [4, 5]. It occurs in 80% to 97% of posterior cross-bite cases. Primary canine involvement is often seen and considered a part of a posterior crossbite. However, a bilateral cross-bite can occur without any functional shift (Fig. **2**).

d. Mixed dentition: **33-34 mm**, Permanent dentition: **35-39 mm** [6].

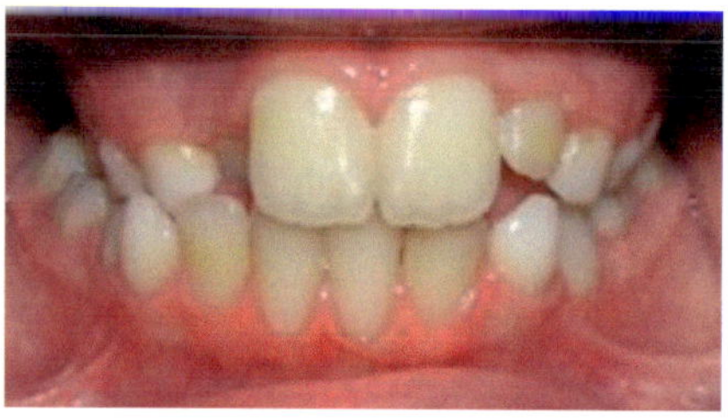

Fig. (1). Posterior cross-bite.

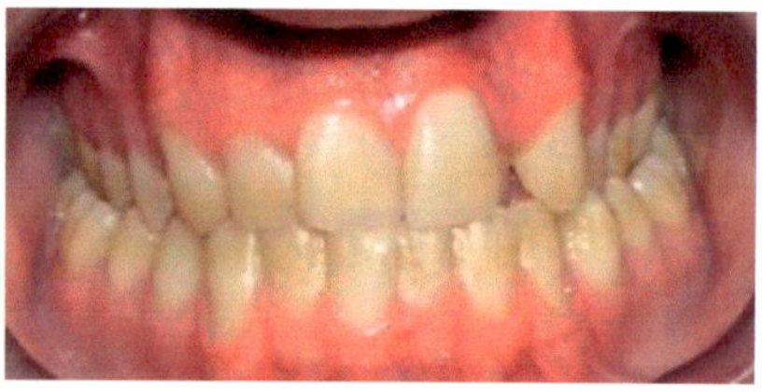

Fig. (2). Posterior cross-bite.

2. Which Other Problems Could be Associated with Maxillary Constriction?

- Malocclusion-aesthetics-functional difficulties
- Narrowing of the pharyngeal airway
- Increased nasal resistance and mouth breathing
- Retroglossal airway narrowing because of alterations in tongue posture [7, 8].

3. How Do You Diagnose the Posterior Cross-Bite?

The proper diagnosis includes **clinical** [2 - 4, 7, 8], **radiographical** [8 - 10] **and study casts** [12, 13] evaluation.

The clinical examination includes the evaluation of the face and the dentition in the frontal view as well as the lateral chin deviation in maximum interdigitation (Figs. **3**, **4**). A functional examination of the mandible's closing pathway from maximum opening to first contact and then to maximum intercuspation must be performed to determine whether a lateral mandible shift occurs following the first contact. *If there is any doubt about a lateral shift, it is prudent to disarticulate the occlusion by bite plate for two weeks before re-examining.*

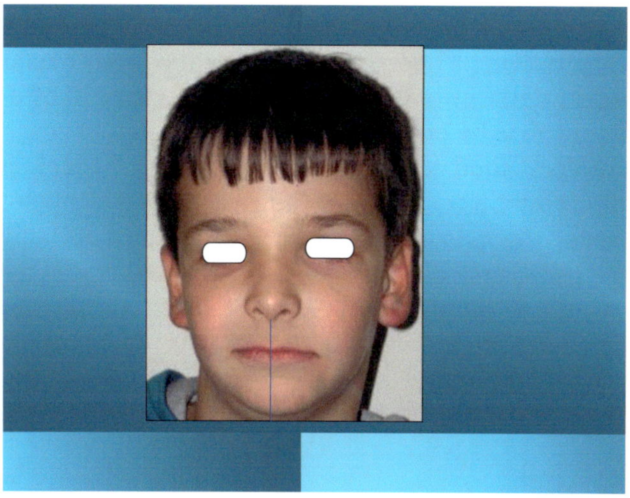

Fig. (3). Extra-oral pictures.

Radiographic Evaluation: In the absence of a lateral shift, findings of unilateral cross-bite establish the presence of a true unilateral skeletal asymmetry. The diagnosis should be based on the **posterior-anterior cephalometric radiograph,** which is the most useful tool in quantifying true maxillary-mandibular skeletal asymmetries. In this radiograph, the left-to-right maxillary jugal width is compared to the left-to-right mandibular antegonial width in order to estimate transverse skeletal discrepancies.

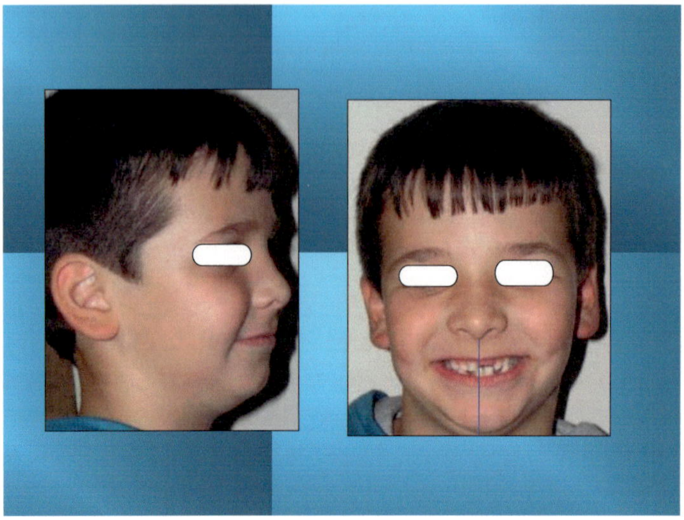

Fig. (4). Lateral chin deviation.

Study Model Examination: The examination of the dental relationships on the study casts is used to determine whether the discrepancy is of dental or skeletal origin. The casts must first be examined for posterior dental compensations of the permanent first molars such as excessive maxillary buccal crown torque or mandibular lingual crown torque as viewed in the frontal plane. Uprighting the molars on the casts, the posterior transverse interarch relationship could be improved, then the transverse discrepancies is of dental origin and can be treated with dental movement. If the transverse interarch relationship worsens, then the discrepancy is of skeletal origin.

4. What Are the Reasons for Correcting the Posterior Cross-Bite with Lateral Shift?

The index of treatment need categorises posterior cross-bite types as severe and requiring treatment [3]. Treatment of the posterior cross-bite with a functional shift should be initiated as soon as it is diagnosed because it could create:

- *Asymmetrical facial growth and chin deviation.* During the growth period, continuous asymmetric condylar displacement in the glenoid fossa induces differential growth of the condyles and of the mandibular ramus, leading to skeletal asymmetry [7 - 9, 11].

- *Abnormal wear patterns, adverse periodontal responses around the affected teeth.*
- *Dental arch space loss and crowding in the permanent dentition* [14, 15].

5. Provide the Relationship Between Cross-Bite and Facial Muscle Activity in Young Patients.

The activity of the temporal and masseter muscles in functional crossbite patients is disturbed. At rest, electromyography activity should be minimal or completely absent. However, in children with functional crossbite, the activity of the anterior temporalis muscle on the non-crossbite side and of the posterior temporalis muscle on the crossbite side is higher in order to counterbalance the force of gravity. Moreover, the asymmetrical mandibular position induces different developments of the elevator muscles of the mandible, leading to a heavier masseter muscle on the non-crossbite side [16 - 19].

6. a. What Are the Criteria for Using the Proper Maxillary Expander? b. Into What Categories Can the Maxillary Expansion Appliances be Generally Divided? What Are the Advantages of Fixed Expansion Appliances?

a. The appliance selection for maxillary expansion could be based on many different criteria such as the age of the patient, skeletal or dental expansion needs, the number of available teeth and the need or not for conjunction with other appliances such as facemask [1, 20, 25].

b. Tooth-borne appliances such as Hyrax, Quad-helix and W-arch, tissue-borne expander such as Haas appliance and a combination of both of the above such as mini-screw implants. The main advantages of fixed expansion appliances are that they are not dependent on the patient's compliance, they have minimal effects on speech and they have continuous action over a long period of time [16, 20 - 25].

7. Describe the Treatment Protocol of the Posterior Dento-Alveolar Cross-Bite with Lateral Shift in the Following Patients

Early treatment by selective grinding of premature contacts in the primary teeth is an effective method in order to prevent a posterior crossbite from being perpetuated to the late mixed and permanent dentition (Figs. **3-6**) [12, 15, 17].

"The greatest chance of correction after selective grinding occurred *when the maxillary inter-canine width is at least 3 mm greater than the corresponding mandibular inter-canine width*". When this procedure is not effective, the dento-alveolar crossbite requires expansion of the maxillary arch. Dental tipping or translation can be used to correct transverse discrepancies in the range of 4 to 5 mm. A high success rate was found and a substantial expansion effect was shown of treatment with Quad Helix and Expansion Plates (Figs. **7** & **8**) [1, 17].

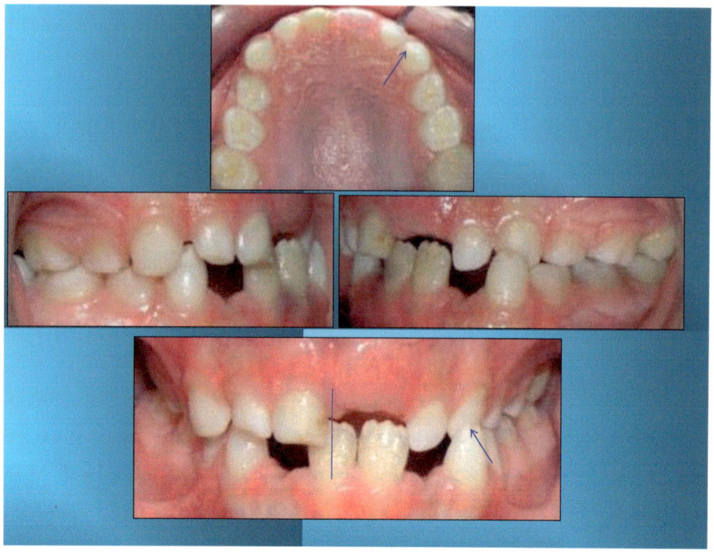

Fig. (5). Intra-oral pictures illustrating the midline deviation. Arrow shows the occlusal (primary canine) interferences to first contact to maximum intercuspation.

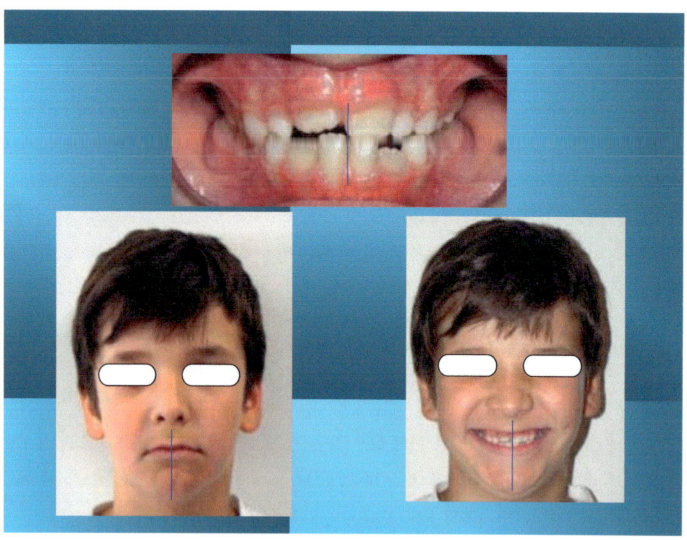

Fig. (6). Dental and skeletal correction after selective grinding of premature contacts.

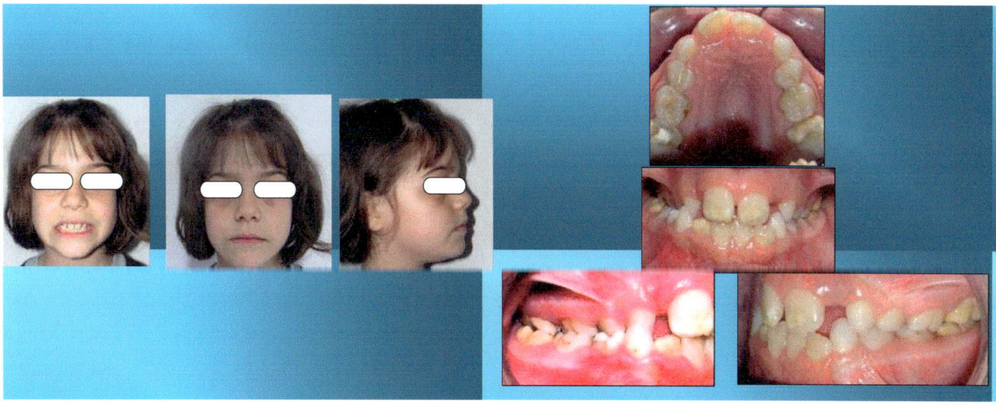

Fig. (7). Extra-oral and intra-oral pictures before treatment.

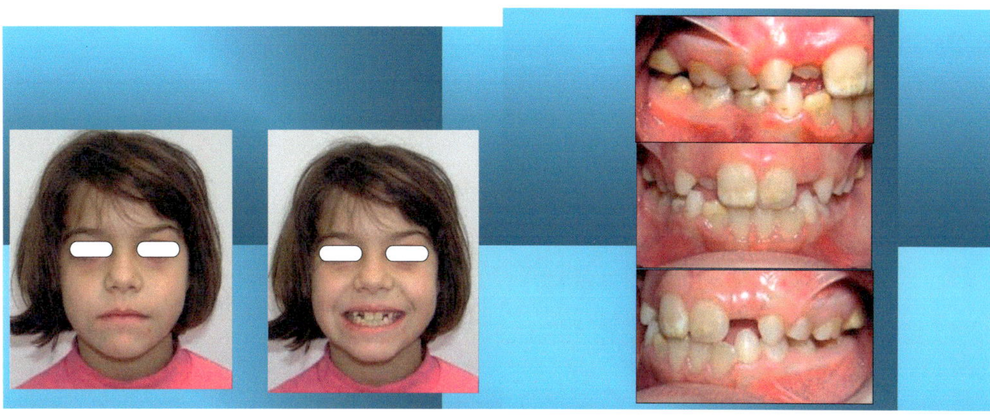

Fig. (8). Extra-oral and intra-oral pictures after treatment.

8. Quad-Helix, Expansion Plate, or Rapid Maxillary Expansion?

In the mixed dentition the Quad Helix appliance (Fig. **9**) seems to be superior to the expansion plate (Fig. **10**) in success rate and treatment time and is considered to be the more cost-effective choice for treatment. It expands the maxillary arch much less aggressively than the RME appliance (Fig. **11**), it is a much more predictable appliance than the removable plate and, finally, it doesn't need the patient's cooperation. However, there is very little evidence to suggest that the **Quad-helix appliance** may be more successful than removable **expansion plates** at correcting posterior crossbites and expanding the inter-molar width for children [24, 26].

Both the rapid maxillary expansion (RME) and semi-rapid maxillary expansion (SRME) protocol during early mixed dentition not only produce an expansion force at the inter-maxillary suture but also cause adverse high forces on various structures in the craniofacial complex [23].

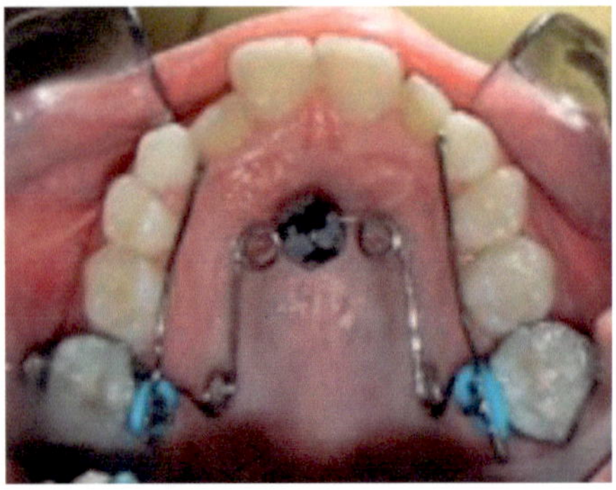

Fig. (9). Quad-Helix.

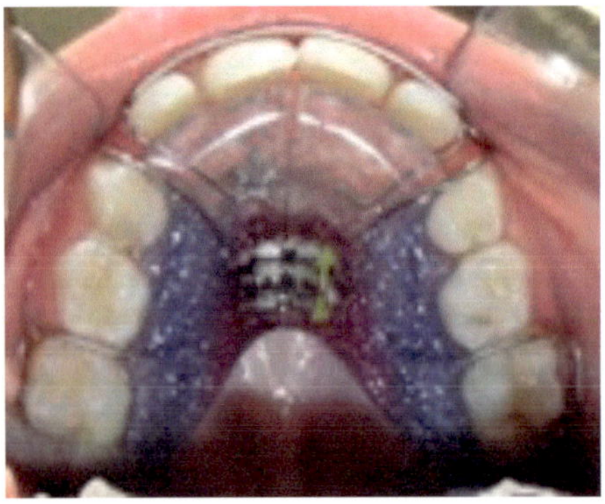

Fig. (10). Removable appliance.

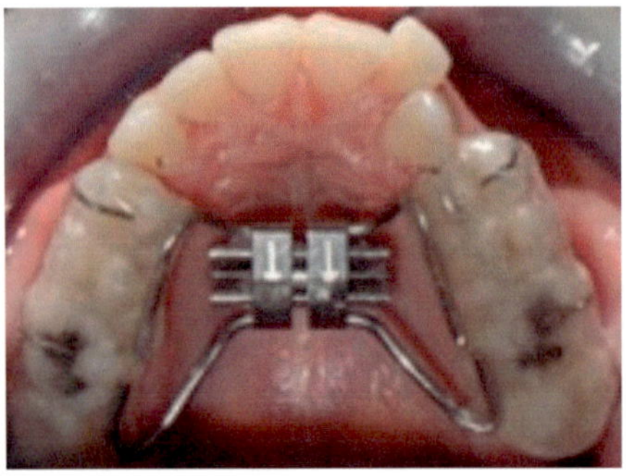

Fig. (11). RME appliance.

9. What's the Difference between Slow and Rapid Palatal Expansion?

Table 1. Slow vs. Rapid palatal expansion.

Slow Palatal Expansion	Rapid Palatal Expansion
- Removable appliance	- Fixed appliance
- Expansion rate: Twice a week, 1 turn: 0.25mm	- Expansion rate: Twice a day, 2 turns: **0.5mm**
- Mixed dentition.	- Adolescent with gross skeletal discrepancy
- Both dental and skeletal changes (1:1)	- Predominantly skeletal effects (8:2) and later dental changes take place after skeletal relapse
- More physiologic to tissues	- More traumatic to tissues

10. Could You Describe Two Methods of Quad-helix Activation?

- 1st Ricketts's method [26]: The clinical steps could be summarised in the following picture (Fig. **12**). He suggested that the clinician should activate the appliance before placing in the mouth with a three-pronged plier to incorporate expansion and molar-rotating force. Although it takes some experience, it is possible to re-activate a quad helix after it has been cemented to the teeth.
- 2nd method: The clinical steps of another method could be summarised in the following principles:

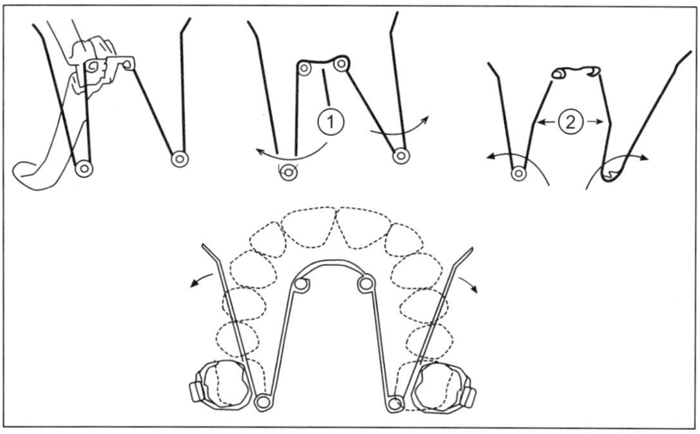

Fig. (12). Quad-helix activation.

The appliance tested passive into the mouth. Prior to cementation, it is expanded out of the mouth 4mm and then inserted and cemented. Expansion should re-activate at the rate of 1mm per side, in 3-5 week intervals till the over-correction of the crossbite. At the end of the treatment, the appliance should remain in the mouth as a retention appliance for another 3 months [1, 14].

11. Name the Indications of the Quad-helix Expansion Appliance During the Mixed Dentition Period

- *In Class II children needing bilateral or unilateral maxillary expansion.* Because most of these patients require maxillary molar derotation, all of the expansion force will be directed at these molars in the initial stages of treatment. The molar derotation effected also causes sufficient molar distalization to resolve most minor Class II end-to-end molar malocclusions [26].
- *In mild maxillary deficient Class III cases.* In addition to maxillary expansion, a .045" wire section could be placed in the headgear tubes of the maxillary molar bands and the Quad-helix appliance may be used in conjunction with a protraction face mask to advance the maxilla.
- *Relieve the anterior crowding*; prevent canine impaction.
- *In tongue-thrusting and thumb-sucking children* after the proper modifications on the anterior bar of the Quad-helix appliance [1].
- *Cleft palate patients* [14].

12. What is the Following Appliance? What Are the Advantages of this Appliance?

NiTi Expander (Fig. **13**). It is a fixed-removable expansion appliance with activation based on shape memory and super-elasticity properties of NiTi. The main advantages of this expander are that it is a self-activated appliance which requires little manipulation by the clinician applying light continuous orthodontic forces [27].

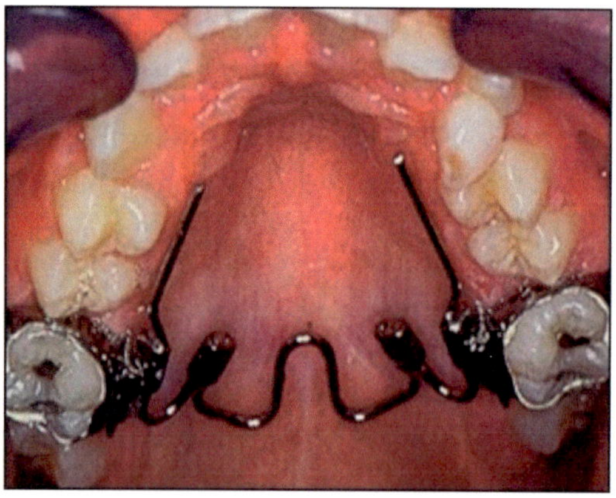

Fig. (13). NiTi expander.

13. How Do You Treat the Skeletal Posterior Cross-bite in the Late Mixed or Early Permanent Dentition?

Patients in this dental stage require greater force and a faster rate of expansion because of growth-related changes in suture biology. Rapid Maxillary Expansion (RME) should be used using **Haas** or **Hyrax** expansion appliances. These appliances consist of a jackscrew in banded or bonded appliances with the presence or absence of an acrylic pad close to the palate. One type is the tooth tissue-borne expander or Haas-type expander and another type is the tooth-borne expander or Hyrax expander [6, 9, 16, 24, 25].

Growing Patients: Two turns each day for the first 4 to 5 days, one turn each day for the remainder of RME treatment.

Adults: Two turns each day for the first 2 days, one turn each day for the next 5 to 7 days, and one turn every other day for the remainder of RME treatment. *Expansion should stop when the maxillary palatal cusps are level with the buccal cusps of the mandibular teeth.*

14. Provide the Indications and the Benefits of RPE Treatment.

Table 2. Indications and the benefits of RPE treatment [22, 24, 25, 28, 29].

Indications RPE	Benefits of RPE
- Skeletal constricted maxilla	- Correction of crossbite
- Bilateral or unilateral cross-bite	- Increasing arch length
- Maxillary retrognathism	- Correction of buccal inclination of posterior teeth
- Borderline space deficient cases (4-5 mm)	- Preparation for functional jaw orthopaedics
- Cleft palate	- Broadening the smile, facilitate canine eruption, improve nasal airflow

15. When is the Proper Time for Skeletal Maxillary Expansion?

Clinicians have commonly reported difficulty in producing palatal separation following the pubertal growth period while favourable orthopaedic responses have been indicated prior to and during pubertal growth. Greater and more stable orthopaedic changes have been reported in patients under the age of 12.

A direct relationship between increased resistance to skeletal expansion and increasing patient age has been quantified and associated with the formation of mechanical interlocking at maxillary articulations as early as 12 to 13 years of age [24].

In addition, the enhanced skeletal response in younger age groups has been associated with a greater cellular activity and increased reparability potential in the growing suture. It seems that the transverse growth pattern of the maxilla follows the body height with similar growth spurt and growth completion [5, 9, 30].

16. a. Provide the Skeletal Versus Dental Effects After Rapid Maxillary Expansion Therapy.
b. Describe some Orthopaedic Effects During RPE Therapy.
c. What Should We Place Within 24 to 48 Hours After the Removal of an RPE?

a. Initial skeletal expansion vs. dento-alveolar expansion is thought to be in the range of 80 to 20, whereas at the end of treatment it is thought to be nearer 50/50 due to tooth movement. This is the reason why over-compensation is necessary to end up with adequate expansion [16, 25].

b. The maxilla displaced inferior and anterior and the mandible rotated clockwise. This bite opening can be favourable when the patient has a Class III, maxillary deficient, low mandibular plane angle skeletal pattern. However, it is more frequently undesirable because Class II high mandibular plane angle patterns predominate.

However, the occlusal acrylic coverage (Fig. **14**), acts as a bite block to inhibit the eruption of the posterior teeth during treatment, thereby making possible the use of this appliance in patients with increased lower anterior facial heights [31].

The design of this appliance is to intentionally infringe upon a patient's freeway space, transferring an apically directed force to the maxillary and mandibular teeth [32]. Finally, during Rapid Maxillary Expansion the alveolar processes bend laterally and the nasal cavity widens as well [9, 11, 22].

c. A removable maintenance plate or a TPA with extensive arms in order to prevent relapse.

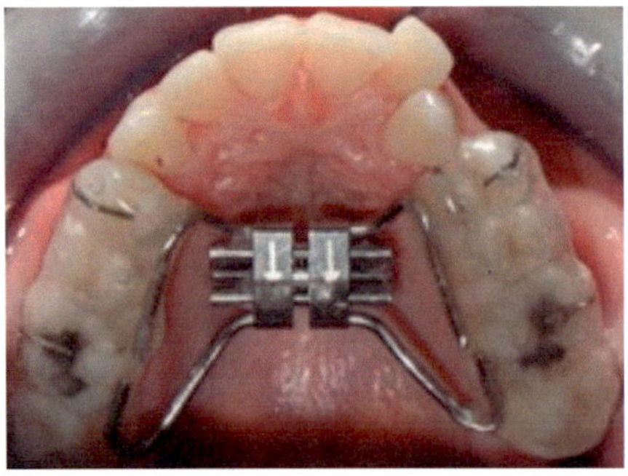

Fig. (14). Hyrax appliance with occlusal coverage.

17. Provide Any Possible Relationship between Rapid Maxillary Expansion Therapy and Breathe Function

Although the purpose of Rapid Maxillary Expansion is to correct dental and skeletal maxillary transverse discrepancies by opening the mid-palatal suture, some investigators have shown that treatment outcomes could also involve increasing nasopharyngeal airway dimensions, leading to improved nasal breathing. RME causes decreased nasal airway resistance, reduction of head elevation resulting in improvement of nasal breathing. Moreover, Rapid Maxillary Expansion provides significant volume increases not only in the upper nasal airways but also in the middle and lower airway compartments, reducing the obstructive sleep apnoea symptoms [5, 7, 9, 11].

18. Name the Indirect Effects on Mandibular Arch Dimensions After Rapid Palatal Expansion Therapy

It was speculated that the position of the mandibular dentition might be influenced more by maxillary skeletal morphology than by the size and shape of the mandible. Some mandibular arch decompensation could be observed during rapid maxillary expansion because the force vector acting on the mandibular posterior teeth is altered by the maxillary expansion [6, 32, 33].

Another possible explanation could be that the pressure from the buccinator muscle is decreased, allowing pressure from the tongue to expand the mandibular teeth in a buccal direction. It was shown that mandibular inter-molar arch width and molar angulation increased significantly in early mixed dentition patients with posterior crossbite after RPE treatment. This increase was followed also by a little effect on inter-canine distance and angulation [6]. However, neither the small gain in mandibular intermolar width northe long-term questionable results justify using maxillary expansion in order to gain mandibular arch width [22].

19. a. Describe the Main Orthopaedic Effect of the RPE Treatment You See in the Following Pictures.
b. Describe Some Dental Effects During RPE Therapy.
c. What Do You See in the Same Patient Four Months After RME Therapy?

a. The Hyrax appliance, opens the mid-palatal suture (triangular radiolucency) and creates a diastema between the maxillary central incisors (Figs. **15 & 16**). It is estimated that the incisors separate approximately half the distance the expansion screw has been opened [2, 9, 16, 24, 25].
b. Midline diastema between central incisors, increased overjet, decreased overbite, buccal tipping of the maxillary posterior teeth and possible uprighting of the mandibular posterior teeth.

c. Four months after the RPE (Fig. **17**) treatment:
   - The midline diastema disappears due to the pulling effect of elastic transeptal gingival fibres. First the crowns contact and then the continued pull of the fibres causes the roots to converge toward their original axial inclinations.
   - Crowding relieve: Maxillary expansion therapy is another method to gain space in the dental arch because of its potential for increasing arch perimeter to alleviate crowding in the maxillary arch without adversely affecting the facial profile. Every 1mm of increase in posterior arch width produced by RPE translates to 0.7mm of increased arch perimeter [28].

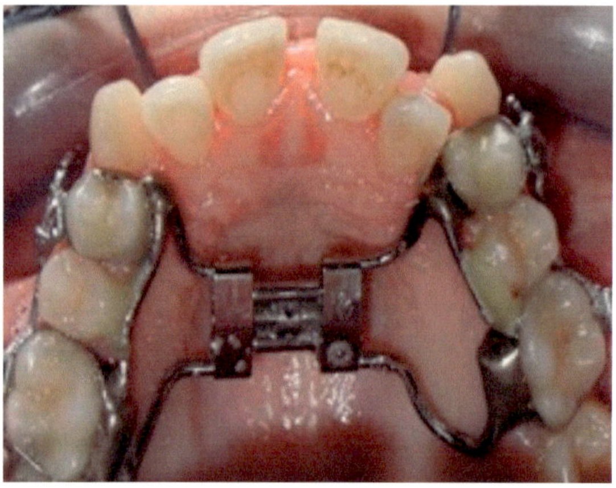

Fig. (15). Hyrax expansion treatment.

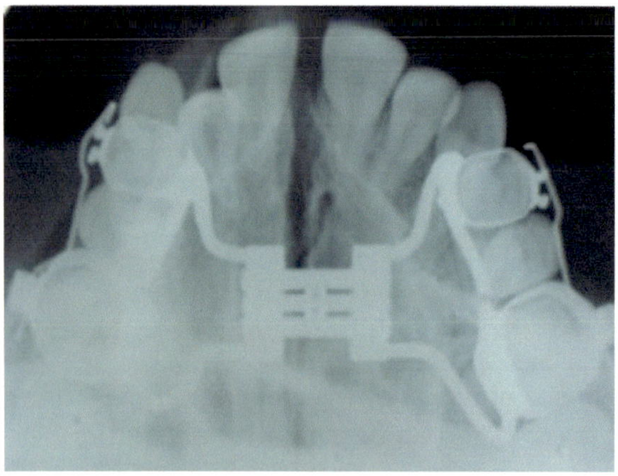

Fig. (16). Triangular radiolucency.

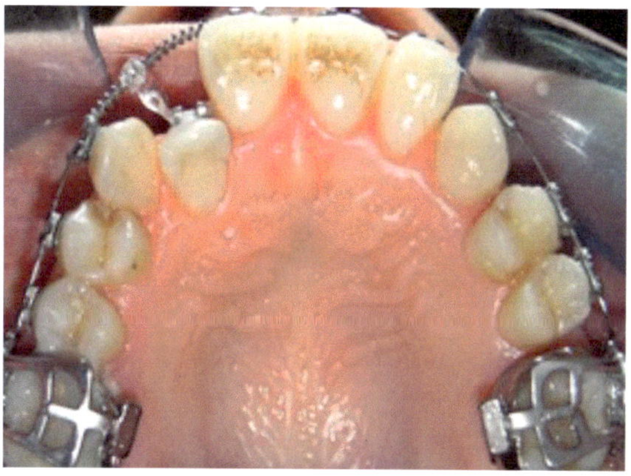

Fig. (17). Four months after Hyrax expansion treatment.

20. Why is this Possible From a Histological Point of View?

Because the mid-palatal suture appears smooth and broadens during the early mixed dentition period, becomes squamous with overlapping sections. This stage is called juvenile. Later, it becomes squamous with overlapping sections (adolescent stage), increasing the interdigitations between two halves of the maxilla, and finally the suture forms numerous bony bridges and synostosis in the adult stage [6, 25].

21. a. What is the Buttressing Effect During RME Treatment? b. Could You Approximate the Location of the Centre of the Maxillary Bone During RME Treatment?

a. The maxilla is articulated to seven facial bones, mostly by sutures superiorly and posteriorly. The only free maxillary segments are the anterior and inferior. The opening of the **sutura media palatina** in the horizontal plane is triangular in shape, with its base on anterior teeth and its tip on the posterior teeth [28]. In the frontal plane, the opening is triangular with the apex being in the fronto-maxillary suture (Fig. **18**). The resisting units on the posterior side are **zygomatic arch** and the **corpus of the sphenoid bone** displacing the maxilla downward and forward [2, 5].
b. It depends on the configuration of the circumaxillary sutures, the interdigitations within the midpalatal suture, the anteroposterior or inferior-superior position of the expansion device and the child's age [5].

22. In the Absence of a Posterior Crossbite, Should Maxillary Expansion be Used to Correct a Class II Relationship?

Any Class II improvement with maxillary expansion in early treatment is probably due to simple unlocking of the occlusion and the greater normal forward growth of the mandible compared with the maxilla. These patients have either end-to-end molar relationship with reasonably well-balanced skeletal structures, or characterised clinically as mild-to-moderate mandibular skeletal retrusion [6]. However, the effect of maxillary expansion on the sagittal dimension of Class II is still controversial and has not been substantially proven yet [32].

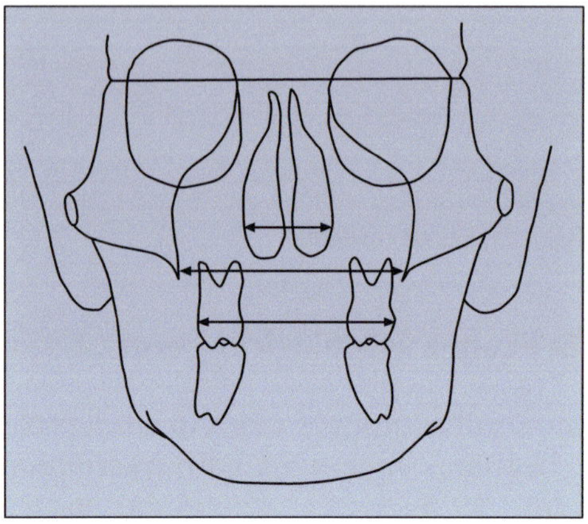

Fig. (18). Triangular opening at the frontal plane.

CONCLUDING REMARKS

The orthodontic treatment for mixed dentition patients with constricted maxilla and tooth/arch size discrepancies is to correct the skeletal discrepancy and to gain additional space in the dental arches to resolve crowding. Maxillary expansion therapy can be used effectively for this treatment approach. This procedure increases the upper arch transverse dimensions either by transverse expansion of the posterior teeth and alveolar processes or by both separation of the two maxillary halves and buccal movement of the posterior teeth.

REFERENCES

[1] Bell RA, LeCompte EJ. The effects of maxillary expansion using a quad-helix appliance during the deciduous and mixed dentitions. Am J Orthod 1981; 79(2): 152-61. [http://dx.doi.org/10.1016/0002-9416(81)90313-4] [PMID: 7008619]

[2] Betts NJ, Vanarsdall RL, Barber HD, Higgins-Barber K, Fonseca RJ. Diagnosis and treatment of transverse maxillary deficiency. Int J Adult Orthodon Orthognath Surg 1995; 10(2): 75-96. [PMID: 9082002]

[3] Brook PH, Shaw WC. The development of an index of orthodontic treatment priority. Eur J Orthod 1989; 11(3): 309-20. [http://dx.doi.org/10.1093/oxfordjournals.ejo.a035999] [PMID: 2792220]

[4] Andrade AdaS, Gameiro GH, Derossi M, Gavião MB. Posterior crossbite and functional changes. A systematic review. Angle Orthod 2009; 79(2): 380-6.

[http://dx.doi.org/10.2319/030708-137.1] [PMID: 19216602]

[5] Björk A, Skieller V. Growth of the maxilla in three dimensions as revealed radiographically by the implant method. Br J Orthod 1977; 4(2): 53-64.
[http://dx.doi.org/10.1179/bjo.4.2.53] [PMID: 273440]

[6] McNamara JA Jr, Sigler LM, Franchi L, Guest SS, Baccetti T. Changes in occlusal relationships in mixed dentition patients treated with rapid maxillary expansion. A prospective clinical study. Angle Orthod 2010; 80(2): 230-8.
[http://dx.doi.org/10.2319/040309-192.1] [PMID: 19905846]

[7] Pinto AS, Buschang PH, Throckmorton GS, Chen P. Morphological and positional asymmetries of young children with functional unilateral posterior crossbite. Am J Orthod Dentofacial Orthop 2001, 120(5): 513-20.
[http://dx.doi.org/10.1067/mod.2001.118627a] [PMID: 11709670]

[8] Pirttiniemi P, Kantomaa T, Lahtela P. Relationship between craniofacial and condyle path asymmetry in unilateral cross-bite patients. Eur J Orthod 1990; 12(4): 408-13.
[http://dx.doi.org/10.1093/ejo/12.4.408] [PMID: 2086261]

[9] Ballanti F, Lione R, Baccetti T, Franchi L, Cozza P. Treatment and posttreatment skeletal effects of rapid maxillary expansion investigated with low-dose computed tomography in growing subjects. Am J Orthod Dentofacial Orthop 2010; 138(3): 311-7.
[http://dx.doi.org/10.1016/j.ajodo.2008.10.022] [PMID: 20816300]

[10] Grummons DC, Kappeyne van de Coppello MA. A frontal asymmetry analysis. J Clin Orthod 1987; 21(7): 448-65.
[PMID: 3476493]

[11] Smith T, Ghoneima A, Stewart K, *et al.* Three-dimensional computed tomography analysis of airway volume changes after rapid maxillary expansion. Am J Orthod Dentofacial Orthop 2012; 141(5): 618-26.
[http://dx.doi.org/10.1016/j.ajodo.2011.12.017] [PMID: 22554756]

[12] Lindner A. Longitudinal study on the effect of early interceptive treatment in 4-year-old children with unilateral cross-bite. Scand J Dent Res 1989; 97(5): 432-8.
[PMID: 2617141]

[13] Ngan P, Fields H. Orthodontic diagnosis and treatment planning in the primary dentition. ASDC J Dent Child 1995; 62(1): 25-33.
[PMID: 7775680]

[14] Petrén S, Bondemark L. Correction of unilateral posterior crossbite in the mixed dentition: a randomized controlled trial. Am J Orthod Dentofacial Orthop 2008; 133(6): 790.e7-790.e13.
[http://dx.doi.org/10.1016/j.ajodo.2007.11.021] [PMID: 18538237]

[15] Petrén S, Bondemark L, Söderfeldt B. A systematic review concerning early orthodontic treatment of unilateral posterior crossbite. Angle Orthod 2003; 73(5): 588-96.
[PMID: 14580028]

[16] Wertz RA. Skeletal and dental changes accompanying rapid midpalatal suture opening. Am J Orthod 1970; 58(1): 41-66.
[http://dx.doi.org/10.1016/0002-9416(70)90127-2] [PMID: 5269181]

[17] Thilander B, Wahlund S, Lennartsson B. The effect of early interceptive treatment in children with posterior cross-bite. Eur J Orthod 1984; 6(1): 25-34.
[http://dx.doi.org/10.1093/ejo/6.1.25] [PMID: 6583062]

[18] Hesse KL, Artun J, Joondeph DR, Kennedy DB. Changes in condylar postition and occlusion associated with maxillary expansion for correction of functional unilateral posterior crossbite. Am J Orthod Dentofacial Orthop 1997; 111(4): 410-8.
[http://dx.doi.org/10.1016/S0889-5406(97)80023-6] [PMID: 9109586]

[19] Kiliaridis S, Katsaros C, Raadsheer MC, Mahboubi PH. Bilateral masseter muscle thickness in growing individuals with unilateral posterior cross-bite. J Dent Res 2000; 79: 497.

[20] Godoy F, Godoy-Bezerra J, Rosenblatt A. Treatment of posterior crossbite comparing 2 appliances: a community-based trial. Am J Orthod Dentofacial Orthop 2011; 139(1): e45-52. [http://dx.doi.org/10.1016/j.ajodo.2010.06.017] [PMID: 21195256]

[21] Kutin G, Hawes RR. Posterior cross-bites in the deciduous and mixed dentitions. Am J Orthod 1969; 56(5): 491-504. [http://dx.doi.org/10.1016/0002-9416(69)90210-3] [PMID: 5261162]

[22] Vanarsdall RL Jr. Transverse dimension and long-term stability. Semin Orthod 1999; 5(3): 171-80. [http://dx.doi.org/10.1016/S1073-8746(99)80008-5] [PMID: 10860069]

[23] Ramoglu SI, Sari Z. Maxillary expansion in the mixed dentition: rapid or semi-rapid? Eur J Orthod 2010; 32(1): 11-8. [http://dx.doi.org/10.1093/ejo/cjp057] [PMID: 19797410]

[24] Schiffman PH, Tuncay OC. Maxillary expansion: a meta analysis. Clin Orthod Res 2001; 4(2): 86-96. [http://dx.doi.org/10.1034/j.1600-0544.2001.040205.x] [PMID: 11553090]

[25] Wertz R, Dreskin M. Midpalatal suture opening: a normative study. Am J Orthod 1977; 71(4): 367-81. [http://dx.doi.org/10.1016/0002-9416(77)90241-X] [PMID: 322499]

[26] Ricketts RM. Bioprogressive technique lecture notes. Scottsdale, AZ: American Institute for Bioprogressive Education 1996.

[27] Arndt WV. Nickel titanium palatal expander. J Clin Orthod 1993; 27(3): 129-37. [PMID: 8496351]

[28] Adkins MD, Nanda RS, Currier GF. Arch perimeter changes on rapid palatal expansion. Am J Orthod Dentofacial Orthop 1990; 97(3): 194-9. [http://dx.doi.org/10.1016/S0889-5406(05)80051-4] [PMID: 2178393]

[29] Gianelly AA. Rapid palatal expansion in the absence of crossbites: added value? Am J Orthod Dentofacial Orthop 2003; 124(4): 362-5. [http://dx.doi.org/10.1016/S0889-5406(03)00568-7] [PMID: 14560264]

[30] Petrén S, Bjerklin K, Bondemark L. Stability of unilateral posterior crossbite correction in the mixed dentition: a randomized clinical trial with a 3-year follow-up. Am J Orthod Dentofacial Orthop 2011; 139(1): e73-81. [http://dx.doi.org/10.1016/j.ajodo.2010.06.018] [PMID: 21195260]

[31] Majourau A, Nanda R. Biomechanical basis of vertical dimension control during rapid palatal expansion therapy. Am J Orthod Dentofacial Orthop 1994; 106(3): 322-8. [http://dx.doi.org/10.1016/S0889-5406(94)70053-2] [PMID: 8074098]

[32] Miller CL, Araújo EA, Behrents RG, Oliver DR, Tanaka OM. Mandibular arch dimensions following bonded and banded rapid maxillary expansion. J World Fed Orthod 2014; 119-23. [http://dx.doi.org/10.1016/j.ejwf.2014.05.003]

[33] Lima AC, Lima AL, Filho RM, Oyen OJ. Spontaneous mandibular arch response after rapid palatal expansion: a long-term study on Class I malocclusion. Am J Orthod Dentofacial Orthop 2004; 126(5): 576-82. [http://dx.doi.org/10.1016/j.ajodo.2004.06.011] [PMID: 15520690]

CHAPTER 7

Dental Anomalies -Tooth Impaction

Abstract: Dental anomalies can be caused by any etiological factor that interrupts odontogenesis. Leaving environmental factors aside, genetics have been found to be a factor at various levels in dental anomalies and the fact that some human dental anomalies are often seen together supports the evidence that there is shared genetic control of disturbances in dental development. Early diagnosis can be assisted by recognition of dental anomalies (*e.g.* peg shape lateral incisors) in early mixed dentition that have a genetic association with canine impaction. Early detection of palatal canine displacement will allow clinicians to focus on prevention of canine impaction. The purpose of this chapter is to approach the early diagnosis and appropriate orthodontic intervention of dental anomalies and tooth impaction.

Keywords: Dental anomalies, Early diagnosis, Palatal canine displacement.

INTRODUCTION

A number of clinical orthodontists who are biologically attuned have focused on associations between dental anomalies. While for the most part they will be asymptomatic, such anomalies may lead to clinical problems and those problems can include delayed eruption or impacted teeth as well as impaired aesthetics, occlusal interference and malocclusion, greater susceptibility to caries and periodontal problems. Orthodontic treatment of impacted teeth causes clinicians difficulties, with treatment usually involving the impacted tooth's surgical exposure after which it is aligned into the dental arch with the aid of orthodontic traction. Common complications include loss of bone, resorption of root, and gingival recession in the same or neighbourhood of the treated teeth. If diagnosis is early enough, patient management and treatment can be optimal with the result that complications are reduced and so is the amount and complexity of treatment.

PART A. DENTAL ANOMALIES

1. What Are the Dental Anomalies?

From orthodontic perspective, dental anomalies could be defined as the interruption of odontogenesis which results in different phenotypic conditions

George Litsas

such as imperfections in the number, size, position and timing of tooth development. Several family and monozygotic twins' studies have suggested a genetic and hereditary background in the etiology of these dental anomalies [1, 2].

2. What is Hypodontia? Provide the Prevalence and the Most Common Affected Teeth

Hypodontia (Tooth agenesis): It is human dentition's commonest developmental anomaly and is characterised by one to six congenital missing teeth [1]. If we exclude third molars, tooth agenesis is present in roughly 4.3% to 7.8% of cases, though, in primary dentition, prevalence is very low at 0.3% [3]. Tooth agenesis may appear in isolation or may exhibit as part of a syndrome. Fig. (**1**) shows the mandibular second premolars, which are the teeth that most commonly fail to appear. Second most common among missing teeth are the maxillary lateral incisors shown in Fig. (**2**) [4]. The tendency is familiar and more females than males are affected [3, 4]. Where only a few teeth are missing, the most distal tooth of any given type will be absent – that is, lateral rather than central incisors and second bicuspids rather than first. There may be an association between tooth agenesis and non-syndromic cleft lip and palate [5, 6].

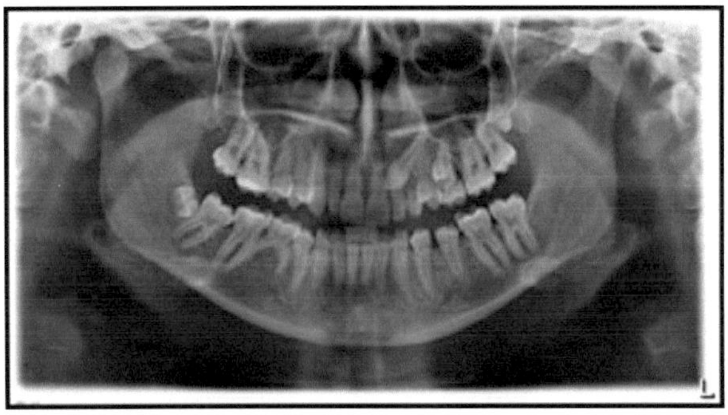

Fig. (1). Congenital missing of right mandibular 2nd premolar.

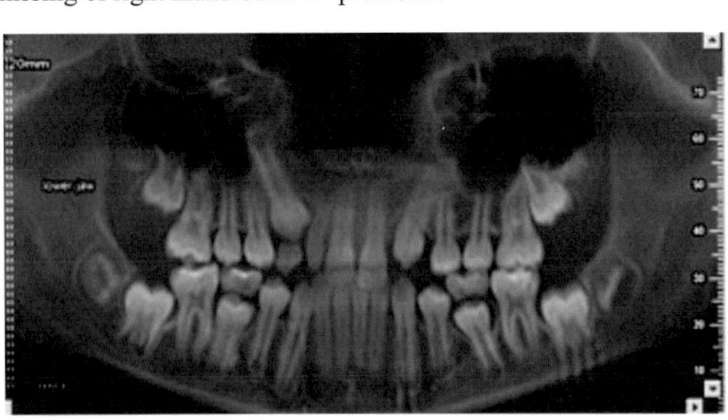

Fig. (2). Congenital missing of left lateral incisor.

3. What is Non-syndromic Hypodontia?

Non-syndromic hypodontia is the congenital absence of a specific number of teeth where no other deformity is present. A familial autosomal dominant hypodontia was demonstrated to be caused by a point mutation in the MSX1 gene [7]. It has been demonstrated that there is an association between the PAX9 gene on chromosome 14 and autosomal dominant, non-syndromic, familial hypodontia and a generalised reduction in teeth sizes [8]. Agenesis of incisors may be due to a mutation of the AXIN2 gene, while mutation of the LTBP3 and EDA genes can be responsible for an autosomal recessive form of familial oligodontia and a congenital absence of maxillary and mandibular incisors, canines and first molars [2, 8 - 10].

4. Which Are the Most Common Syndromes Associated With Tooth Agenesis?

Tooth agenesis could be associated with a number of syndromes indicating that both the teeth and certain organs development is controlled by the same molecular mechanisms. *Ectodermal dysplasia, orofacial digital syndrome type 1 (hypodontia of the lower incisors), syndromic cleft lip and palate like Pierre Robin and Van Der Woude* are some of the disorders associated with tooth agenesis [4, 6].

5. What Dental Anomaly Do You see Here? Provide the Etiology and the Characteristics of the Rest of the Dentition in Patients With this Kind of Dental Anomaly

Peg shaped and congenital missing upper lateral incisors: Genetics has been shown by recent studies to play a predominant role in this condition's aetiology. It is possible that patients with congenital tooth agenesis may show a reduction in tooth size, other than for first molars, that is both generalised and significant (Fig. **3**). An obvious example would be agenesis of the maxillary lateral incisor and the contralateral teeth's peg shape [3, 4]. There is an incomplete expression (peg-shaped) resulting from a genetic defect that caused agenesis of the lateral incisor in the right side of the dental arch (Fig. **4**) [10]. It should be noted, though, that agenesis of one or two teeth has been suggested to be associated with the presence of larger remaining teeth. This increase in size could be caused by a compensatory mechanism on the part of the teeth next to the missing teeth [11].

6. What is Oligodontia, Microdontia and Hyperodontia?

Oligodontia: More than six missing permanent teeth (excluding the third molars). It is often associated with a number of oral-facial syndromes such as ectodermal dysplasia. In patients with oligodontia, the reduction of tooth size is remarkable

[11 - 14].

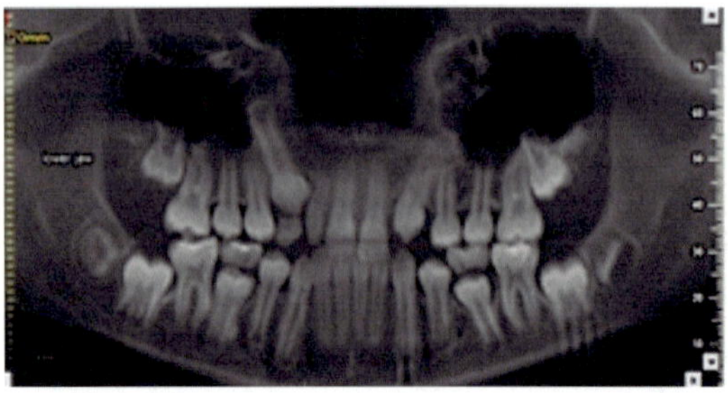

Fig. (3). Congenital missing of left lateral incisor.

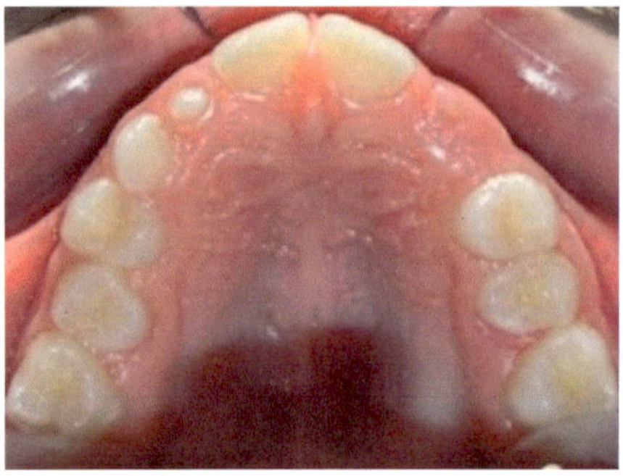

Fig. (4). Congenital missing of left lateral incisor and peg-shaped right lateral incisor.

Microdontia: The term microdontia (microdentism, microdontism) is defined as the condition of having abnormally small teeth. In generalized microdontia, the teeth are small with short crowns and roots, and missing contact points (Fig. **5**). It is frequently associated with short cranial base length and maxillary length, class III tendency and reduced vertical facial dimensions [5, 6, 15 - 18].

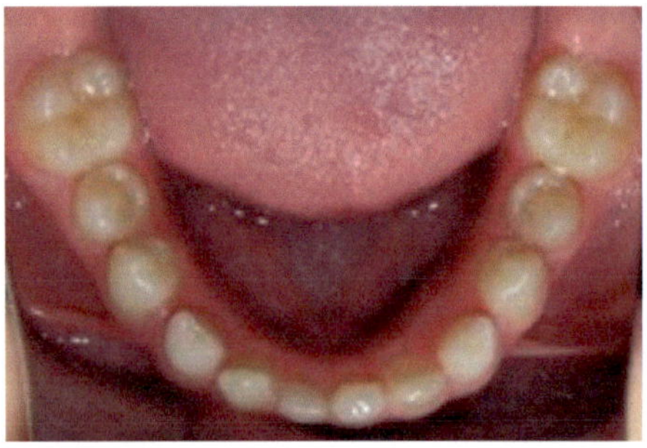

Fig. (5). Microdontia.

Hyperdontia: A supernumerary tooth in the permanent dentition called mesiodens is the most common type of hyperdontia. Evidence from twin and family studies supported the genetic basis of hyperdontia. The mode of inheritance of hyperdontia has been proposed as autosomal dominant [19 - 21].

7. Which Other Dental Anomalies Could be Associated With the Non-Syndromic Hypodontia?

Tooth agenesis is associated [3, 10, 22] with.

a. Palatal canine displacement/impaction.
b. Tooth transposition.
c. Infraocclusion of primary mandibular molars.
d. Mesial path of eruption of first molars.

8. a. What Dental Anomaly Do You See Here?
b. Which Other Dental Anomaly is Normally Confused With This?

a. **Gemination.** Gemination describes an enlarged tooth or joined teeth, when the anomalous tooth is counted as one, the tooth count is normal [2]. It is regarded as an attempt by a single tooth bud to divide, resulting in the formation of a tooth that has a bifid crown and, usually, a shared root and root canal (Fig. **6**).
b. **Fusion.** Fusion is what happens when two tooth germs combine to form a single enlarged tooth. Literature suggests that geminated teeth have single root canal and fused tooth has separate root canals [2].

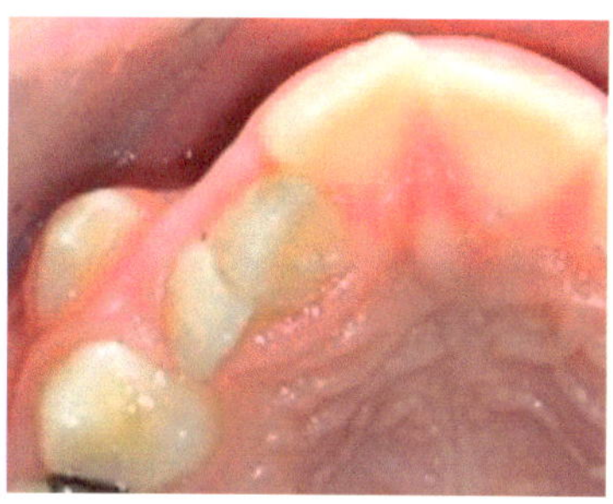

Fig. (6). Gemination.

9. a. What Dental Anomalies Do You Recognize Here?
b. Name any Prognostic Factors of these Anomalies
c. Provide Any Early Clinical Intervention

a. Maxilla right: Congenital missing lateral permanent incisor (Fig. **7**). Maxilla left: Palatal canine displacement **(PDC)**.
b. A palatal displaced canine **(PDC)** is a more common developmental disorder

with a prevalence of 0.8-2.8% [3]. Palatal canine impaction may be prevented if anomalies such as a peg shape or congenital missing of lateral incisors in early mixed dentition are recognised. A palatal displaced canine and hypodontia is likely to occur at the same time in 19% to 20% of first- and second-degree relatives, and this is 2½ times greater than the rate of occurrence in the normal population [22, 24]. Where tooth disturbances like a peg shape, the absence of lateral incisors, enamel hypoplasia, aplasia of second premolars, and infraocclusion of primary molars are recognised in early mixed dentition, they could predict canine impaction. Palatal canine displacement will frequently result in impaction [21, 25].

There can be other indicative factors in early mixed dentition including:

1. It has been reported that the dimensions of the mesiodistal crown of maxillary and mandibular incisors are markedly smaller in **PDCs** [25].
2. Half of **PDCs** patients have Class II, Division II malocclusion, maxillary width excess and a low angle vertical growth pattern [26, 27].
3. Maxillary deficiency patients have a higher prevalence of unilateral PDCs [27].

c. A success rate of between 50% and 62.5% has been reported for extraction of the primary canine to prevent palatal canine displacement **(PDC)** [29]. The canine erupts successfully in 87.5% of cases of subjects treated by headgear in addition to primary canine extraction [26]. Another option for treatment in early mixed dentition would be Rapid Maxillary Expansion therapy. The prevalence rate of canine eruption after rapid maxillary expansion is 65.7% in maxillary deficient patients [27].

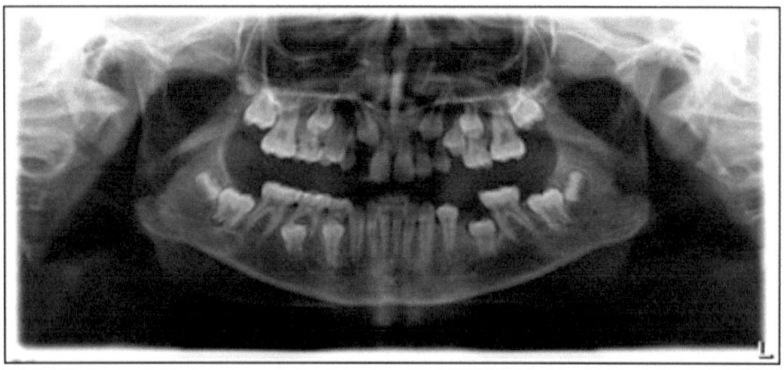

Fig. (7). Panoramic X-Ray.

10. a. What Dental Anomalies Do You Recognize Here?
b. What is the Etiology of Mesial Molar Eruption Disturbance?
c. How Do You Diagnose this Dental Anomaly?
d. Provide Any Early Orthodontic Intervention

a. Mesial path of eruption of maxillary permanent molars, peg-shaped lateral incisors and third molar agenesis (Fig. **8**).
b. Mesial eruption of the maxillary first permanent molar is caused by factors that are not well documented and probably has a multifactorial aetiology. Before the tooth erupts, the germ points downward, backward, and outward, but the tooth takes on a more vertical position during eruption. The prevalence in the members of the same family is approximately 20%, whereas prevalence in the general population is only 4% [30]. Among the factors that could cause the mesial molar eruption were related to space deficiency in the posterior region of the maxilla because of discrepancies in bone growth at the tuberosity region and tooth size. However, the higher frequency in siblings or in cleft lip palate children than in normal children as well as the association with other dental anomalies of genetic etiology such as tooth agenesis and palatal displaced canines **(PDC)** add the mesial eruption of first maxillary molars to the list of the genetically determined dental anomalies [22].
c. The diagnosis should be diagnosed both clinical and radiographical. A mesial path of eruption of first permanent maxillary molars should be suspected if the distal cusps of the permanent molar are emerging before the mesial cusps or a unilateral-bilateral delay of tooth eruption was observed. Radiographic examination may appear to show a superimposed image and impaction in the primary second molar's distal-buccal root.
d. Early treatment of this anomaly is recommended to avoid premature loss of the second primary molars and reduction in the arch perimeter. Clinical intervention needs only the application of a distal force on the first molar, but pathological resorption of the distal root could result in early exfoliation of the primary second molars, mesial migration of the first molar and arch length loss (Fig. **9**). Space regaining procedures seems mandatory (Fig. **10**). Maxillary molar distalization was completed in 5 months. Space gained in each side was 5 mm. The rate of distalization was almost 1 mm per month.

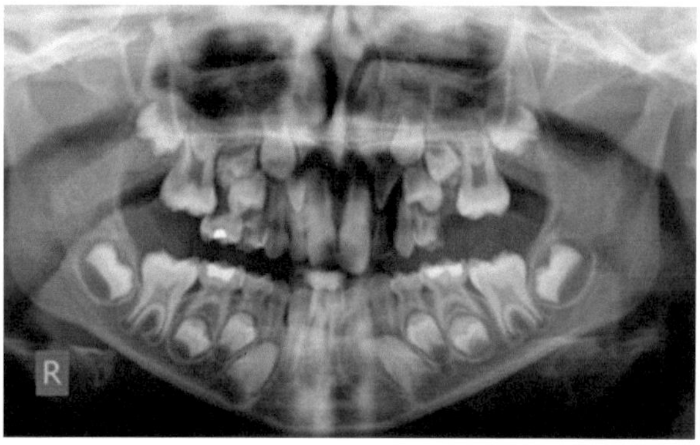

Fig. (8). Panoramic X-Ray.

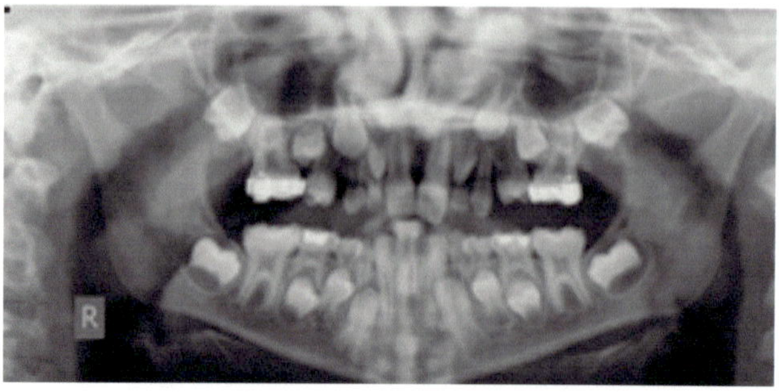

Fig. (9). Panoramic X-Ray.

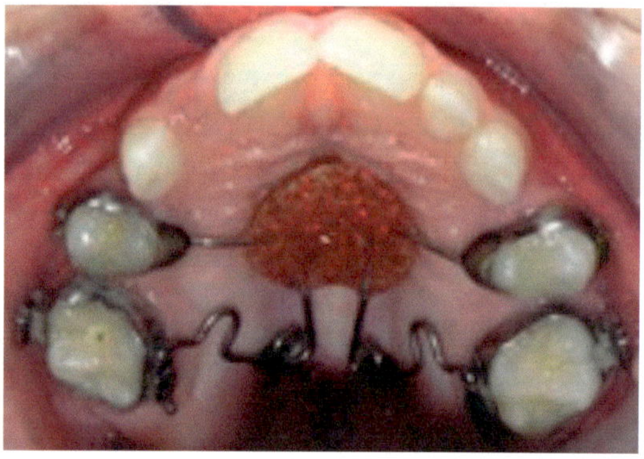

Fig. (10). Space regaining.

11. What Dental Anomalies Do You Recognize Here?

a. Maxillary right: Mesial path of eruption of the right permanent molar, agenesis of the third molar and peg-shaped lateral incisor (Figs. **11** & **12**).
b. Maxillary left: Palatal canine displacement (PDC) and agenesis of the third molar.
c. Mandibular left: Third molar agenesis.

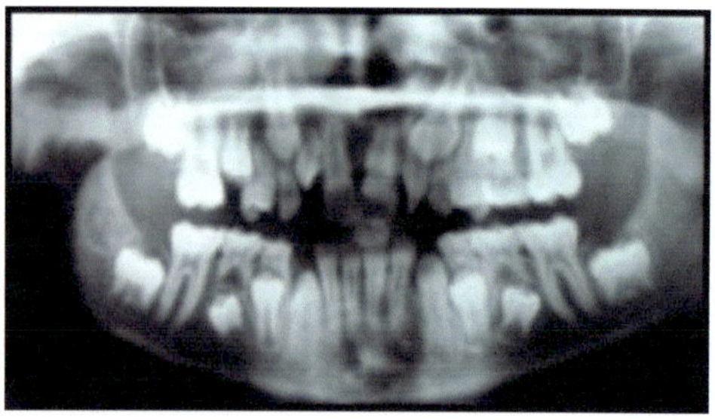

Fig. (11). Panoramic X-Ray.

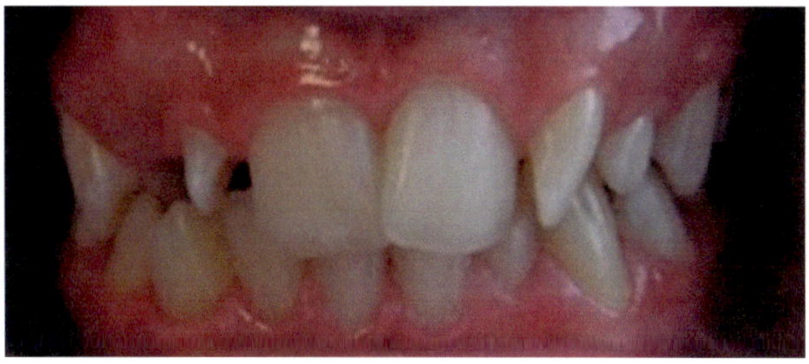

Fig. (12). Anterior occlusal view.

12. a. What Dental Anomaly do you Recognize Here?
b. Name the Etiology and the Most Common Types of This?
c. How Do You Manage this Dental Anomaly?

a. Tooth transposition between the maxillary left canine (Fig. **13**) and the first premolar. Transposition is a unique and an extreme form of ectopic eruption in which a permanent tooth develops and erupts in the position which is normally occupied by other permanent teeth. It may present as complete or incomplete transposition. Complete transposition occurs when the position of the whole dental structure including root and crown is ectopic [31]. Incomplete transposition is where the crowns are ectopic but the roots are in the correct position. The commonest transposition is that of maxillary canine/first premolar transposition [32].

b. A number of aetiological factors are associated with tooth transposition; they include genetics, trauma, mechanical interference, and positional interchange by developing tooth buds [31, 32]. The maxillary canine, 1st premolar transposition is associated with:

   i. High prevalence of third molar agenesis,
   ii. Palatal canine displacement **(PDC)**,
   iii. Congenital missing or peg-shaped lateral incisors (Fig. **14**).

   The most common types [32] of maxillary tooth transposition are:

   - Maxillary canine-first premolar (Fig. **14**)
   - Maxillary canine-lateral incisor (Fig. **15**)
   - Maxillary canine to first molar site
   - Maxillary lateral incisor-central incisor
   - Maxillary canine to central incisor

   iv. When treating maxillary canine premolar transposition, many factors that affect the treatment results must be considered, such as age of the patient, dental crowding, occlusal characteristics, esthetic demands and patient comfort. Extraction of the first premolar could be an alternative treatment when a severe arch length deficiency exists.

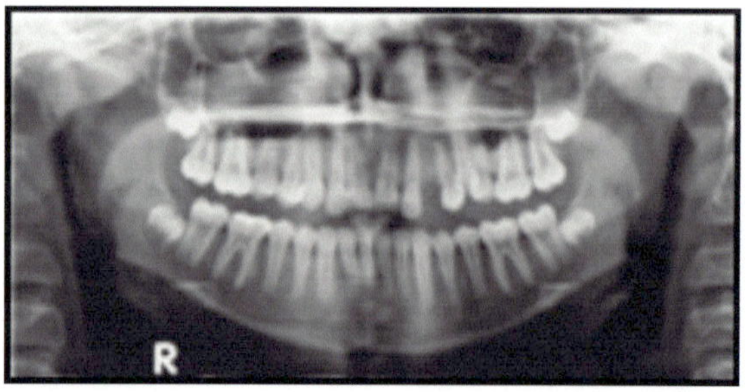

Fig. (13). Panoramic X-Ray.

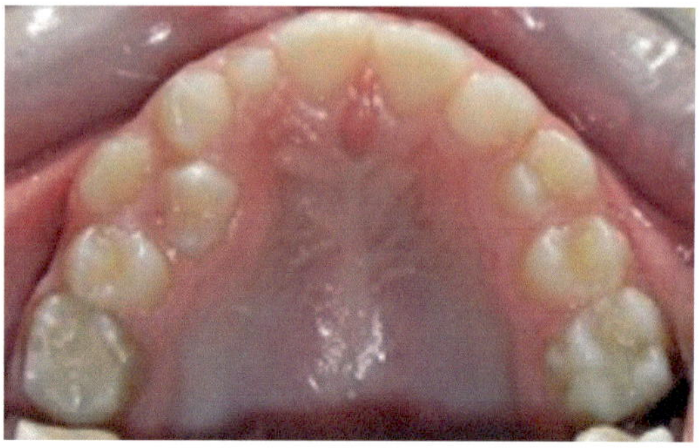

Fig. (14). Peg-shaped lateral incisor and maxillary canine-first premolar transposition.

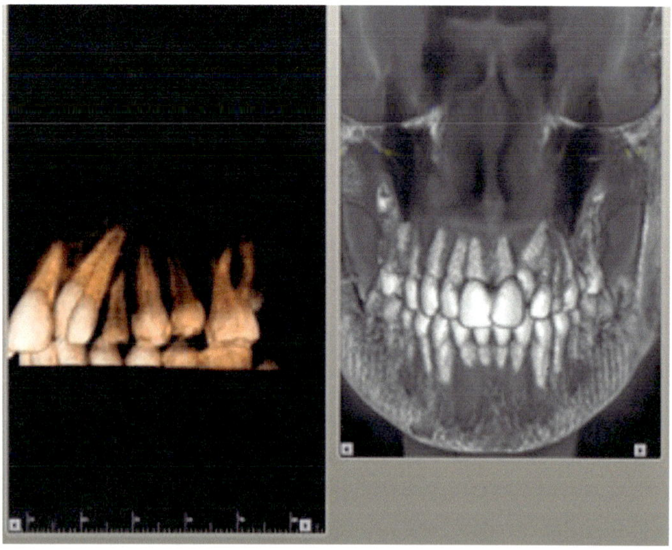

Fig. (15). Maxillary canine-lateral incisor transposition.

13. a. What Dental Anomalies Do You Recognize Here?
b. What is the Etiology?
c. How Do You Manage this Dental Anomaly?

a. Complete tooth transposition between the mandibular right canine (Fig. **16**) and the lateral incisor.

b. The etiology of a transposition is still obscure. It seems to share similar genetics mechanisms such as tooth agenesis and peg-shaped maxillary lateral incisors. Third molar agenesis and palatal canine displacement **(PDC)** was found to be strongly associated with mandibular incisor-canine [26]. A number of other factors have also been suggested; they include: genetic interchange in the position of the developing tooth buds; lack of primary canine root resorption; mechanical interferences; early loss; or prolonged retention of primary teeth [21].

c. Treatment of this dental transposition depends on their eruption stages. In the early mixed dentition period, the mandibular lateral incisor crown deviates distally and rotated mesiolingually while the apex is located at the normal position (Fig. **17**).

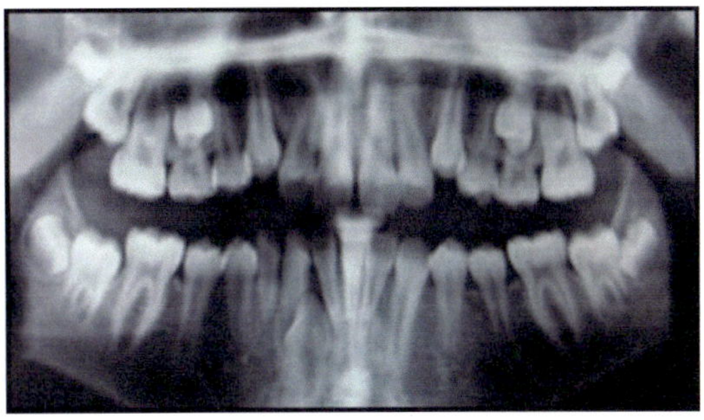

Fig. (16). Panoramic X-Ray.

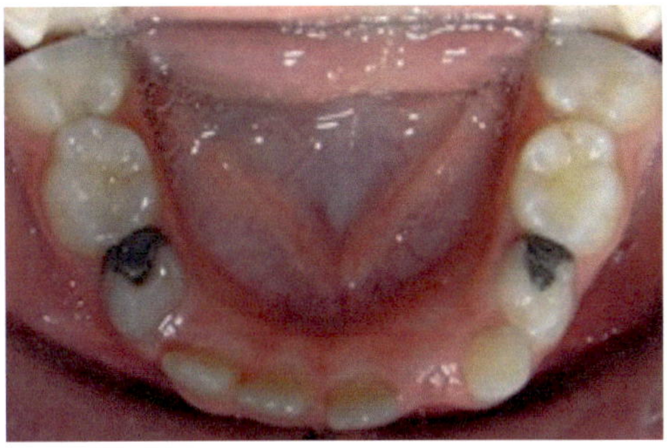

Fig. (17). Lower occlusal view.

If the transposition is in an early stage (before the eruption of the permanent canine), the orthodontic upright of mandibular lateral incisor mechanics can prevent the lateral incisor-canine transposition (Fig. **18**). If the transposition is recognized after the transposed teeth have erupted, the roots of the involved teeth are parallel in a dense thin facio-lingual alveolar bone and it is preferred to maintain their interchanged position.

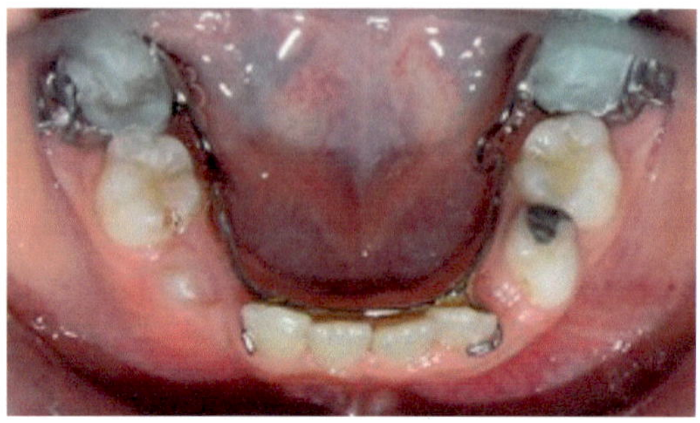

Fig. (18). Lower occlusal view.

14. Name the Dental Anomalies in the Following Figures

Figure 19

a. Maxilla right: Congenital missing of the second premolar, palatal displaced canine (PDC) and peg-shaped maxillary right lateral incisor.
b. Maxilla left: Palatal displaced canine (PDC).
c. Mandible: Congenital missing of the second premolars. All third molars are missing.

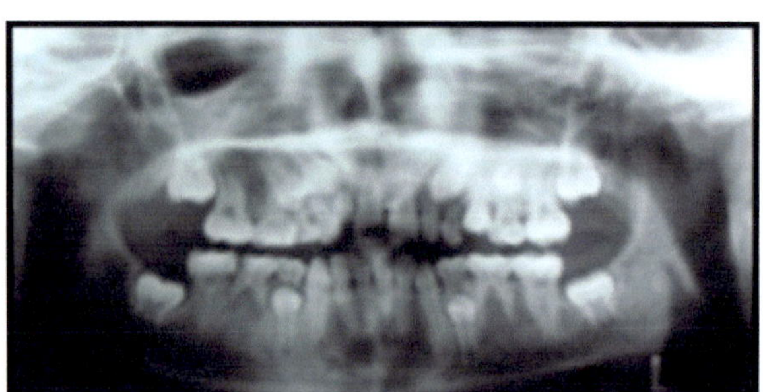

Fig. (19). Panoramic X-Ray.

Figure 20

a. Maxilla right: Peg-shaped lateral incisor and missing third molar.
b. Maxilla left: Impacted canine.
c. Mandibular Right: agenesis of the second premolar.
d. Mandibular Left: agenesis of the third molar.

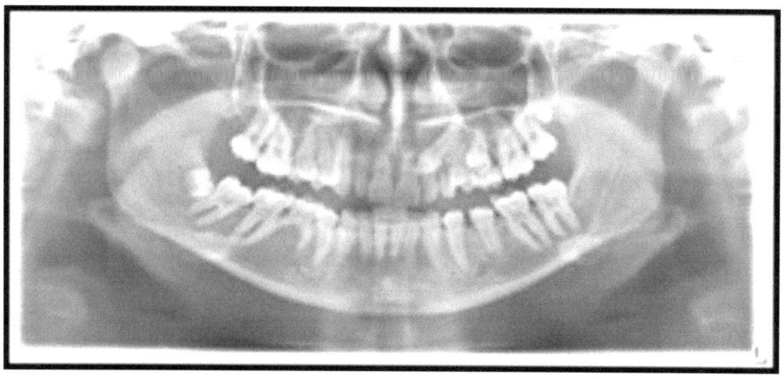

Fig. (20). Panoramic X-Ray.

Figure 21

a. Maxilla right: Missing lateral incisors
b. Maxilla left: Palatal canine displacement (PDC)
c. Mandible left: Delayed development of second premolar
d. All third molars are missing

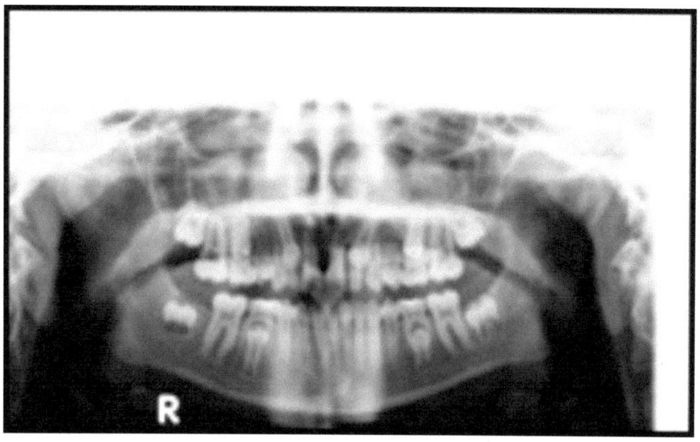

Fig. (21). Panoramic X-Ray.

Figure 22

Maxilla right: Congenital missing lateral incisor BUT Palatal canine impaction on the left side.

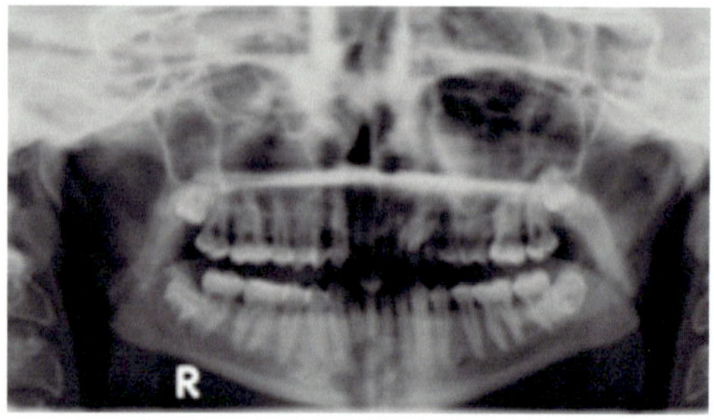

Fig. (22). Panoramic X-Ray.

Figure 23

Congenital missing maxillary right lateral incisor BUT palatal canine impaction on the left side.

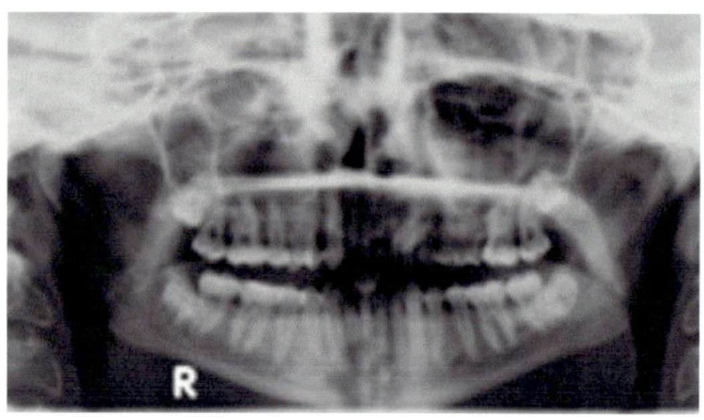

Fig. (23). Panoramic X-Ray.

Figure 24

Very rare condition of congenital missing of the maxillary permanent right canine

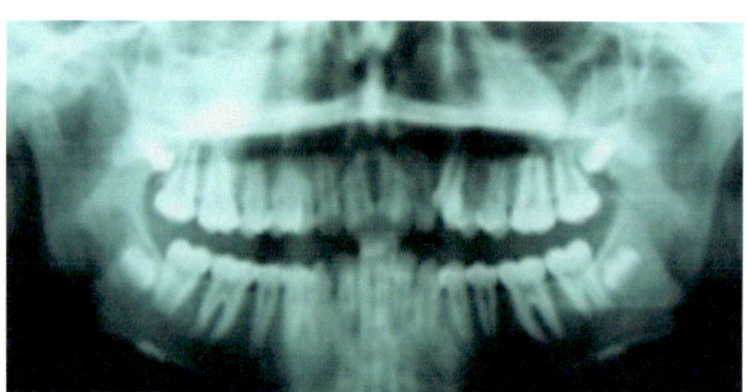

Fig. (24). Panoramic X-Ray.

PART B. TOOTH IMPACTION

1. In the Absence of Trauma or Extraction Which Are the Most Common Causes of the Unerupted Permanent Incisor?

A supernumerary tooth called mesiodens is the most likely cause of the unerupted permanent incisor. 80% to 90% of all supernumerary teeth occur in the maxilla and half of them located in the maxillary central incisor region [20, 21].

2. a. In Which Cases Should be Suspected Mesiodens?
b. Could You Classify the Mesiodens According to their Morphology?
c. Do You Know the Prevalence of Mesiodens?

a. A mesiodens should be suspected [19, 33] in cases of:
   - Asymmetric eruption pattern of one or both permanent maxillary incisors
   - Significant ectopic eruption of one or both permanent maxillary incisors
   - Over retained one or both primary incisors

b. *Conical:* Peg-shaped-complete root formation-located palatally between the centrals-displaced centrals labially.
   Tuberculate: Barrel shaped-incomplete or abnormal root formation-located palatal-delay eruption of centrals.
   Molariform: Premolar shaped-rare type [24].

c. 0.45% in Caucasian population, 0.40 in Finnish, 1,43% in Norwegians and 2.2% in Hispanic population [21].

3. List Some Complications of *Mesiodens* to the Rest of the Dentition

a. They are frequently interfering with the eruption and alignment (crowding or diastema) of the maxillary incisors.
b. They may cause ectopic eruption, rotation or labial displacement of one or both permanent incisors.
c. Radicular resorption of adjacent teeth.
d. Dentigerous cyst.
e. Intra-oral infection [19].

4. Provide the Etiology of Mesiodens

It is a common finding in syndromes which linked to hyperactivity of dental lamina like *Apert, Crouzon, Gardner and Down syndrome* as well as to *cleidocranial dysplasia.* A genetic basis for supernumerary teeth could also be suggested considering higher rate observation of hyperdontia among related families. Furthermore, an X-linked inheritance has been documented which can explain sex dominance in this anomaly [21].

5. Describe the Most Diagnostic Radiographic Method to Identify and Locate Them

Occlusal or Periapical X-Rays. Provide details of the crown and the root morphology of the unerupted teeth the presence of the mesiodens and their relationship to the incisor roots. *The parallax (horizontal or vertical) technique is the most commonly used method in localized maxillary mesiodens.* This technique requires two intra-oral films for horizontal parallax or one intra-oral (anterior occlusal) and the panoramic radiograph for vertical parallax method.

Dental Panoramic Radiograph. Serves as a screening aid and provides additional information about the presence of the supernumerary teeth as well as the presence and the position of the unerupted teeth. Panoramic radiography may yield limited evidence for the mesiodens because there is insufficient clarity in the midline region [33].

6. Why and How You Manage this Dental Condition in the Early Mixed Dentition Period?

Mesiodens can cause significant alteration in occlusion and in appearance by altering the eruption path and the permanent incisor's position. Significant mesiodens complications involving the permanent incisors include: dilaceration of the developing roots; root resorption; and loss of tooth vitality [19].

If the arch space is available (Fig. **25**) extraction of a supernumerary mesiodens is recommended for promoting self-eruption of permanent central incisors. *The earlier the extraction of the mesiodens in early mixed dentition (Fig. **28**) the more immature the root of the permanent incisor (Figs. **26** & **27**) and the greater the chance for spontaneous eruption (Fig. **29**). Six months' recall is recommended to determine clinical and radiographical the position of the unerupted tooth* [19, 20].

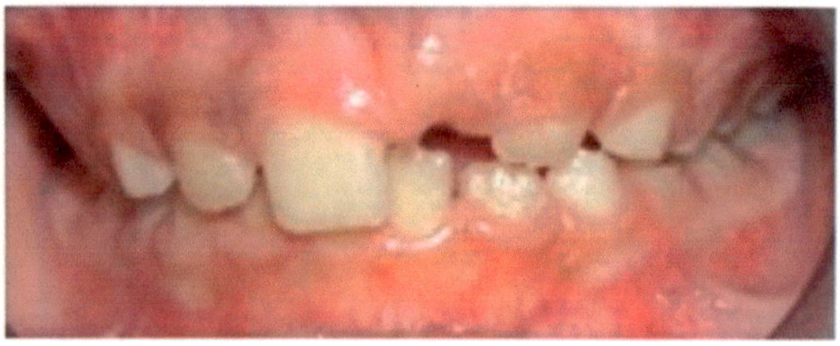

Fig. (25). Anterior occlusal view.

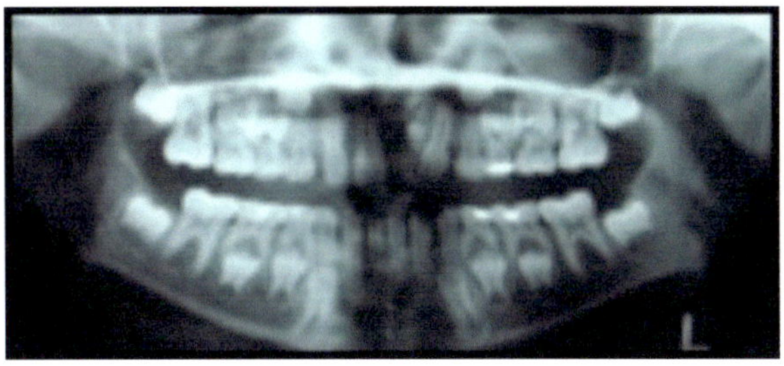

Fig. (26). Panoramic X-Ray.

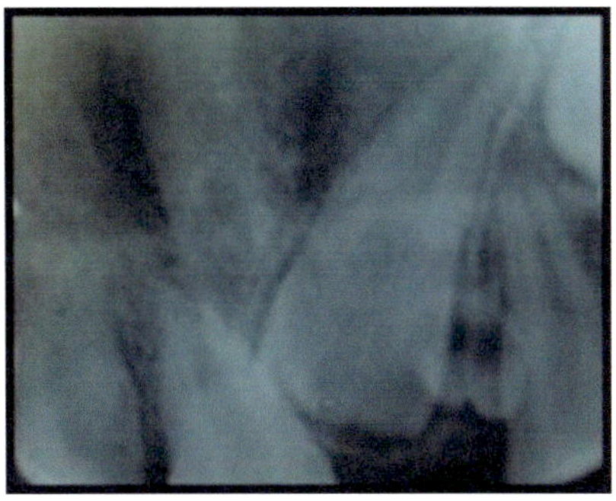

Fig. (27). Periapical X-Ray.

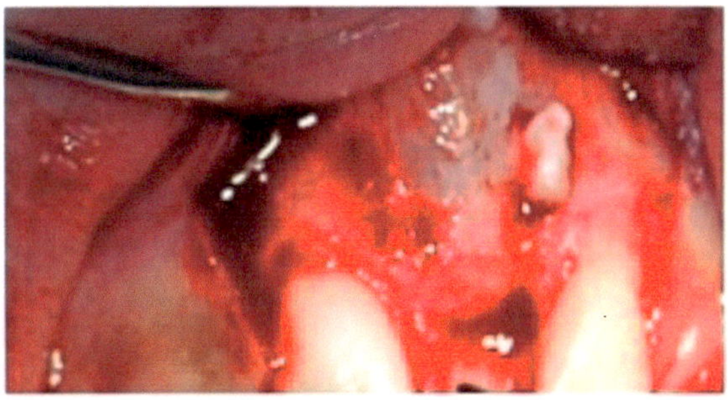

Fig. (28). Extraction of the mesiodens.

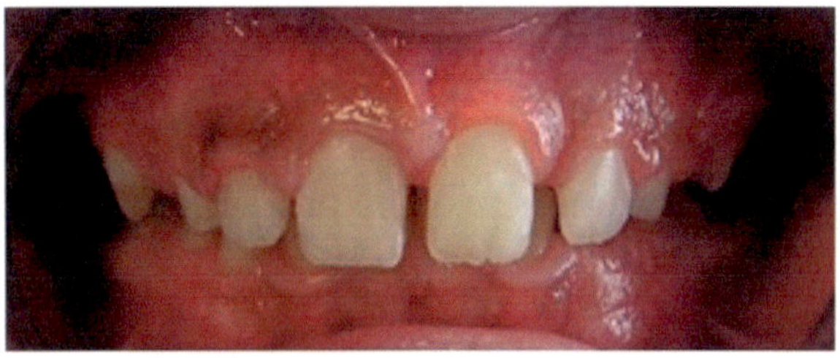

Fig. (29). Spontaneous eruption of central incisor.

If a tooth does not start erupting within a year after extraction of the mesiodens and sufficient arch space is provided, surgical exposure and **orthodontic traction** of the unerupted incisor are suggested (Figs. **30-34**).

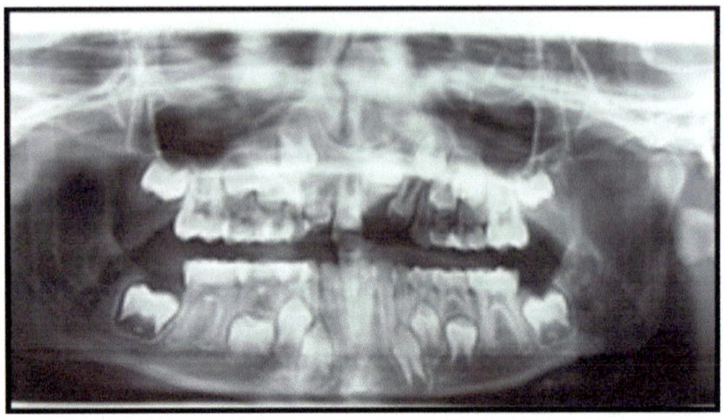

Fig. (30). Panoramic X-Ray.

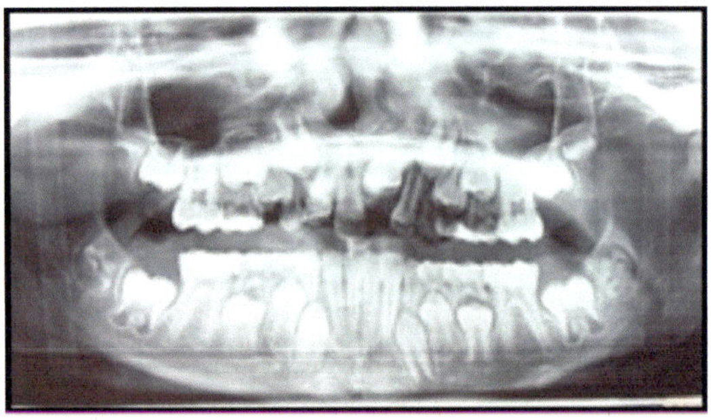

Fig. (31). Panoramic X-Ray.

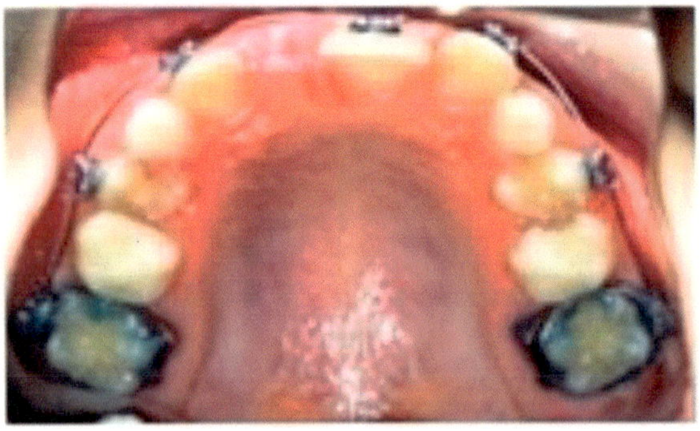

Fig. (32). Upper occlusal view.

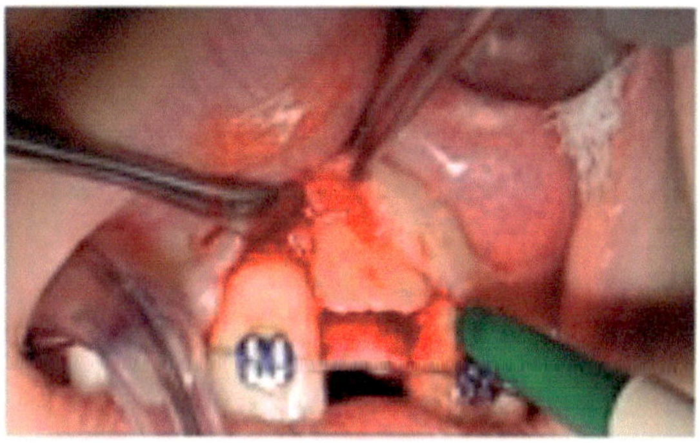

Fig. (33). Surgical exposure.

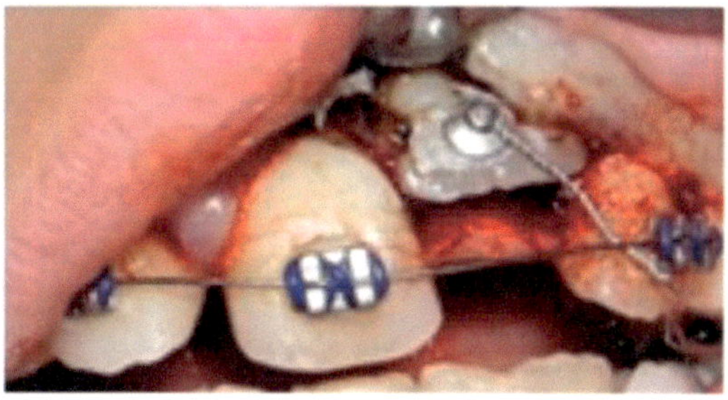

Fig. (34). Orthodontic traction.

7. How Do You Treated in the Late Mixed Dentition Period?

If the mesiodens diagnosed in the late mixed or early permanent dentition clinical and radiographic evaluation is an important requisite for the patient prior to combined surgical/orthodontic treatment of the unerupted teeth [18, 28]. While the radiographical considerations are the same as described above, **some clinical key points** should be mentioned:

i. Arch Space

If the arch space is available (Fig. **35**) alignment and leveling should have progressed to a S.S. arch wire before the surgical exposure and the orthodontic treatment of the unerupted teeth. If the arch space is not available, should be created by orthodontic means.

ii. Anchorage

Orthodontic appliances should be placed on as many maxillary teeth as possible to support the anchorage during orthodontic traction of the unerupted teeth. Removable Cetlin type TPA sometimes is strongly recommended.

iii. The Closed Surgical Technique

In this technique a mucoperiosteal flap is reflected, the mesiodens and the bone covering the crown of the unerupted teeth is removed, an attachment is bonded and the flap is repositioned and sutured (Fig. **36**). The closed surgical technique is superior to the other techniques **because the tooth is exposed with minimum tissue removal,** rapid healing and immediate orthodontic traction of the unerupted incisor (Figs. **37** & **38**).

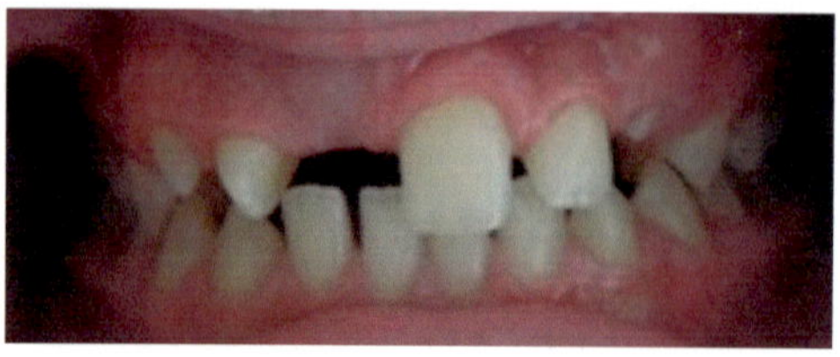

Fig. (35). Anterior occlusal view.

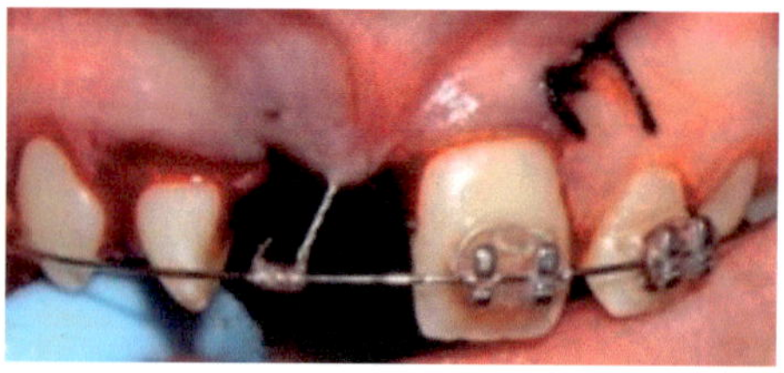

Fig. (36). Closed surgical technique.

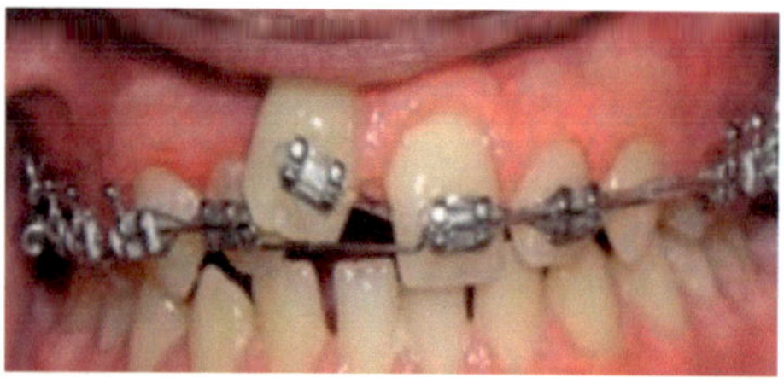

Fig. (37). Eight months after surgery.

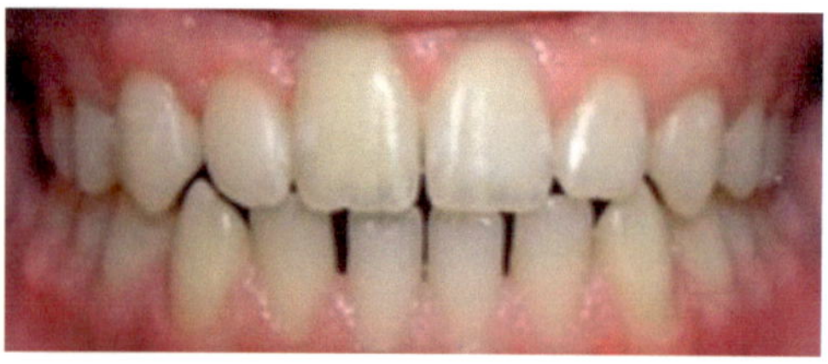

Fig. (38). Eighteen months treatment.

8. Maxillary Canine Impaction. Give the Definition, Prevalence, Incidence and the Possible Causes

It could be defined as the infra-osseous position of the tooth after the expected time of eruption. The maxillary canine is second only to 3rd molars as most frequently impacted tooth; it occurs in 0.8% to 5.2% of subjects, depending on what population is under discussion. Canine impaction occurs twice as often in the maxilla as in the mandible, and there is an 8:1 ratio of palatal to buccal impaction. 8% of canine impactions are bilateral and it is seen twice as often in girls as in boys. The most common theories explaining palatal impacted maxillary canines are the guidance theory and the genetic theory [23].

9. Describe the "Guidance Theory" and the "Genetic Theory"

According to the guidance theory, in its simplest form, the canine lacks the guide during the eruption pathway because of extra space in the apical part of the maxilla, owing to hypoplastic or missing lateral incisor. This theory supports that palatal displaced canines are frequently found in dentitions with **peg- shaped or missing laterals, spaced or late developed dentitions.** Even if these anomalies are genetically determined, the guidance theory states that the palatal canine impaction has not a similar genetic association but occurs as a result of these local environmental disturbances [28, 29, 34].

The genetic theory assigns the eruption anomaly of the upper permanent canine as a result of a developmental disturbance of the dental lamina. This theory indicates **multiple evidential categories for the genetic origin of palatal impacted canines,** such as familial and bilateral occurrence, sex differences, as well as an increased occurrence of other significant reciprocal dental associations such as ectopic eruption of first molars, infraocclusion of primary molars, aplasia of premolars and one third molar [22, 24, 26, 27].

10. What is the Difference Between "Canine Impaction" and "Canine Displacement?"

Canine impaction can be defined as the infra-osseous position of the tooth after the expected time of eruption.

The anomalous infra-osseous position of the canine before the expected time of eruption can be defined as a **displacement**. Frequently, palatal displacement results in impaction.

11. How do you Evaluate the Position of the Impacted Maxillary Canine?

Several radiographic methods have been suggested to evaluate the position of the impacted maxillary canines. The parallax (horizontal or vertical) technique is the most commonly used method in localized impacted maxillary canines [35]. This technique requires:

- Vertical parallax method: panoramic radiograph (Fig. **39**) and anterior occlusal radiograph (Fig. **40**).
- Horizontal parallax: two intra-oral films.

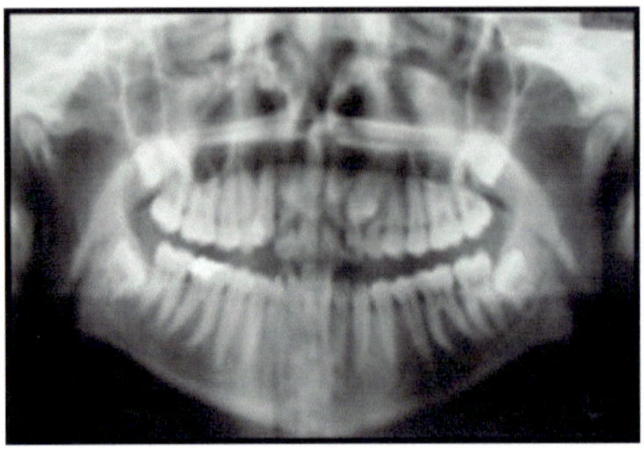

Fig. (39). Panoramic X-ray.

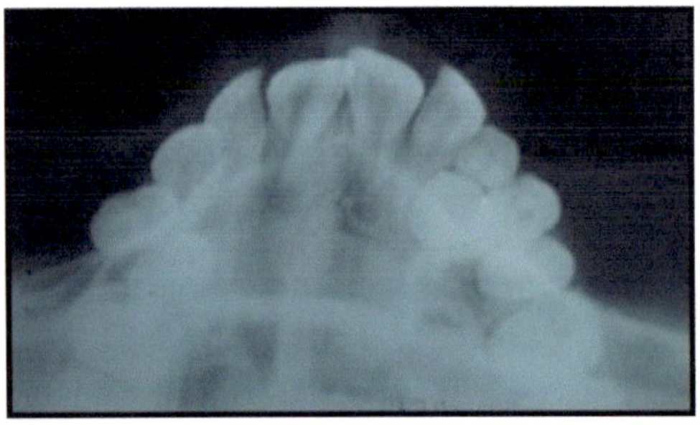

Fig. (40). Occlusal X-Ray.

12. Describe the Advantages of CBCT Image Compared to Panoramic Radiographs

a. 3D images increase the precision in the localization of the canines improving the diagnosis and the treatment planning
b. CBCT provides elements for the impacted teeth such as the size of follicle, the amount of the bone covering the tooth and 3D proximity of adjacent teeth [36].
c. Efficient and less time consuming orthodontic treatment.

13. Describe the most Important Variables During the Early Mixed Dentition that Could Predict Possible Maxillary Canine Impaction?

I. Clinical Evaluation

- Recognition in early mixed dentition of such anomalies as peg shape or missing lateral incisors, enamel hypoplasia, aplasia of second premolars, and infra-occlusion of primary molars could predict possible canine impaction [10, 22].
- The maxillary transverse arch dimension is significantly wider in the palatal displacement canine patients [23].
- Horizontal facial growth pattern and Angle II/II malocclusion. When associated with an increased transverse dimension of the upper arch, deep bite, upright and small incisors, this heritable malocclusion could be regarded as a risk factor for canine impaction [23, 37].

II. Radiographic Evaluation

- Overlapping canine and lateral incisors in a panoramic X-Ray may be a sign of early canine displacement after the incisor's root development [35].
- If the permanent canine's crown is distal to the midline of the later incisor root, then in 91% of cases extraction of the primary canine will normalise the erupting position of the permanent canine. This success rate falls to 64% where the permanent canine crown is mesial to the midline of the lateral incisor root [38].
- The rate of eruption increased if the patient treated by headgear or rapid maxillary expansion in addition to primary canine extraction [26, 27].

14. a. Describe the Radiographic Variables in the Following Picture b. Provide the Relationship Between Treatment Timing and These Radiographic Variables

a. Three variables are visible on this panoramic radiograph (Fig. **41**):
   - Angle (a) measured between the long axis of the impacted canine and the midline,
   - Distance (d) between the canine cusp tip and the occlusal plane (from the first molar to the incisal edge of the central incisor)
   - Sector (s) where the cusp of the impacted canine is located [38].

b. The treatment time is proportional to the *d-distance* and the *sector (s).* When the canines cusp located medially to the long axis of the lateral incisor 10 more visits required than the distally located canines. Regarding the *sector of impaction*, when the impacted canine belongs in *sector 1*, six more weeks of active orthodontic traction was required comparing to impaction in *sector 3* [38 - 40].

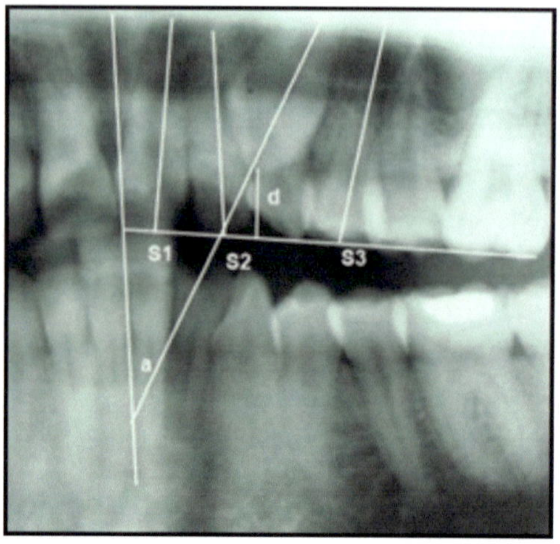

Fig. (41). Panoramic X-ray.

15. a. Which is the Most Important Sequel of Maxillary Canine Impaction? b. Name Some Predisposing Factors of this Sequel

a. Palatal impacted teeth can cause migration of the neighbouring teeth, loss of arch length, cystic lesions and infection, but the most important consequence is root resorption of the nearby lateral incisors jeopardizing their longevity. The mid root level of lateral incisors is more affected than the apical or the cervical regions. It is, unfortunately, almost impossible to clinically diagnose resorption of the incisor roots because there will usually be no symptoms. Cone beam computer tomography (CBCT) has allowed new and much more documented light to be focused on root resorption following canine displacement. Resorption on the roots of maxillary incisors due to impaction of the maxillary canines is a more common phenomenon than previously believed [36, 41].

b. Where the developed canine's cusp is mesially positioned to the lateral incisor, there is a threefold increase in the risk of complications. The risk of resorption increases 50% when the canine's angulation is greater than 25 degrees [39]. Resorption of the lateral incisor root is three times more usual in girls than in boys.

16. Which Are the Most Commonly Used Surgical Methods for Exposing the Palatal Impacted Maxillary Canines?

The three most commonly used surgical methods [42, 43] for exposing palatal impacted maxillary canines are:

i. *The open surgical exposure and spontaneous eruption.* This method is most useful only when the impacted canine has a correct axial inclination.

ii. *The open surgical technique with subsequent bonding of an auxiliary orthodontic attachment.* The advantages of this method are the faster eruption and the continuing access to the impacted teeth during the eruption process whereas bone loss, gingival recession and decreased width of keratinized tissue have been reported as the main disadvantages.

iii. *The closed surgical technique.* In this technique a mucoperiosteal flap is reflected, the bone covering the crown of the impacted teeth is removed, an attachment is bonded and the flap is repositioned and sutured.

Many authors supported that the closed surgical technique is superior to the other techniques because the tooth is exposed with minimum tissue removal, *rapid healing and immediate orthodontic traction.* However, an increase in pocket depth at the distal-buccal surface of the impacted canines and at the mesial-lingual, distal-lingual, and mesio-labial surfaces of the adjacent lateral incisors and first premolars has been reported.

17. a. How Do You Describe the Position of the Right Maxillary Cuspid in this Patient?
b. What is the Possible Cause of this Clinical Situation and How Do You Treat this?
c. What Surgical Method Would you Consider in this Case?

a. Unerupted, rotated upper right permanent canine at the middle of the bone (Figs. **42** & **43**).

b. From the mesial inclination of the first premolar and the class II molar relationship (Fig. **44**), we can assume that the major etiological cause of the unerupted maxillary canine should be the space deficiency.

c. Orthodontic treatment with fixed mechanisms, the open surgical exposure and spontaneous eruption. This method is most useful when the impacted canine has a correct axial inclination.

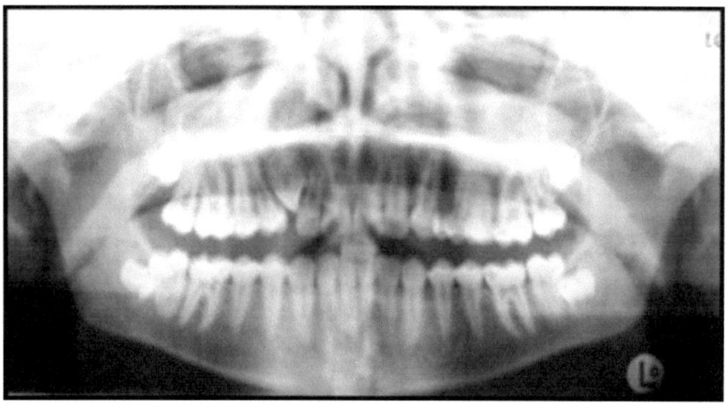

Fig. (42). Panoramic X-Ray.

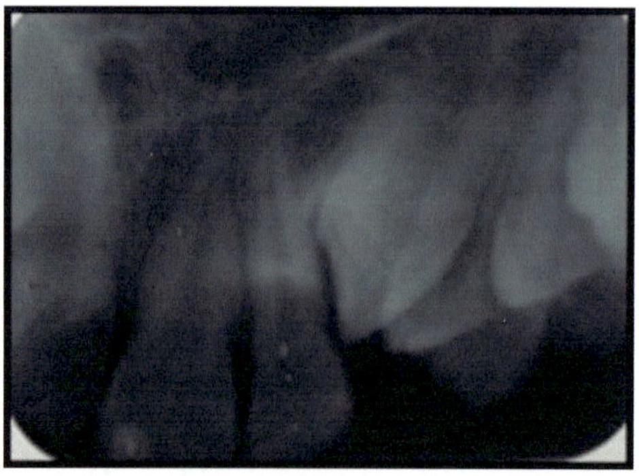

Fig. (43). Periapical X-Ray.

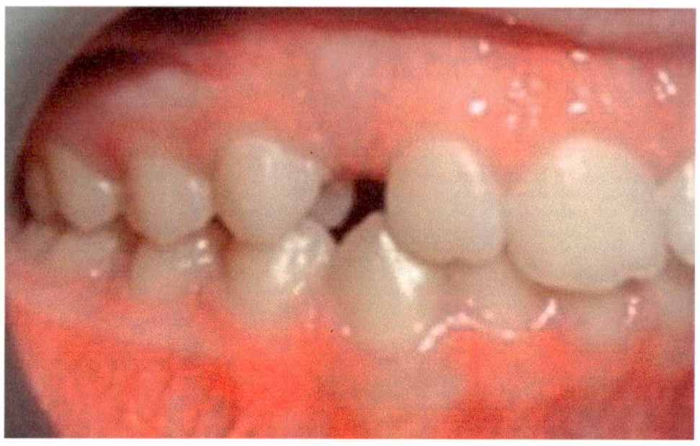

Fig. (44). Lateral occlusal view.

18. a. At What Stage of Dental Development is this Child?
b. How Do You Diagnose the Position of the Canine Clinical?
c. Provide Your Interceptive Orthodontic Treatment

a. The child is in the late mixed-early permanent dentition period (Fig. **45**).

b. The clinical key point at this age is that the upper permanent cuspids should be palpable on the buccal sulcus.

c. Extraction of the primary canine, in the mixed dentition period, as an interceptive treatment to prevent permanent canine impaction, has been supported on the assumption that persistence of the primary tooth would represent a mechanical obstacle for the emergence of the permanent tooth. Where the crown of the permanent canine is distal to the midline of the lateral incisor root, extraction of the primary canine normalises the eruption position of the permanent canine in 91% of cases [35, 38, 42]. This success rate falls to 64% when the permanent canine crown is mesial to the midline of the lateral incisor root. In this patient, in order to prevent the impaction of the left permanent canine the primary canine was extracted and fixed orthodontic treatment begins to improve the intra-osseous position of the permanent canines. The position of the upper left canine improved dramatically (Fig. **46**), whereas one year later (Fig. **47**) erupting in their normal position in the maxilla.

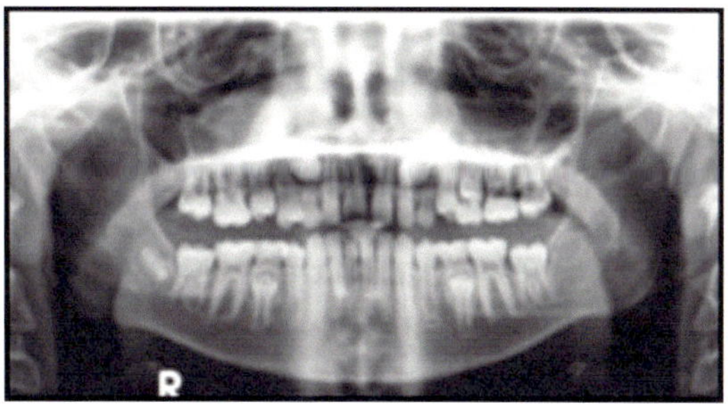

Fig. (45). Panoramic X-Ray.

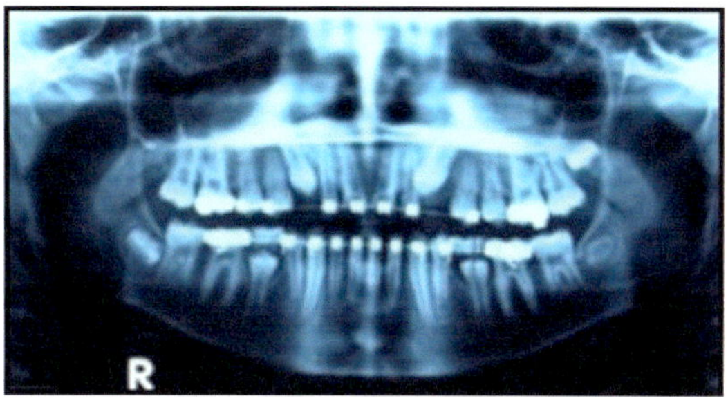

Fig. (46). Panoramic X-Ray.

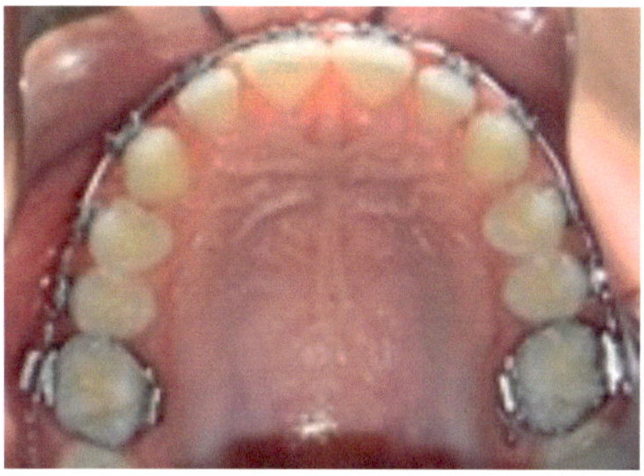

Fig. (47). Upper occlusal view.

19. What Other Orthodontic Procedures Would You Consider to Manage the Cuspids Position at this Stage?

a. Canines erupt successfully in 80% of subjects treated by headgear in addition to the extraction of the primary canine.

b. Rapid Maxillary Expansion has been reported to be effective in interceptive treatment of maxillary canine impaction. Intra-osseous improvement of the position of the canine after rapid maxillary expansion may be the mechanism by which eruption proceeds favourably.

Canines erupt successfully in 65.7% of subjects treated by RPE in addition to extraction of the primary canine.

20. a. At What Stage of Dental Development Are these Children?
b. Which Surgical Method Do You Consider in this Case?

a. Permanent dentition (Figs. **48** & **49**)
b. Orthodontic treatment with fixed mechanisms and the closed surgical technique. However, in the second patient (Fig. **50**) space regaining orthodontic procedures are required because of the space deficiency.

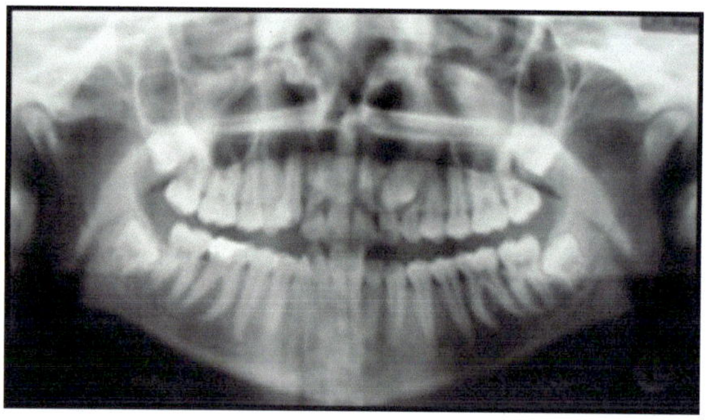

Fig. (48). Panoramic X-ray.

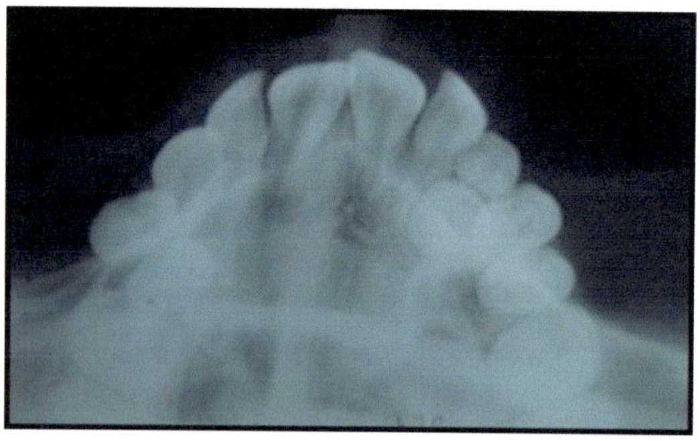

Fig. (49). Upper occlusal view.

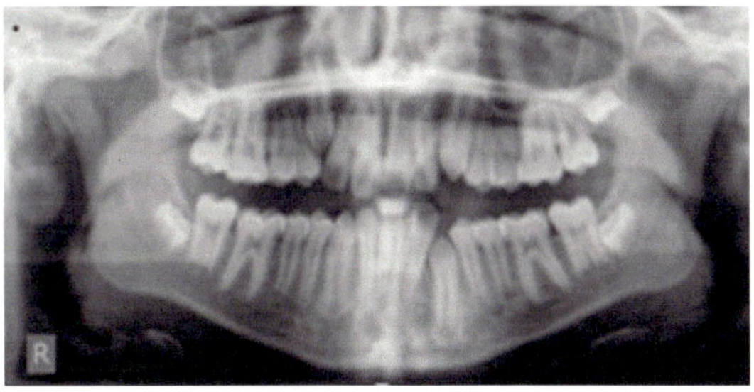

Fig. (50). Panoramic X-ray.

21. a. What Do You See Here?
b. How Do You Manage the Problem?

a. Figs. (**52 & 53**). Both the maxillary canines are palatal impacted. Class II/II malocclusion associated with an increased transverse dimension of the upper arch, deep bite, and upright incisors could be regarded as a risk factor for canine impaction [4, 8, 17]. Closed surgical technique and orthodontic traction are required.

b. Figs. (**53 & 54**). Left maxillary canine impaction. The extra space in the apical part of the anterior maxilla during clinical examination should make us suspicious for the position of the permanent canines because the canine could lack the guide during the eruption pathway [7, 8]. Extensive orthodontic treatment, surgical exposure and orthodontic traction are required.

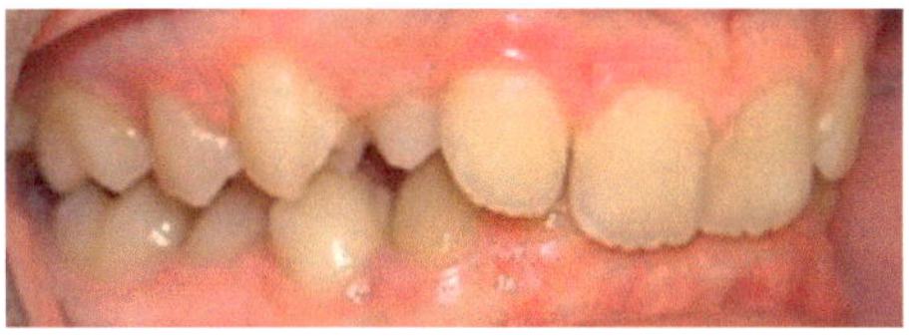

Fig. (51). Lateral occlusal view.

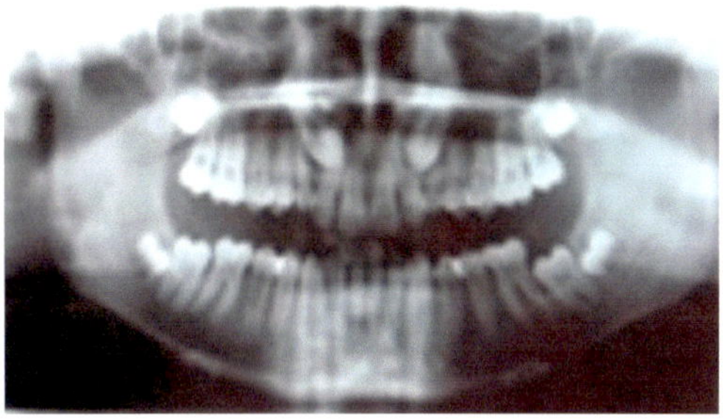

Fig. (52). Panoramic X-Ray.

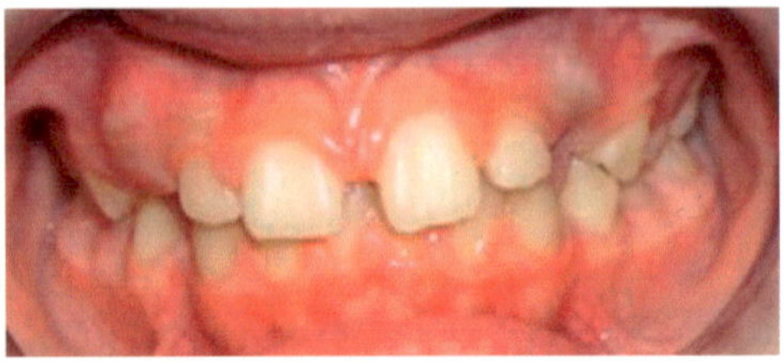

Fig. (53). Anterior occlusal view.

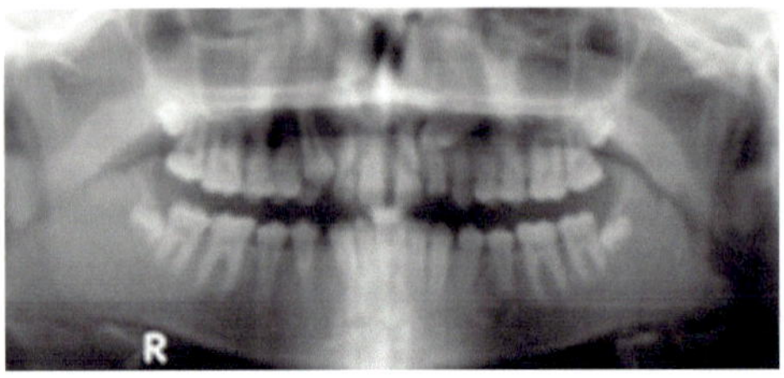

Fig. (54). Panoramic X-ray.

CONCLUDING REMARKS

Human permanent dentition can be affected by variations in the number, size, position and form of the teeth. These variations may be caused by local or systemically acting environmental factors, may be genetic, or may spring from a combination of those two factors. Displaced and impacted maxillary canines are often associated with other dental anomalies and this frequent association has led some researchers to suggest they be used as markers indicating that further clinical analysis is necessary to facilitate an early diagnosis.

REFERENCES

[1] Arte S, Nieminen P, Apajalahti S, Haavikko K, Thesleff I, Pirinen S. Characteristics of incisor-premolar hypodontia in families. J Dent Res 2001; 80(5): 1445-50. [http://dx.doi.org/10.1177/00220345010800051201] [PMID: 11437217]

[2] Brook AH, Jernvall J, Smith RN, Hughes TE, Townsend GC. The dentition: the outcomes of morphogenesis leading to variations of tooth number, size and shape. Aust Dent J 2014; 59 (Suppl. 1): 131-42. [http://dx.doi.org/10.1111/adj.12160] [PMID: 24646162]

[3] Baccetti T. A controlled study of associated dental anomalies. Angle Orthod 1998; 68(3): 267-74. [PMID: 9622764]

[4] Polder BJ, Van't Hof MA, Van der Linden FP, Kuijpers-Jagtman AM. A meta-analysis of the prevalence of dental agenesis of permanent teeth. Community Dent Oral Epidemiol 2004; 32(3): 217-26. [http://dx.doi.org/10.1111/j.1600-0528.2004.00158.x] [PMID: 15151692]

[5] Endo T, Ozoe R, Yoshino S, Shimooka S. Hypodontia patterns and variations in craniofacial morphology in Japanese orthodontic patients. Angle Orthod 2006; 76(6): 996-1003. [http://dx.doi.org/10.2319/082905-303] [PMID: 17090161]

[6] Tavajohi-Kermani H, Kapur R, Sciote JJ. Tooth agenesis and craniofacial morphology in an orthodontic population. Am J Orthod Dentofacial Orthop 2002; 122(1): 39-47. [http://dx.doi.org/10.1067/mod.2002.123948] [PMID: 12142896]

[7] Vastardis H, Karimbux N, Guthua SW, Seidman JG, Seidman CE. A human MSX1 homeodomain missense mutation causes selective tooth agenesis. Nat Genet 1996; 13(4): 417-21. [http://dx.doi.org/10.1038/ng0896-417] [PMID: 8696335]

[8] Brook AH, Elcock C, Aggarwal M, *et al.* Tooth dimensions in hypodontia with a known PAX9 mutation. Arch Oral Biol 2009; 54 (Suppl. 1): S57-62. [http://dx.doi.org/10.1016/j.archoralbio.2008.05.017] [PMID: 18653171]

[9] Fekonja A. Hypodontia in orthodontically treated children. Eur J Orthod 2005; 27(5): 457-60. [http://dx.doi.org/10.1093/ejo/cji027] [PMID: 16043466]

[10] Garib DG, Alencar BM, Lauris JR, Baccetti T. Agenesis of maxillary lateral incisors and associated dental anomalies. Am J Orthod Dentofacial Orthop 2010; 137(6): 732.e1-6. [http://dx.doi.org/10.1016/j.ajodo.2009.12.024] [PMID: 20685523]

[11] Mirabella AD, Kokich VG, Rosa M. Analysis of crown widths in subjects with congenitally missing maxillary lateral incisors. Eur J Orthod 2012; 34(6): 783-7. [http://dx.doi.org/10.1093/ejo/cjr094] [PMID: 21911843]

[12] Nowak AJ. Dental treatment for patients with ectodermal dysplasias. Birth Defects Orig Artic Ser 1988; 24(2): 243-52. [PMID: 3052619]

[13] Hobkirk JA, Nohl F, Bergendal B, Storhaug K, Richter MK. The management of ectodermal dysplasia and severe hypodontia. International conference statements. J Oral Rehabil 2006; 33(9): 634-7. [http://dx.doi.org/10.1111/j.1365-2842.2006.01628.x] [PMID: 16922735]

[14] Alcan T, Basa S, Kargül B. Growth analysis of a patient with ectodermal dysplasia treated with endosseous implants: 6-year follow-up. J Oral Rehabil 2006; 33(3): 175-82. [http://dx.doi.org/10.1111/j.1365-2842.2005.01566.x] [PMID: 16512883]

[15] Yamada H, Kondo S, Hanamura H, Townsend GC. Tooth size in individuals with congenitally missing teeth: a study of Japanese males. Anthropol Sci 2010; 118: 87-93. [http://dx.doi.org/10.1537/ase.090706]

[16] Alexandersen V, Nielsen OV. Generalized microdontia probably associated with intrauterine growth retardation in a medieval skeleton. Am J Phys Anthropol 1970; 33(3): 389-401. [http://dx.doi.org/10.1002/ajpa.1330330313] [PMID: 4321404]

[17] Zhu JF, Marcushamer M, King DL, Henry RJ. Supernumerary and congenitally absent teeth: a literature review. J Clin Pediatr Dent 1996; 20(2): 87-95. [PMID: 8619981]

[18] Thesleff I. Genetic basis of tooth development and dental defects. Acta Odontol Scand 2000; 58(5): 191-4. [http://dx.doi.org/10.1080/000163500750051728] [PMID: 11144868]

[19] Hyun HK, Lee SJ, Lee SH, Hahn SH, Kim JW. Clinical characteristics and complications associated with mesiodentes. J Oral Maxillofac Surg 2009; 67(12): 2639-43. [http://dx.doi.org/10.1016/j.joms.2009.07.041] [PMID: 19925984]

[20] Primosch RE. Anterior supernumerary teeth--assessment and surgical intervention in children. Pediatr Dent 1981; 3(2): 204-15. [PMID: 6945564]

[21] Van Buggenhout G, Bailleul-Forestier I. Mesiodens. Eur J Med Genet 2008; 51(2): 178-81. [http://dx.doi.org/10.1016/j.ejmg.2007.12.006] [PMID: 18262485]

[22] Peck S, Peck L, Kataja M. Concomitant occurrence of canine malposition and tooth agenesis: evidence

of orofacial genetic fields. Am J Orthod Dentofacial Orthop 2002; 122(6): 657-60.
[http://dx.doi.org/10.1067/mod.2002.129915] [PMID: 12490878]

[23] Litsas G, Acar A. A review of early displaced maxillary canines: etiology, diagnosis and interceptive treatment. Open Dent J 2011; 5: 39-47.
[http://dx.doi.org/10.2174/1874210601105010039] [PMID: 21566691]

[24] Peck S, Peck L, Kataja M. Site-specificity of tooth maxillary agenesis in subjects with canine malpositions. Angle Orthod 1996; 66: 473-6.
[PMID: 8974184]

[25] Becker A, Sharabi S, Chaushu S. Maxillary tooth size variation in dentitions with palatal canine displacement. Eur J Orthod 2002; 24(3): 313-8.
[http://dx.doi.org/10.1093/ejo/24.3.313] [PMID: 12143095]

[26] Baccetti T, Leonardi M, Armi P. A randomized clinical study of two interceptive approaches to palatally displaced canines. Eur J Orthod 2008; 30(4): 381-5.
[http://dx.doi.org/10.1093/ejo/cjn023] [PMID: 18524761]

[27] Baccetti T, Mucedero M, Leonardi M, Cozza P. Interceptive treatment of palatal impaction of maxillary canines with rapid maxillary expansion: a randomized clinical trial. Am J Orthod Dentofacial Orthop 2009; 136(5): 657-61.
[http://dx.doi.org/10.1016/j.ajodo.2008.03.019] [PMID: 19892281]

[28] Becker A, Gillis I, Shpack N. The etiology of palatal displacement of maxillary canines. Clin Orthod Res 1999; 2(2): 62-6.
[PMID: 10534981]

[29] Becker A. In defense of the guidance theory of palatal canine displacement. Angle Orthod 1995; 65(2): 95-8.
[PMID: 7785811]

[30] Kurol J, Bjerklin K. Ectopic eruption of maxillary first permanent molars: familial tendencies. ASDC J Dent Child 1982; 49(1): 35-8.
[PMID: 6948834]

[31] Peck S, Peck L, Kataja M. Mandibular lateral incisor-canine transposition, concomitant dental anomalies, and genetic control. Angle Orthod 1998; 68(5): 455-66.
[PMID: 9770104]

[32] Peck L, Peck S, Attia Y. Maxillary canine-first premolar transposition, associated dental anomalies and genetic basis. Angle Orthod 1993; 63(2): 99-109.
[PMID: 8498708]

[33] Russell KA, Folwarczna MA. Mesiodens--diagnosis and management of a common supernumerary tooth. J Can Dent Assoc 2003; 69(6): 362-6.
[PMID: 12787472]

[34] Becker A, Chaushu S. Dental age in maxillary canine ectopia. Am J Orthod Dentofacial Orthop 2000; 117(6): 657-62.
[http://dx.doi.org/10.1016/S0889-5406(00)70174-0] [PMID: 10842108]

[35] Ericson S, Kurol J. Radiographic examination of ectopically erupting maxillary canines. Am J Orthod Dentofacial Orthop 1987; 91(6): 483-92.
[http://dx.doi.org/10.1016/0889-5406(87)90005-9] [PMID: 3473928]

[36] Alqerban A, Jacobs R, Souza PC, Willems G. In-vitro comparison of 2 cone-beam computed tomography systems and panoramic imaging for detecting simulated canine impaction-induced external root resorption in maxillary lateral incisors. Am J Orthod Dentofacial Orthop 2009; 136(6): 764.e1-764.e11.
[http://dx.doi.org/10.1016/j.ajodo.2009.03.036] [PMID: 19962592]

[37] Leonardi R, Peck S, Caltabiano M, Barbato E. Palatally displaced canine anomaly in monozygotic

twins. Angle Orthod 2003; 73(4): 466-70.
[PMID: 12940569]

[38] Warford JH Jr, Grandhi RK, Tira DE. Prediction of maxillary canine impaction using sectors and angular measurement. Am J Orthod Dentofacial Orthop 2003; 124(6): 651-5.
[http://dx.doi.org/10.1016/S0889-5406(03)00621-8] [PMID: 14666077]

[39] Zuccati G, Ghobadlu J, Nieri M, Clauser C. Factors associated with the duration of forced eruption of impacted maxillary canines: a retrospective study. Am J Orthod Dentofacial Orthop 2006; 130(3): 349-56.
[http://dx.doi.org/10.1016/j.ajodo.2004.12.028] [PMID: 16979493]

[40] Zasciurinskiene E, Bjerklin K, Smailiene D, Sidlauskas A, Puisys A. Initial vertical and horizontal position of palatally impacted maxillary canine and effect on periodontal status following surgical-orthodontic treatment. Angle Orthod 2008; 78(2): 275-80.
[http://dx.doi.org/10.2319/010907-8.1] [PMID: 18251594]

[41] Ericson S, Kurol PJ. Resorption of incisors after ectopic eruption of maxillary canines: a CT study. Angle Orthod 2000; 70(6): 415-23.
[PMID: 11138644]

[42] Becker A, Chaushu G, Chaushu S. Analysis of failure in the treatment of impacted maxillary canines. Am J Orthod Dentofacial Orthop 2010; 137(6): 743-54.
[http://dx.doi.org/10.1016/j.ajodo.2008.07.022] [PMID: 20685529]

[43] Crescini A, Nieri M, Buti J, Baccetti T, Pini Prato GP. Orthodontic and periodontal outcomes of treated impacted maxillary canines. Angle Orthod 2007; 77(4): 571-7.
[http://dx.doi.org/10.2319/080406-318.1] [PMID: 17605500]

Recent Advances in Dentistry, 2018, *Vol. 2*, 178-214

CHAPTER 8

Class II, Class III Malocclusion

Abstract: Class II malocclusion is a much more frequent type of skeleton-dental disharmony than a class III malocclusion. The nature of these malocclusions is not a result of a single component, but a variety of different dental and skeletal combinations such as maxillary-mandibular skeletal and dental position, as well as the vertical components. The more severe the malocclusion at the young ages, the greater the psychosocial and functional problems present. The disharmony could become more pronounced during the pubertal peak period and continue until growth is completed. As a result, it is important to understand the aetiology of these malocclusions so that orthodontic treatments can focus on possible prevention or early intervention in order to avoid any related craniofacial deformities. The timing of treatment varies from early intervention during the pre-pubertal stages of growth or intervention during the peak-growth stage after the patient has completed their active growth.

Keywords: Functional appliances, Orthopaedic treatment, Skeletal discrepancy.

INTRODUCTION

The Class II malocclusion is a common skeletal problem seen in orthodontics. Approximately 15% of the Caucasian population has a Class II malocclusion greater than 5 mm. On the other hand, the prevalence of Class III malocclusions differs between different ethnic groups. Class III malocclusions are seen less often in Caucasian than Chinese or Japanese populations. Both skeletal imbalances are established early in life and are not self-correcting during development. In both malocclusions, there is a discrepancy between the maxillary and the mandibular dentition, which may or may not be accompanied by skeletal discrepancy. However, sagittal changes are largely due to the differential growth of the mandible rather than the maxilla. There are various techniques to correct Class II malocclusions, including functional and fixed appliances, extra-oral forces, elastics, extractions and even surgery.

PART A. CLASS II MALOCCLUSION

1. What is a Class II Malocclusion?

Angle describes Class II malocclusions as dental relationships where the lower

George Litsas

first molars are locked distally to the upper first molars by at least half a cusp width on both the left and right sides of the jaw when compared to Class I. Angle's definition was based on the upper first molar, which was the "key to occlusion." Although the classification by Angle is restricted to dental relationships, it is still widely used because of its simplicity as well as a method of communication between dental professionals. Angle subdivided the Class II malocclusion into two types based on the inclination of the maxillary central incisors [1].

The Angle Class II/I is characterised by protruding and flaring upper incisors, increased overjet and deep bite in some cases (Figs. **1 & 2**), and more or less "V" shaped maxillary arch [1 - 4].

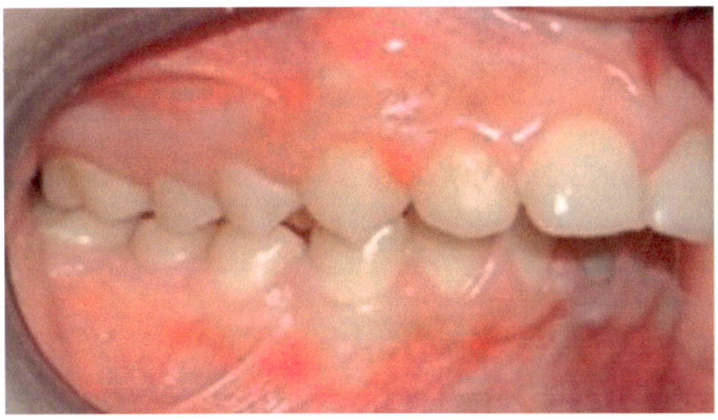

Fig. (1). Angle class II/I lateral view.

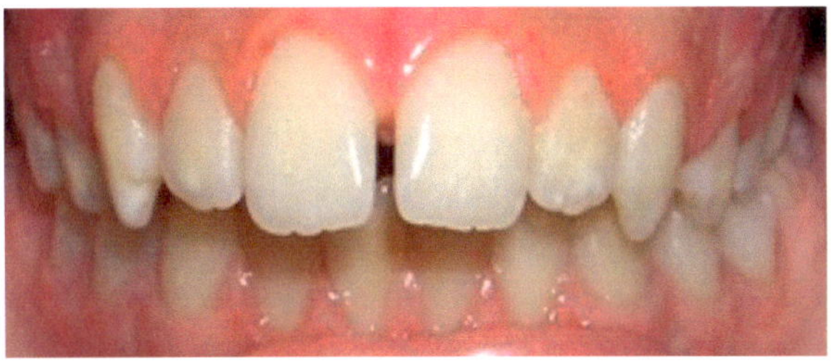

Fig. (2). Angle class II/I frontal view.

The class II/II malocclusion is characterised by less narrowing of the upper arch, retroclined maxillary central incisors, overlapped on the labial by the lateral incisors deep bite and minimal overjet (Fig. **3**). Sometimes, both the central and the lateral incisors are lingual inclined and overlapped by the labial inclined canines (Fig. **4**). The mandibular incisors are either retroclined or normal [5 - 7].

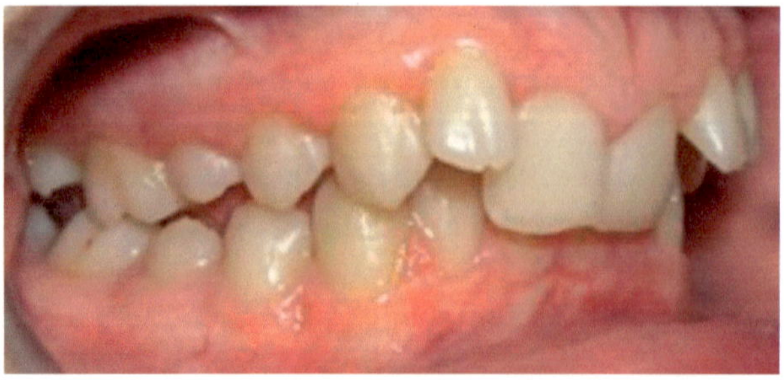

Fig. (3). Angle class II/II lateral view.

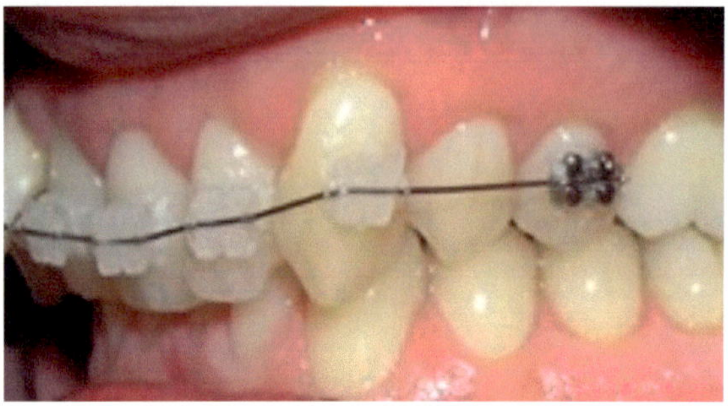

Fig. (4). Angle class II/II lateral view.

2. What is the Aetiology of Class II Malocclusion?

Heredity: Craniofacial structures are developed from complex processes of tissue interactions, cell migrations and coordinated growth. Part of Class II malocclusion is heritability and is consistent with a polygenic mode of inheritance. Neural crest cells are thought to be controlled by homeobox genes (Msx-1 and Msx-2) and their derivations include the maxilla, mandible, zygomatic, nasal bones and bones of the cranial vault. Disruption in the migration of the neural crest cells can produce dento-alveolar abnormalities and skeletal asymmetries. Due to the significant genetic complexity in the formation of the face and jaws, it is difficult to ascertain what genes are affecting various features in a particular malocclusion case [8 - 10].

Environment: Nose allergies, premature loss of maxillary primary molars, mouth breathing, pacifier thumb and lip sucking [4, 11]. Heredity and environment have variable influences on the development of malocclusion in each individual. However, the percentage of genetics contribution *versus* environmental factors has never been clearly defined and is often different between individuals and such influences must be evaluated and taken into consideration when developing a treatment plan

3. How Could an Abnormal Swallowing Pattern Exaggerate the Class II/ Division 1 Malocclusion?

During swallowing, an abnormal mentalis muscle activity, increased buccinator muscle activity and lower tongue position could cause changes in the dentofacial structures such as constriction of the maxillary arch, protrusion and spacing of the maxillary incisors and abnormal inclination of the mandibular incisors [13, 14].

4. What Do You See In the Following Figures?

Lip trap: The lower lip is positioned palatal to the upper incisors at rest (Fig. **5**). The lip trapped is a common soft tissue characteristic of skeletal class II malocclusion which enhances the overjet, remains or even accentuates the Class II malocclusion and prevents normal deglutition as well. 'Lip sucking' during swallowing, together with hyperactive mentalis muscle activity and the tongue position and function, could also cause spaced and proclined upper incisors (Fig. **6**) as well as retroclined lower incisors [12 - 14], (Fig. **7**).

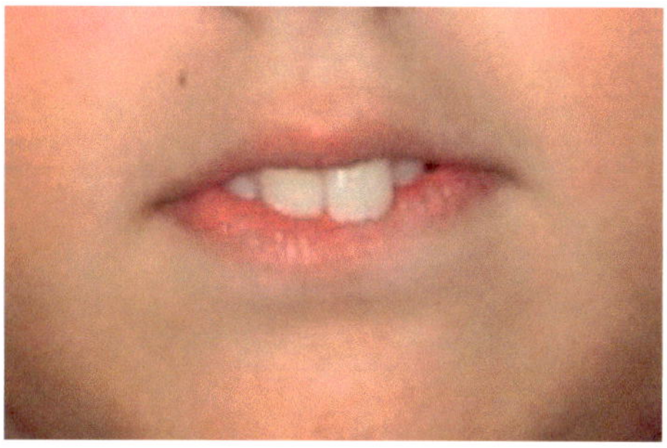

Fig. (5). Lip trap.

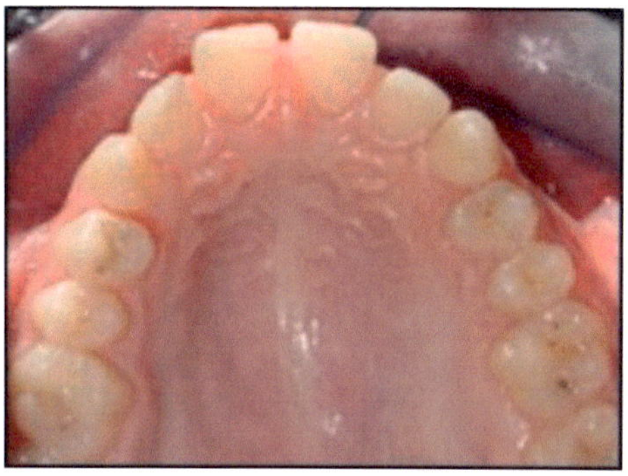

Fig. (6). Spaced and proclined upper incisors.

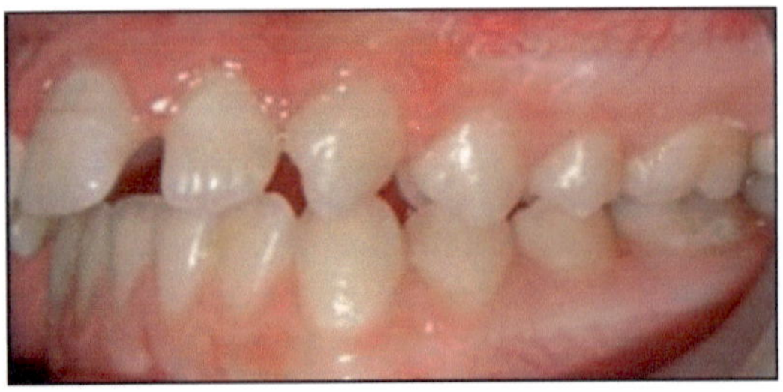

Fig. (7). Retroclined lower incisors.

Finger Sucking (Fig. **8**): The duration of force is more important than its magnitude (Fig. **6**). Children with prolonged finger sucking exhibit:

a. Decreased maxillary arch width and posterior crossbite
b. Increased overjet
c. Decreased overbite
d. Anterior open bite
e. Increased facial height

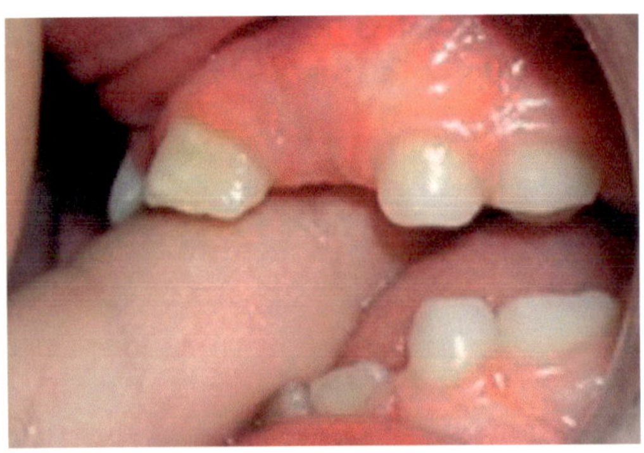

Fig. (8). Thumb sucking.

5. What is the Dental Arch Shape in Class II Individuals?

Many Class II/I individuals were characterised by a V-shaped maxillary arch (Fig. **9**), posterior cross-bite, excessive curve of Spee and increased overbite and overjet. Dentally, maxillary incisors were found to be at a normal inclination; however, the lower incisors were more proclined than the Class I controls. Anterior arch length was found to increase during the transition period in Class II/I individuals, whereas the maxillary arch width has been shown to have more constriction than those of Class I malocclusion [2, 15 - 17].

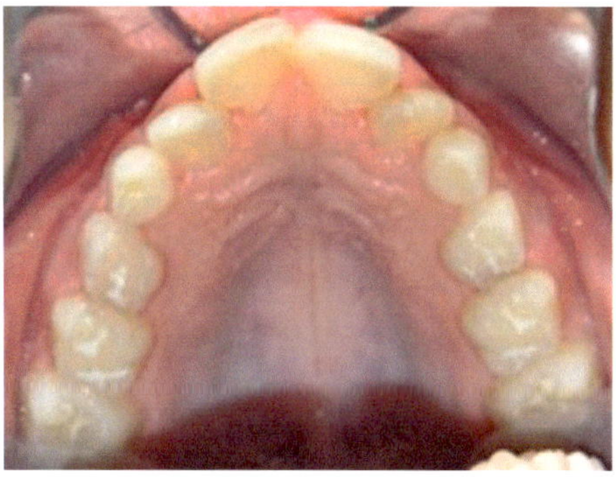

Fig. (9). V maxillary arch.

In class II/II individuals, the maxillary incisors are retroclined and the mandibular incisors are either retroclined or normal. Although the maxillary dental arch is wider (Fig. **10**) in the division II subjects, the anterior arch length was not increased during the transition period. It seems that the anterior dentition in both males and females was smaller than in the controls [4 - 7].

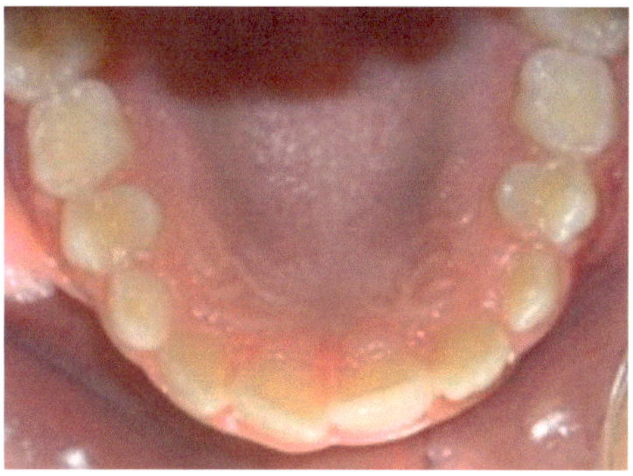

Fig. (10). Maxillary arch in class II/II.

6. What are the Main Skeletal Components of Skeletal Class II/ Division 1 and Class II/ Division 2 Malocclusion (Table 1)?

Table 1. Components of skeletal Class II/ division 1 and Class II/ division 2 malocclusion [2, 4, 5, 15 - 19].

Class II/I	Class II/II
The maxilla bone and the upper teeth are cited anterior to cranial base	Orthognathic maxilla
The maxillary teeth are cited anterior but the maxilla bone size is normal	Retrognathic mandible Short mandibular body length

(Table 1) contd.....

Class II/I	Class II/II
The mandible bone size is normal but positioned posterior	A hypodivergent facial pattern Acute gonial angle
The mandibular bone is underdeveloped	Flat mandibular plane Prominent chin
Short ramus height **Increase in the mandibular plane angle** **Anterior vertical excess**	Increased ramus height, Increased posterior facial height Decreased anterior facial height

7. Assess the Facial Characteristics of Class II/ I and Class II/II Malocclusion (Table 2)

Table 2. Facial characteristics of Class II malocclusion [2 - 4, 7, 15].

Class II/ I (Fig. 11)	Class II/II (Fig. 12)
The facial profile could be convex or straight	A convex profile, obtuse nasio-labial angle
Prominent chin	Soft tissue pogonion positioned posterior
Deep mentolabial sulcus	Incompetent lips
Excessive overbite	Excessive overjet
High upper lip positioned (Gummy smile)	Short upper lip
The lower lip line is high relative to the upper incisors	Trapped lower lip

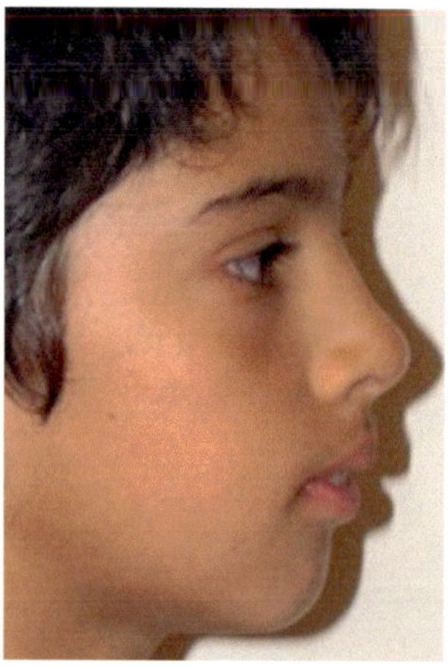

Fig. (11). Class II/I facial profile.

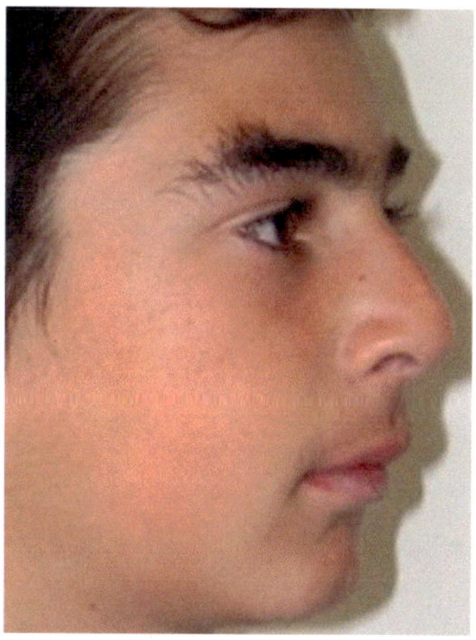

Fig. (12). Class II/II facial profile.

8. Describe the "six" Horizontal Phenotypical Characterizations of Class II Relationship, as Presented by Moyers, and the possible Orthodontic Treatment Procedures

Horizontal Group A

Group A represents the "pseudo Class II" which has normal skeletal relations of maxilla and mandible to cranial base and to each other (Fig. **13**). However, maxillary dentition is protracted, **resulting in a class II canine** relationship, increased overjet and overbite (Fig. **14**).

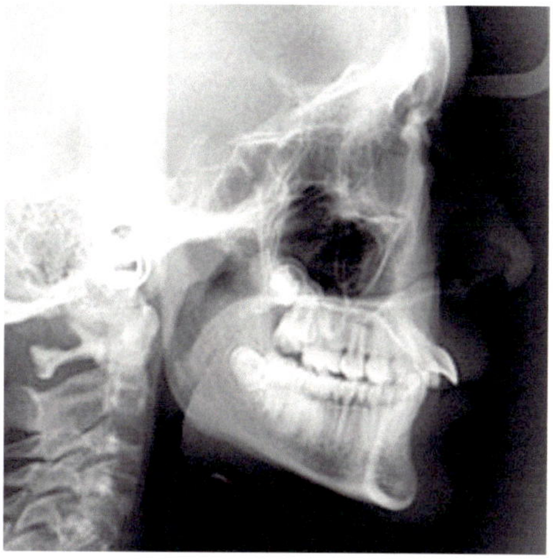

Fig. (13). Lateral cephalometric X-Ray in "pseudo Class II".

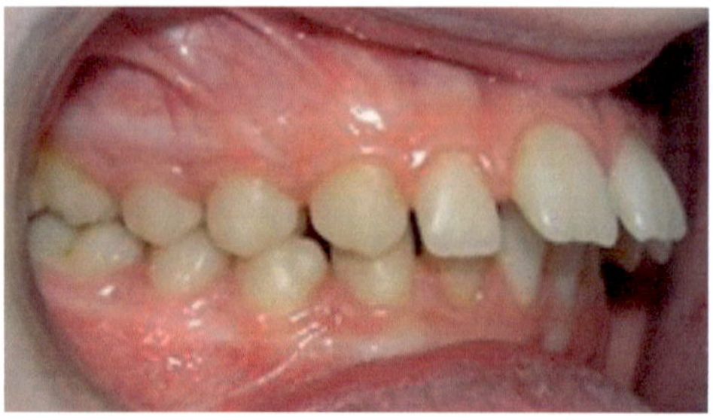

Fig. (14). Lateral occlusal view in "pseudo Class II".

Treatment: Tooth extraction or orthodontic distalization treatment [20 - 22].

Horizontal Group B

Group B has both skeletal and dental maxillary protrusion. Mandible displayed normal position and size (Figs. **15** & **16**).

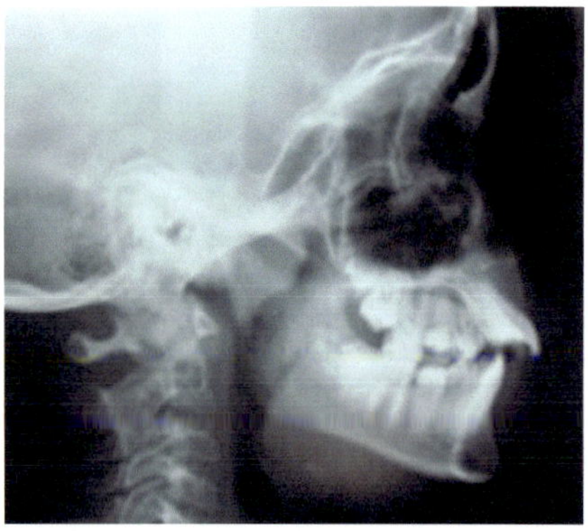

Fig. (15). Lateral Cephalometric X-Ray in maxillary protrusion.

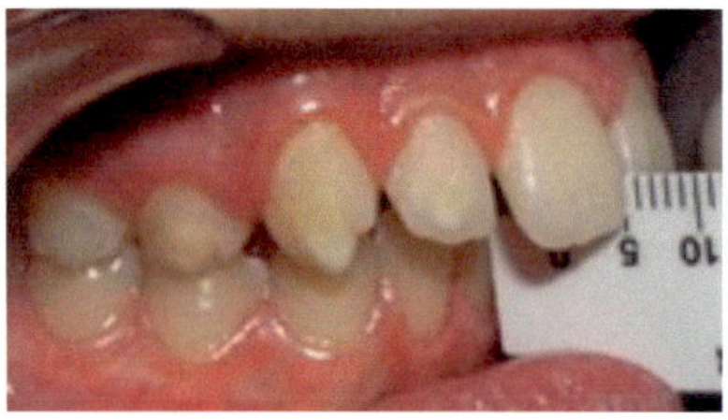

Fig. (16). Lateral occlusal view in maxillary protrusion.

Treatment:

a. Headgear growth modification treatment protocol [4, 20, 23, 24].
b. Extraction of upper first bicuspids and retraction of six anterior teeth [8, 31].

c. Distalization of the upper dentition into class I relationship [20 - 22].
d. Orthognathic surgery. Maxillary alveolar osteotomy set back combined with first bicuspid extraction treatment protocol [4].

Horizontal Group C

Group C had bimaxillary retrusion beneath the anterior cranial base (Fig. **17**), maxillary dental upright or protrusion depending on the vertical relationship and mandibular dental protrusion.

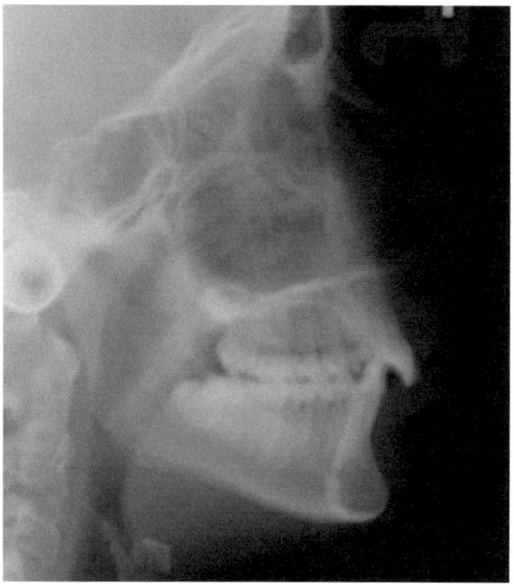

Fig. (17). Lateral cephalometric X-Ray in bimaxillary retrusion.

Treatment:

a. Orthodontic extraction treatment. Extraction of four first bicuspids combined with extensive orthodontic treatment [4].
b. Orthodontic extraction treatment plus orthognathic surgery. Extraction of upper second and lower first bicuspids combined with mandibular advancement orthognathic surgery treatment [28].

Horizontal Group D

Group D displayed maxillary and mandibular retrognathism but mandibular dental upright (lip trapped cases). The mandible is smaller than the normal size (Fig. **18**).

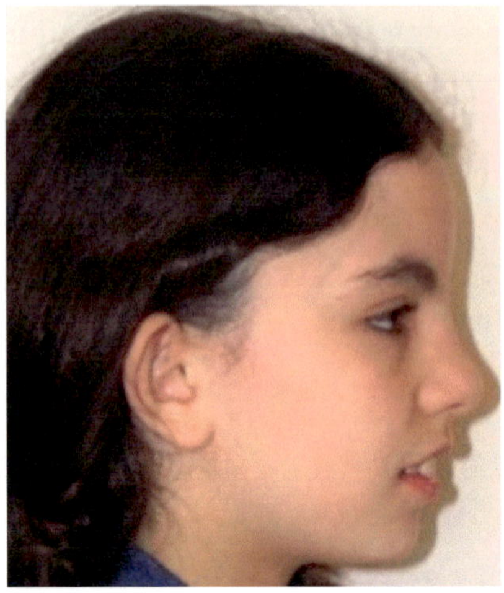

Fig. (18). Facial profile in lip trapped.

Treatment:

a. Functional jaw orthopaedic treatment [25 - 27].
b. Orthognathic surgery. Mandibular advancement orthognathic surgery procedures [4, 28, 29].

Horizontal Group E

Group E represented the severe class II relationship.

Maxillary-mandibular prognathism with bimaxillary dental protrusion (Fig. **19**).

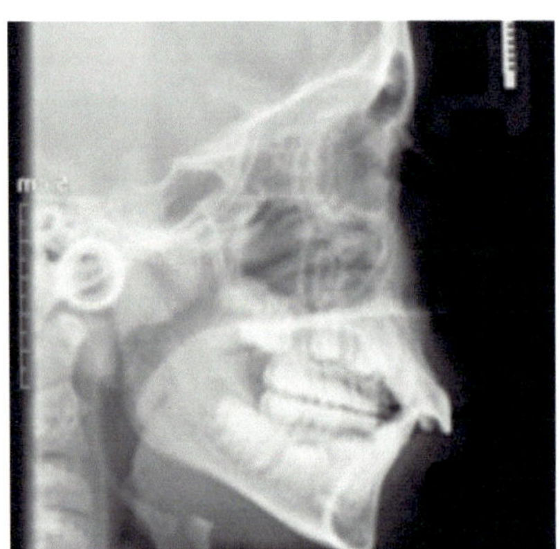

Fig. (19). Lateral Cephalometric X-Ray in bimaxillary protrusion.

Treatment:

a. Growth modification treatment protocol [4, 11, 25, 30].
b. Orthodontic extraction treatment protocol. Extraction of first bicuspids and extensive orthodontic treatment [4, 11].
c. Orthodontic extraction treatment plus orthognathic surgery [29].

Horizontal Group F

Group F displayed mandibular retrusion with upright anterior dentition (Fig. **20**).

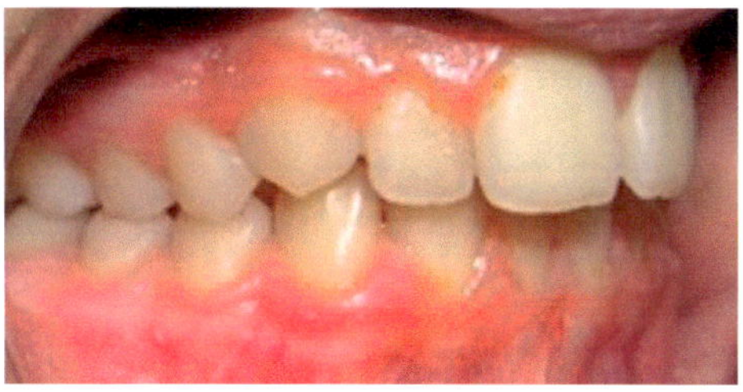

Fig. (20). Lateral occlusal view.

Treatment:

a. Functional jaw orthopaedic treatment [25 - 27].
b. Mandibular advancement orthognathic surgery procedures [28, 29].

9. Describe the Five Vertical Phenotypic Characterisations of the Class II Relationship, as Presented by Moyers

Vertical Type 1

Right: Long face. The anterior facial height is larger than the posterior facial height. The mandibular plane angle is steeper than normal and the anterior cranial base tends to be upward (Fig. **21**).

Vertical Type 2

Left: In this type of face the mandibular, maxillary planes and the anterior cranial base tend to be horizontal. It has a small gonial angle, skeletal deep bite and square face (Fig. **22**).

Vertical Type 3

Right: Open bite type with steep mandibular plane, short upper anterior facial

height, long lower anterior facial height and counter-clockwise rotation of maxillary plane (Fig. **23**).

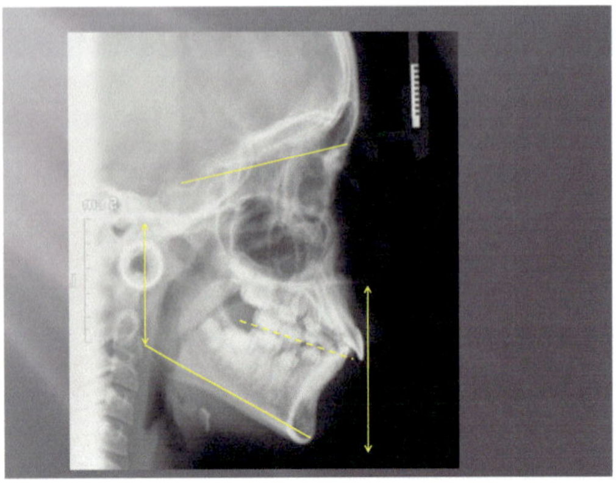

Fig. (21). Skeletal long face.

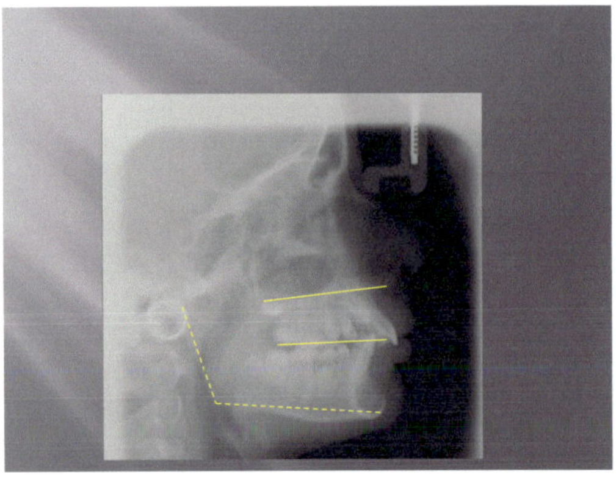

Fig. (22). Skeletal short face.

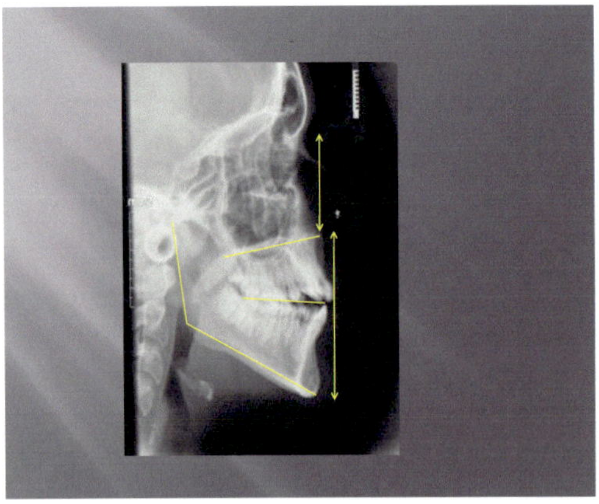

Fig. (23). Skeletal open-bite.

Vertical Type 4

Left: Gummy smile patient. Maxillary and mandibular plane rotated clockwise with obtuse gonial angle (Fig. **24**). Upper incisors are tipped labially.

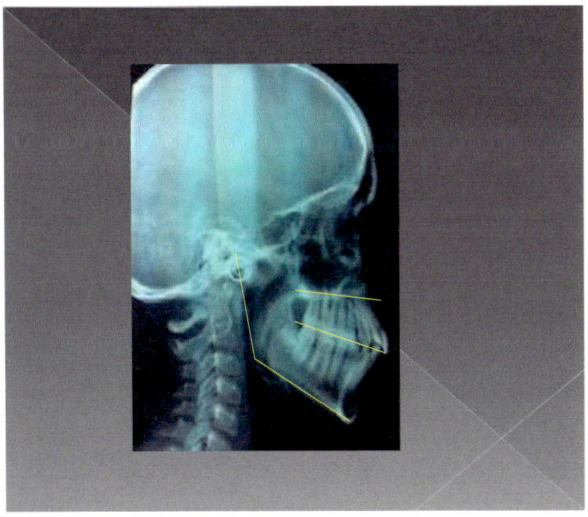

Fig. (24). Skeletal gummy smile.

Vertical Type 5

The maxillary plane rotated clockwise but the mandibular plane is normal (Fig. **25**). Skeletal deep bite exists and the upper incisors are tipped lingually and lower incisors are normal or tipped labially.

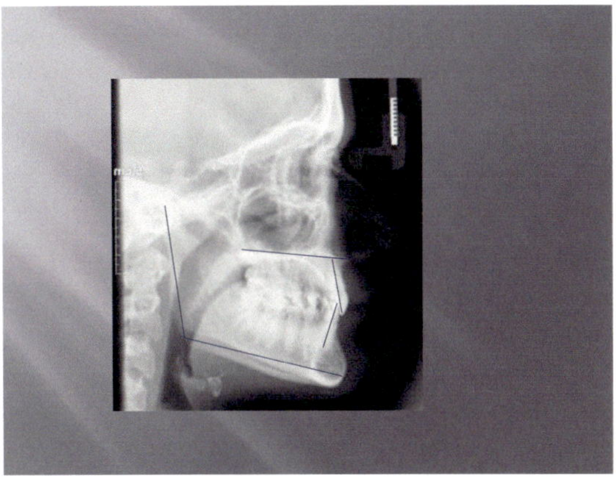

Fig. (25). Skeletal deep bite.

10. How Early Can You Detect the Pattern of Class II Skeletal Growth and Why is it not Self-corrected?

The sagittal and vertical maxilla-mandibular skeletal difference in skeletal class II growth pattern is established early in life and remains either the same or worsening during the growth period. The reasons are that during the transition period from early mixed to late mixed dentition, the posterior facial height decreases relative to the anterior facial height and the mandibular plane angle opens every year, contributing to the more retrusive mandibular position. In addition, the mandibular growth rate in skeletal Class II individuals is smaller during the pubertal growth period and the direction is in a generally more downward and backward direction. There is shorter mandibular ramus height because there is less vertical condyle growth and less gonial remodelling among Class II skeletal patterns compared with Class I individuals [4, 11, 25 - 27, 31].

11. What is Growth Modification Treatment?

Growth modification treatment is considered the orthodontic-orthopaedic approach attempting to minimize dental movements while maximizing skeletal correction. Growth modification appliances can affect not only skeletal and dento-alveolar structures, but also soft tissues of the face, providing significantly more attractive facial appearance of the patient [4, 11, 22, 25 - 27, 31]. Both extra-oral headgears and functional appliances could be considered as growth modification appliances. Extra-oral appliances include a variety of headgears that transmit force to the maxilla *via* the teeth [20, 21, 24, 30]. Functional appliances, on the other hand, are intraoral appliances that transmit forces *via* the teeth and/or soft tissues to distract the mandibular condyles, in order to accelerate mandibular growth [4, 11, 25]. However, some functional appliances also have a headgear effect on the maxilla.

12. What is "Early Orthodontic Treatment"?

If we accept that the most common characteristic in Class II patients is mandibular skeletal retrusion, treatment modalities that promote mandibular growth are very important in orthodontic practice. Early orthodontic treatment is based on the concept that orthodontic-orthopedic management of skeletal Class II discrepancies should be initiated in the early mixed dentition period, rather than waiting for the pubertal growth spurt [22, 26, 27, 31].

13. What are the Possible Benefits of Early Orthodontic Treatment?

- Modify the growth and normalise morphology at a young age [22, 33].
- Avoid potential trauma of protruded maxillary incisors, improved patient self-

esteem and parental satisfaction [26, 27].

- Reduce the risk of enamel decalcification, root resorption and bicuspid extraction in the second phase of treatment [31].

14. Why Do Most Clinicians Support the "One-phase Treatment"?

a. Two-phase orthodontic treatment increases the total treatment time [4].
b. Two-phase treatment does not improve the skeletal pattern compared to phase I treatment [31, 34].
c. Two-phase orthodontic treatment appears to be inefficient in reducing the complexity of the second phase of treatment (need for extraction or orthognathic surgery) [26, 27].
d. Lack of cooperation because of long treatment time [34].

15. What is Functional Orthodontic Treatment?

Functional treatment could be defined as the use of "functional appliances" for the treatment of facial skeletal discrepancies. Functional appliances are intraoral appliances that transmit forces *via* the teeth and/or soft tissues to distract the mandibular condyles, in order to accelerate mandibular growth. The purpose of these appliances is to bring the mandible forward, to enlarge the oral space in hopes of maximising the patient's growth potential, achieving a more orthognathic profile and an improved relationship of the tongue, dentition, lips and surrounding soft tissues. Although functional appliances have been used for over half a century, the treatment value of these appliances has been a topic of debate, and there has been considerable discussion in the orthodontic literature regarding the biological and clinical advantages and disadvantages of functional orthodontic treatment. Animal studies have shown a significant long-term increase in mandibular length associated with the use of functional appliances, but human studies have been less conclusive [4, 11, 25, 32].

16. a. List the Possible Mechanisms of Class II/ Division 1 Correction by Functional Orthodontic Treatment (Table 3)
b. Provide the Pre-treatment Predictors for a Good Treatment Result with Functional Appliances (Table 4)

Table 3. Possible mechanisms of Class II/ division 1 correction [4, 11, 25, 32, 35].

a. **Mandible is positioned forward and elongated due to additional growth in the condyles (1-3 mm)**
b. **Fossa displacement, growth and adaptation (3-5 mm)**
c. **Maxillary sagittal growth (1-1.5mm) is inhibited due to the distally directed forces acting on the maxilla**
d. **Upper posterior teeth erupt more distally and the lower molars more mesial (2-2.5mm)**

(Table 3) contd.....

e. **Lingual tipping of the upper incisors and labial of the lower incisors**

Table 4. Pre-treatment predictors for an effective treatment outcome [11, 25, 26].

a. **Increased ANB because of mandibular retrusion**
b. **Horizontal growth pattern**
c. **Well aligned dental arches**
d. **Pubertal growth spurt**
e. **Labial tipping of the upper incisor crowns and lingual tipping of lower incisors.**

17. Why do Functional Protrusive Appliances Increase the Mandibular Growth Rate?

The functional protrusive appliances increase the mandibular growth rate because of the mandibular condylar cartilage. It is a unique cartilage in several respects. The condylar cartilage, which is designated as a secondary cartilage, differs from other primary cartilage in histological organisation, modes of proliferation, differentiation and calcification as well as response in environmental factors (*e.g.* biomechanical stress, hormones and growth factors) [37 - 39].

In addition, condylar cartilage contains chondroid bone (a specialised calcified tissue with morphological properties intermediate between those of bone and cartilage) which plays an important role in regulating different rates of bone formation in intramembranous and endochondral ossification. The histological composition of the temporomandibular joint has been shown to be susceptible to local extrinsic factors such as functional protrusive appliances. The hyper-propulsion of the mandible causes contraction of the lateral pterygoid muscle inducing cellular proliferation in the pre-chondroblast zone and endo-chondral bone growth. All of the proliferative process produces the upward and backward growth of the condyle, whereas endo-chondral growth occurs at the articular contact part of the condyle [32, 35, 36].

18. List the Criteria for a Good Treatment Result with Functional Appliances

a. Class I molar and canine relationship
b. Overjet and overbite within the normal range of 1-3 mm
c. Acceptable soft-tissue profile as defined by the upper and lower lips and chin position
d. Minor relapse of the anterior and posterior relationships when assessed 2 to 5 years after therapy.

19. Pros and Cons of Functional appliances (Table 5)

Table 5. Pros and Cons of Functional appliances [11].

Advantages	Disadvantages
Treatment in mixed dentition period	Needs patient cooperation
Long interval appointments > 2 months	Only in growth active period
Night-time wearable appliances	No clinical value on crowding
Eliminate mouth breathing and non-nutritive habits	Not precise forces

20. Name the Following Appliances and their Components?

Activator

The Activator appliance (Figs. **26** & **27**) shifts the mandible into a protrusive position, generating muscle actions that create the orthodontic force needed to correct the dental arch relationship and aiming to improve the patient's facial profile. The activator prevents the mandible from sliding backward and transfers the force to the maxilla, which is essentially the anchorage unit for the anteriorly displaced mandible. It consists of a lingual flange to position the mandible forward and a labial bow to control the maxillary anterior teeth. Lower incisor coverage (acrylic cap) prevents the vertical eruption or labial tipping of the lower incisors, and it also stabilizes the appliance in the mouth. In the current activator an acrylic shelf impedes the eruption of upper posterior teeth, while allowing the eruption of lower posterior teeth [11].

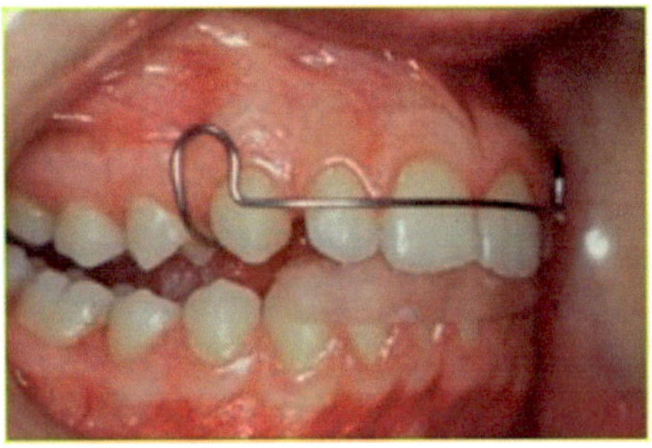

Fig. (26). Activator appliance lateral view.

Balters Bionator Appliance (Fig. **28**): It is a tooth-borne (passive) functional appliance designed and introduced by Balters. This appliance moves the mandible anteriorly so that over time a new position is achieved, producing dento-skeletal changes and improvement of the facial profile. The main components of this appliance are a 1.2 mm thick Palatal Coffin spring, which stabilizes and orientates the tongue anteriorly to contact the palate and a labial-buccal bow (0.9 mm thick) screening wire that could be adjusted during the course of treatment. A lower horseshoe-shaped flange brings the mandible in a forward position and an acrylic capping to control the lower incisors position [11].

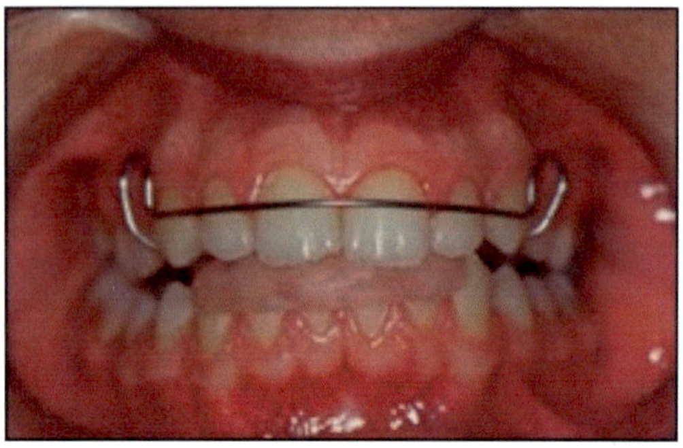

Fig. (27). Activator appliance frontal view.

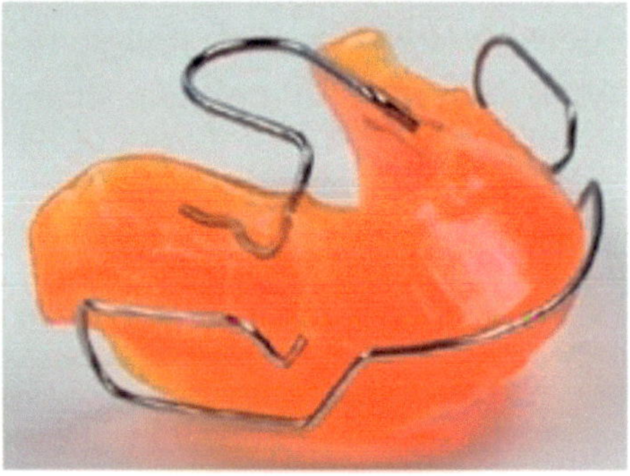

Fig. (28). Balters bionator.

Modern Bionator Appliance (Fig. **29**): An upper labial wire (0.040") is bent in a Hawley configuration with adjustment loops at the same width as the canines and extending upwards 7 to 8 mm above the gingival margin. An upper lingual wire (0.036") provides support for the appliance by using the lingual surfaces of the upper anterior teeth for anchorage. Palatal wire or "Coffin spring" 0.045" is constructed to lie 2 to 3 mm off the palatal tissue for comfort and can be activated for lateral arch development if needed. Eruption facets are made from the inter-occlusal acrylic to facilitate the eruption of both the upper and lower posterior teeth if desired. These pathways or channels are oriented so that the posterior teeth erupt either vertically or laterally. Lower incisor coverage prevents the vertical eruption or labial tipping of the lower incisors, and it also stabilizes the appliance in the mouth [11].

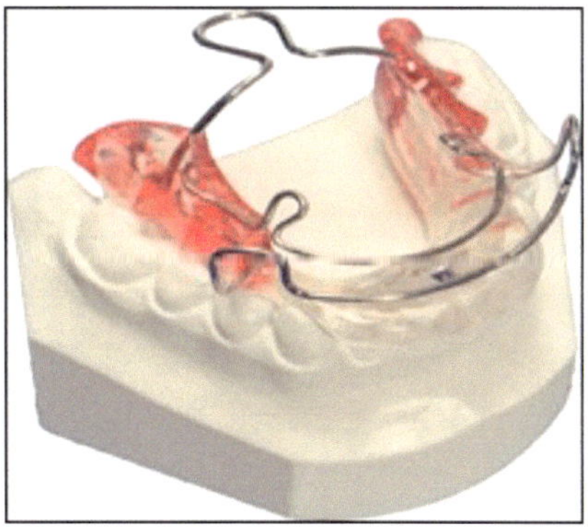

Fig. (29). Modern Bionator.

21. What is the Rationale for the Use of the Activator-Bionator Appliance in Skeletal Class II Malocclusion?

The rationale for the use of the Activator-Bionator appliance in skeletal class II malocclusion [26, 34 - 36, 40] was based on the premise that correction could be achieved by the following:

- Inhibition of forward growth of the maxilla and mesial migration of maxillary teeth.
- Inhibition of maxillary alveolar height increase and extrusion of mandibular molars.
- Increased growth of the mandible and mesial movement of mandibular teeth.
- Anterior relocation of the glenoid fossa.

22. Name the Following Appliances and their Components

Teuscher Activator (Figs. **30** & **31**): The Teuscher activator is used in conjunction with high-pull headgear and incorporates torquing springs. Torquing springs contact the incisors near the cervical line, creating a moment to counteract lingual incisor tipping [11]. A short or moderate length outer bow must be bent upward and connected to the head cap so that the extra oral force vector will pass through the estimated centre of resistance of the maxilla and it will be opposite to the direction of maxillary growth. The amount of extra oral force is about 450 gm per side. The high pull headgear withholds the maxillary forward growth and provides vertical control of both dental and skeletal relationship. The functional appliance enhances the forward displacement of the mandible and the fossa. It is generally accepted that when the restraint on the maxillary growth of a headgear is combined with a stimulation of mandibular growth with a functional appliance, effective antero-posterior skeletal correction of a Class II discrepancy could be achieved [42]. The skeletal effect of the Teuscher appliance is mainly limited to the maxilla, where it restrains forward growth [30, 33].

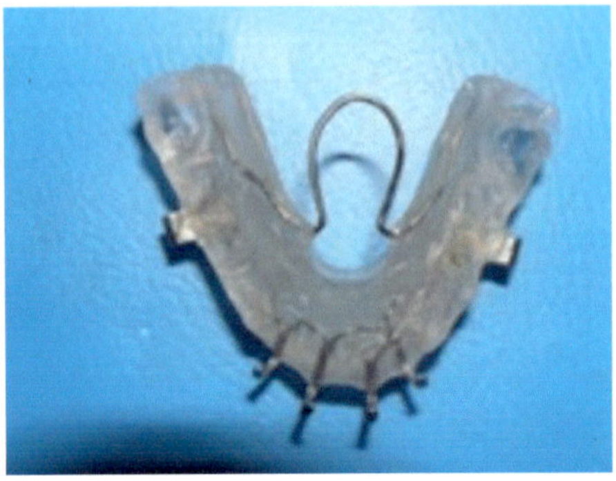

Fig. (30). Teuscher Activator.

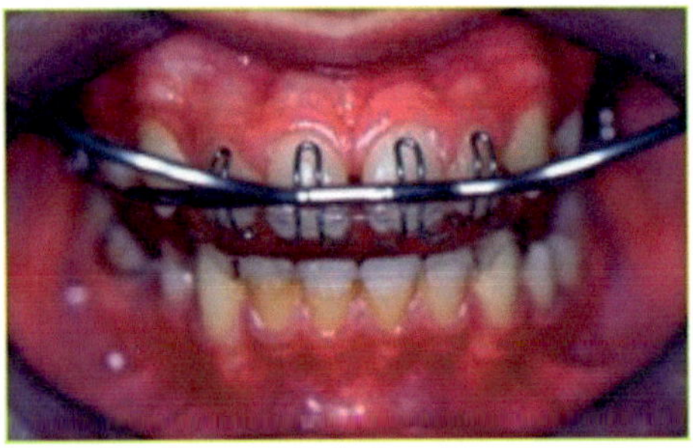

Fig. (31). Teuscher Activator into the mouth.

Twin Block Appliance (Figs. **32** & **33**): The basic design of the appliance is a two-piece system of bite blocks with sloping vertical ramps that encourage forward positioning of the mandible. The design of the twin-block appliance is constructed with acrylic palatal coverage and clasps for retention. The mandibular appliance has a lingual flange at the anterior and also clasps the teeth. The two pieces fit together *via* bite blocks covering the occlusal surfaces of the posterior teeth at the incline plane of approximately 70 degrees. The purpose is to promote protrusive mandibular function for the correction of skeletal Class II malocclusion. It was stated that in comparison to other functional appliances, occlusal inclined planes of the twin–block appliance could have given greater freedom of movement in anterior and lateral excursion and would cause less interference with normal function. An additional motivating factor could be the absence of lip, cheek, or tongue pads [25, 27, 41].

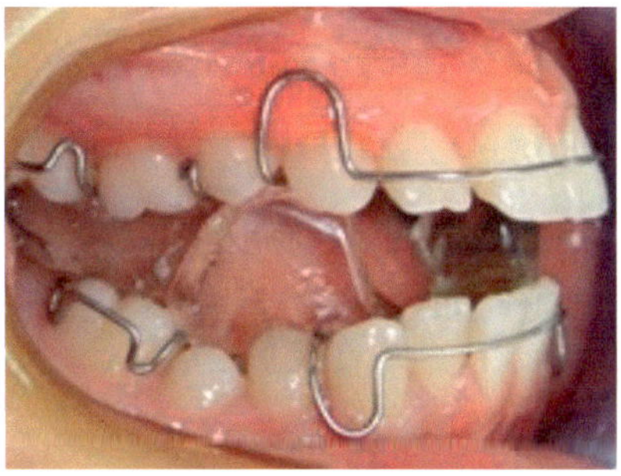

Fig. (32). Twin Block appliance lateral view.

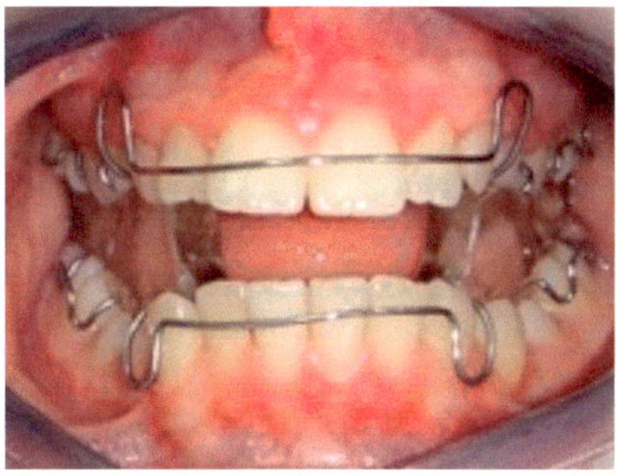

Fig. (33). Twin Block appliance frontal view.

23. Describe the Bite-Registration on Functional Appliances

Although bite registration requires case-specific parameters, a posterior clearance of 3.5 mm, an anterior clearance of 2.5 mm and guidance into Angle's Class I occlusal relation should be followed. If the sagittal discrepancy is not too great (<10mm), the forward posturing of the mandible would be so that the upper and lower incisors would come to an edge-to-edge relationship. If the sagittal discrepancy is >10mm, the anterior mandibular advancement should be 3 mm or more from the most posterior condylar position in the fossa. The second advancement should be made at 3- to 4- month intervals. Vertical opening should be within the limits of the free-way space or only a few millimeters exceeding it [4, 11].

24. What is a Compliance-free Class II Appliance? What Are their Treatment Effects on the Class II Correction (Table 6)?

Compliance-free Class II appliances or fixed-functional appliances are attached to the maxilla and the mandible in order to correct class II malocclusion when a limited amount of compliance is required [31]. The main disadvantage with these appliances is that they are attached only to the teeth. Consequently, the dentition is exposed to greater forces and is far more likely to displace. Some of these appliances are the Herbst, MARA, MPA, Jasper Jumper, and Forsus appliance [43 - 45].

Table 6. Treatment effects of compliance-free class II appliances.

Restriction of the maxillary skeletal growth
Maxillary molar distal tipping
Maxillary incisor uprighting
Mandibular skeletal protraction
Mandibular molar mesial movement
Mandibular incisor proclination

25. a. What is Extra-oral Traction? b. What Are the Main Clinical Applications of Headgears?

a. Extra-oral tractions are the forces exerted on the maxillary dentition or the whole maxilla through the use of headgears. Headgear force is transmitted to the maxillary complex *via* the molars [20].
b. The clinical applications of headgears are:
   1. Anchorage control
   2. Tooth movement
   3. Orthopaedic changes

The main application in mixed dentition patients is to aid in correcting Class II malocclusions by restraining maxillary growth, distalizing maxillary teeth or both. By restraining forward growth of the maxilla, headgear promotes differential growth in favor of the mandible, leading to an improvement or correction of a Class II relationship [20, 21].

26. Give the Relationship between Head-gear Force and Tooth Movement

The relationship between the headgear's resultant force and the tooth's centre of resistance determines the direction of force on the molars. If the *resultant force passes below the centre of resistance*, the maxillary molar crown will tip distally. If the *resultant force passes above the centre of resistance*, the maxillary molar root will tip distally. Finally, *if the resultant force passes directly through the tooth's centre of resistance,* translation of the tooth will occur. Cervical-pull and high-pull headgears produce different effects and are there for prescribed based on which resultant force the clinician desires [20, 21, 24, 30].

27. What Are the Effects of Cervical-pull, High-pull or Combi Headgear?

Cervical-pull headgear (Fig. **34**) inhibits the forward growth of the maxilla, slightly tips the anterior maxilla downward, rotates the mandible clockwise, and increases the eruption and distalization of the maxillary molars. The unwanted side effects, such as maxillary molar extrusion and distal crown tipping, can be controlled by bending the outer bow **10° to 20°** above the occlusal plane every **8 weeks**. However, more recent studies have observed only minor extrusion of maxillary first molars with cervical pull headgear alone when compared to normal eruption [4].

From the skeletal point of view, cervical-pull headgear caused a relative restraint of forward growth of the maxilla and a downward tipping of the anterior maxilla. The longer the time that the appliance is used, the more effective the treatment will be. *It is indicated for Class II patients in the late mixed dentition period who have a flat mandibular plane and a short lower anterior facial height (FMA≤25°).*

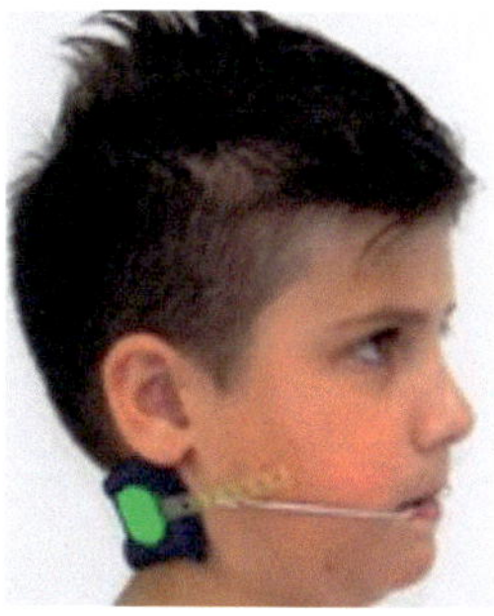

Fig. (34). Cervical-pull headgear.

High-pull headgear (Fig. **35**) can cause the relative restriction of horizontal and vertical maxillary growth, as well as the distalisation and intrusion of the maxillary molars. The applied force of 500g for a minimum of 12 hours a day for 6 months is sufficient to initiate maxillary orthopaedic changes, including the relative restriction of horizontal and vertical maxillary growth. Most of the time the high pull headgear should be combined with activator therapy because it:

a. Restricts the forward growth of the maxilla
b. Inhibits the mesial displacement and eruption of the maxillary teeth
c. Increases the horizontal growth of the mandible
d. Moves mesial the mandibular teeth

However, the skeletal effect of the headgear-activator appliance is mainly limited to the maxilla, where it restrained forward growth. *It is indicated in the mixed dentition for Class II patients with a steep mandibular plane (FMA>25°).* A side effect of the use of the high-pull headgear is the compensatory eruption of the mandibular molars which could be controlled by using a fixed lingual arch at the same time.

Combi headgear (Fig. **36**) is *indicated for cases in which the vector of force application needs to be altered depending on the desired effect.*

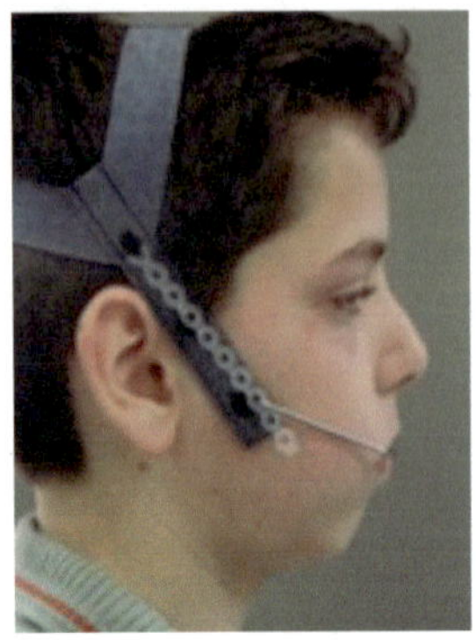

Fig. (35). High-pull headgear.

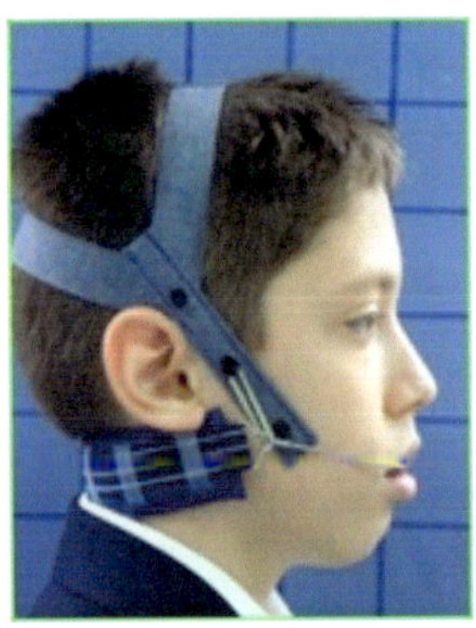

Fig. (36). Combi headgear.

PART B. CLASS III MALOCCLUSION

1. a. Classify this Malocclusion
b. Why is Angle classification not Enough to Describe the Class III Orthodontic Anomalies?

a. Class III malocclusion (Figs. **37** & **38**). According to Angle, Class III molar relationship refers to a condition where the mesiobuccal cusp of the upper first molars occludes between the lower first and second molars. Crowding of the upper anterior teeth and lingual inclination of the lower anterior teeth compose the mosaic of Angle's classification [1].

b. The classification by Angle is restricted to dental relationships without considering other factors such as skeletal, functional, and dental factors which may or may not be associated with each other. Although Angle's classification has been used for many years, his assumptions on aetiology and diagnosis of the malocclusion lack definitive evidence. Conversely, most of the Class III malocclusion cases are caused by a skeletal imbalance due to deficient maxillary growth, excessive mandibular growth or both of the above [46, 47].

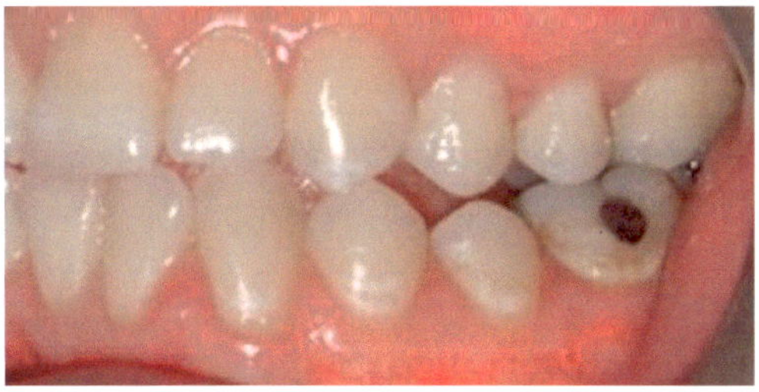

Fig. (37). Class III malocclusion.

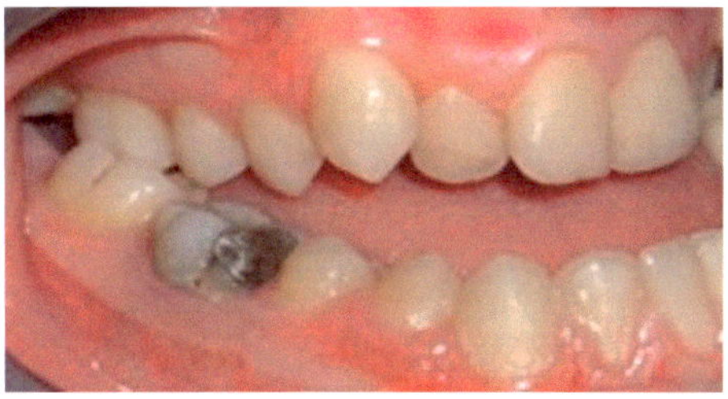

Fig. (38). Class III malocclusion.

2. a. What is the Aetiology of Class III Malocclusion? b. Could You Mention Why Severe Class III Malocclusion Affects Physical Health?

a. Although environmental factors such as trauma, hormonal imbalances, pituitary gland diseases, muscle dysfunction, illness, mandibular posture habits, premature loss of primary teeth, mouth breathing and enlarged tonsils contribute to class III malocclusion the frequent observation of familial tendency in class III malocclusion shows that genetic factors play a substantial role [4, 46 - 48]. The most well-known example of this is the Hapsburg family; the former Austro-Hungarian royal family. Generally speaking, dental variation is more dependent upon environmental factors, whereas class III skeletal characteristics have a stronger heritability-genetic estimate.
b. Severe Class III malocclusion could affect physical health causing speech and mastication problems, temporomandibular joint disorders, negatively impact self-concept attractiveness and intelligence in their social life [4, 11, 25].

3. Describe the Basic Characteristics of the Class III Orthodontic Anomalies

In the early orthodontics, an individual exhibiting a Class III malocclusion was diagnosed routinely as having mandibular prognathism (Fig. **39**). Mandibular prognathism may be present in individuals with a Class III malocclusion but this represents only one part of the spectrum of the different components of the malocclusion. The most common combination of variables is mandibular prognathism, maxillary retrognathism (Fig. **40**), retrusive mandibular dentition, protrusive maxillary dentition, and a combination of the above (Fig. **3** & **4**) [4, 47, 50].

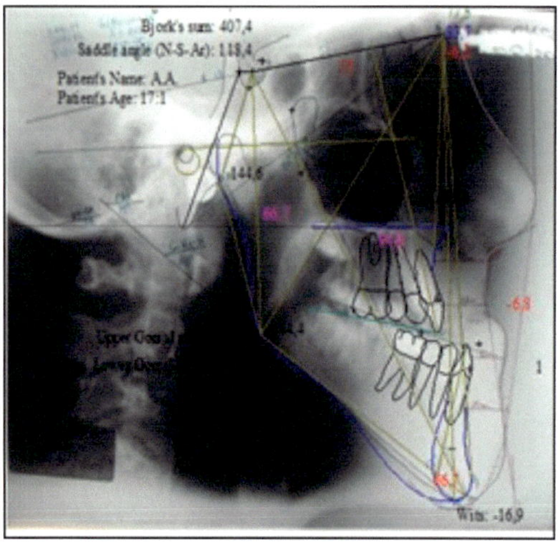

Fig. (39). Skeletal Class III.

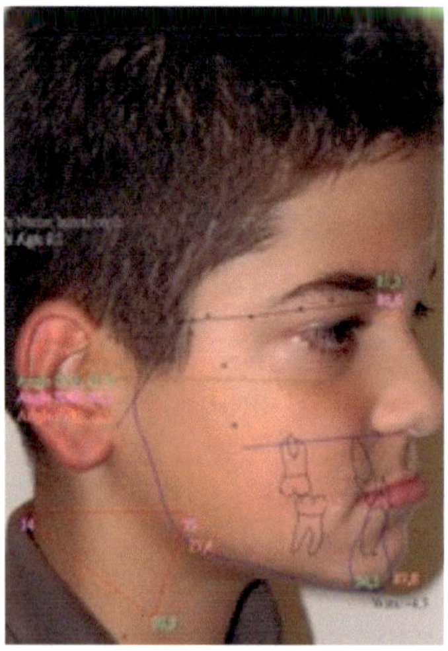

Fig. (40). Maxillary retrognathism.

4. Name the Cephalometric Components of Class III Malocclusion (Table 7)

Table 7. Craniofacial structures of Class III malocclusion [23, 36].

- Long mandibular body or forward placement of the glenoid fossa positioned the mandiblemore forward
- Large mandibular plane and gonial angles
Short and / or retrognathic maxilla
- Superior - posterior tip of the palatal plane (ANS - PNS).
- Short anterior cranial base and /or a higher position of sella relative to nasion and longer posterior cranial base
- Acute saddle angle (N - S - Ar or N - S - Ba)
- Protrusive upper incisors and retrusive lower incisors

5. In Which Age Does the Class III Craniofacial Pattern Appear?

Class III malocclusion develops early in age development and becomes progressively more severe with time [46]. In females, the position of the maxilla is retrusive from the early years of life and remains retrusive till adulthood over time [48]. On the other hand, the mandibular length as well as the lower anterior face height and the mandibular plane continue to increase with time. These differences are more pronounced in males, particularly during the peak and post-peak periods [50].

6. Name the Current Treatment Modalities for Class III Malocclusion

a. Dental-facial orthopaedic therapy such as facemask mask treatment or chin cup therapy
b. Miniplate supported treatment
c. Distraction osteogenesis
d. Orthognathic surgery [4, 47, 51, 52]

7. What is Pseudo-class III Malocclusion? Name Some Skeletal, Dental and Cephalometric Characteristics of this Malocclusion

a. Pseudo-Class III malocclusion is characterized by the presence of an anterior cross-bite due to a forward functional displacement of the mandible because of carious primary molars, palatal tipping or the palatal eruption of the maxillary permanent incisors or abnormal tooth contact that forces the mandible forward. The skeletal/dental characteristics of pseudo-class III malocclusion are characterized by class I skeletal pattern, class I molar relation in centric relationship, but Class III dental pattern in centric occlusion [48]. Elimination of the CR-CO shift reveals that it is a Class I malocclusion. Maxillary incisors are retroclined and mandibular incisors do not show the typical Class III compensatory inclinations. Cephalometrical measurements of pseudo-class III malocclusion (Fig. **41**).

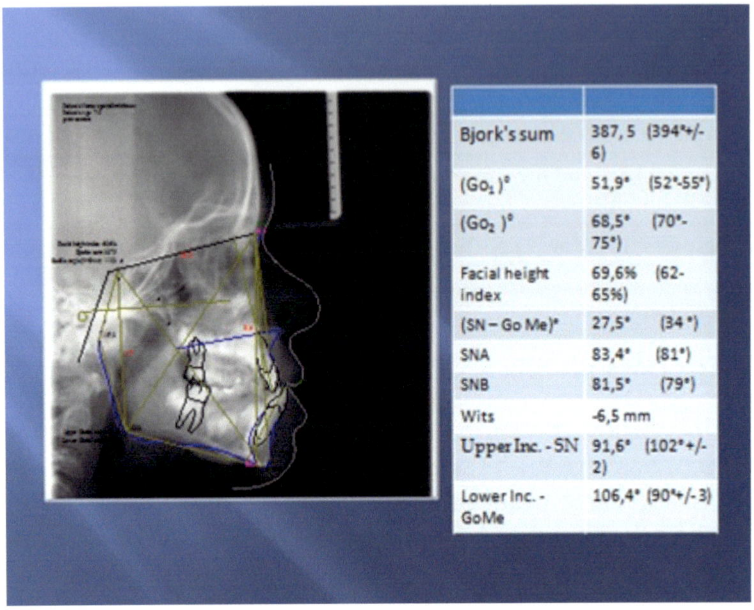

Fig. (41). Cephalometric values of pseudo-class III malocclusion [48].

8. How Do You Differentiate the True from the Pseudo-class III?

The following chart (Fig. **42**) shows a useful tool for differential diagnosis of the true from pseudo-class III malocclusion.

9. What is the Treatment Protocol for Class III Malocclusion During the Mixed Dentition Period? Describe in Detail the Clinical Protocol of Face Mask Treatment

Seventy-five percent of skeletal Class III malocclusions are caused by maxillary retrognathism or a combination of maxillary retrognathism and mandibular prognathism. With expanding accentuation on repositioning the maxilla, as opposed to the mandible in orthognathic surgery, the attention on maxillary orthopaedics and face mask treatment in the early mixed dentition period is of paramount importance [7]. A face mask (FM) is the preferred appliance for the treatment of skeletal Class III patients with maxillary deficiency and normal or short facial height. The face mask is adjusted to rest on the forehead and the chin of the patient (Fig. **7**). Elastics (5/16 inch by 14 ounces) should be worn from a horizontal bar located 2-3 cm in front of the lips to the intraoral attachments located at the gingival level of the primary canine. The force generated by the elastics should be about 300-600 gr bilaterally, 20 hours a day for 4-6 months [52, 54]. Maximal reaction happens in the initial 3 to 4 weeks after the face mask is delivered. Patient compliance is critical and must be emphasized in these first weeks of treatment (Fig. **43**). Overjet overcorrection to envision extra mandibular development is eager objectives

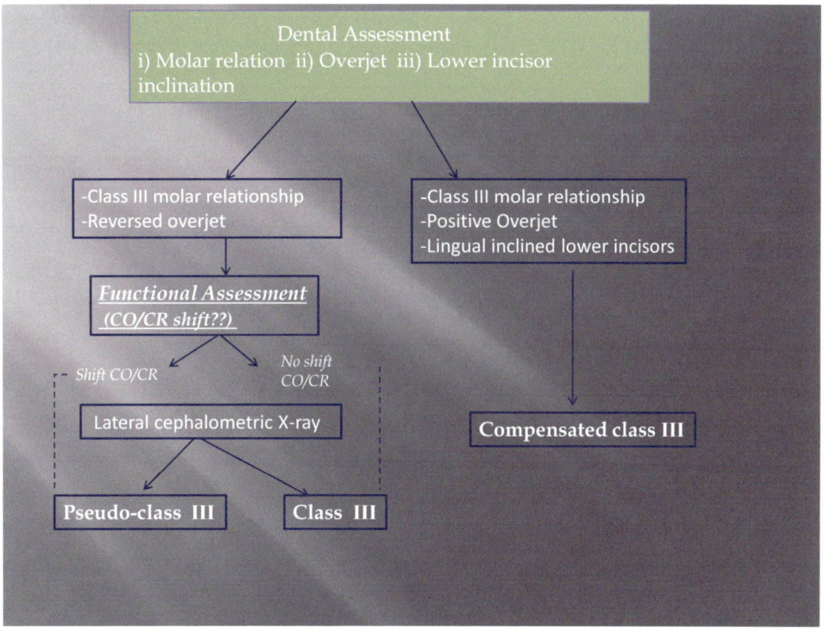

Fig. (42). Diagram for differential diagnosis of the true from the pseudo-class III [22, 23].

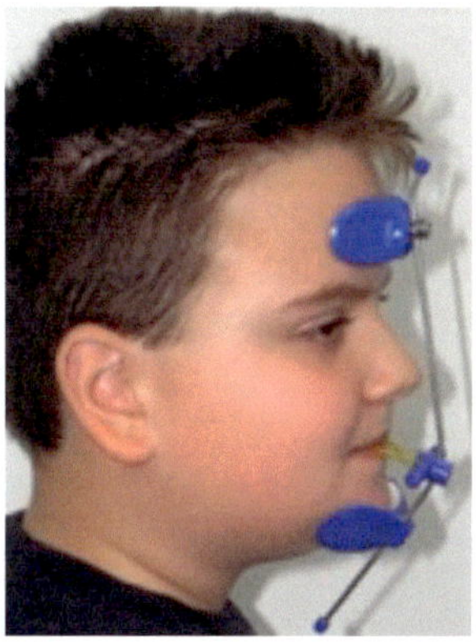

Fig. (43). A face mask.

10. Name the Potential Benefits and the Desirable Skeletal Changes of the Early Face Mask treatment (Table 8)

Table 8. Benefits and skeletal changes of Face Mask treatment.

Benefits of Face Mask	Skeletal Changes
Improve the skeletal discrepancies and provide a more favorable environment for future growth.	Acceleration of forward growth of the maxilla (with an anti-clockwise rotation)
Increase the dental arch length	Forward movement of the maxillary dentition
Avoid enamel abrasion and gingival dehiscence	Backward movement of the mandible (with a clockwise rotation)
Improve the dental, facial aesthetics and the psychological development of the child.	Backward movement of the mandibular dentition
Improve the dental, facial aesthetics and the psychological development of the child.	

11. Describe the Rationale for Rapid Maxillary Expansion (RME) in the Face Mask Treatment

Rapid maxillary expansion (RME) may enhance the protraction effect of the face mask by disrupting the maxillary suture system and it is widely accepted among the orthodontic community in the mid-face deficient class III patients even if there is no deficiency in the transverse dimension [51 - 54]. The rationale for expansion is to reduce the resistance of bony buttresses around the maxilla and to facilitate the forward movement of the maxilla. Moreover, maxillary expansion by acrylic bonded Hyrax appliance minimizes the downward and backward rotation of the mandible and the possible increase of anterior facial height [53 - 55].

12. Describe the Rapid Maxillary Expansion (RME) Activation in the Face Mask Treatment

The appliance should be activated once (1/4 turn each 0.25 mm) or twice (0.50 mm) a day for 7 to 10 days.In alternate rapid maxillary expansion and constriction method **(Alt-RAMEC)** daily alternate expansion (morning) and constriction (night) should be applied for 7 to 9 weeks and face mask treatment (12 or 14 oz)for 4 months .

13. How Can the Skeletal Effect of RPE be Increased in Maxillary Deficiency Patients?

In order to increase the skeletal effect of RPE in maxillary deficiency patients [13, 31] we should increase the rigidity of the appliance by:

a. Include maximum number of teeth.
b. Increase amount and speed of expansion.
c. Open bite: Acrylic occlusal coverage (3mm), preventing tooth eruption.
d. Deep bite: Hyrax appliances allowing tooth eruption.

14. When is the Proper Age to Start Face Mask Treatment and Why?

The application of protraction facemask therapy to the maxilla produces significant tension in the circummaxillary sutures and the maxillary tuberosity area. The tension produced within the sutures causes an increase in vascularity with a concomitant differentiation of the cellular tissues, resulting in an increase in osteoblastic activity in the region. In the pre-peak period, the palatine bone is separated from the adjacent bones by a wide fissure containing loose connective tissue, and a pronounced forward displacement of the maxilla can be obtained with reverse headgear therapy. At later maturational stages, the heavy interdigitations can be expected to exhibit a pronounced [4, 56]. Clinically speaking, the optimal time to intervene in a class III malocclusion is at the stage of eruption of the maxillary incisors.

15. Provide the Short-term Orthopaedic Effects of Chin-cup Treatment in the Mixed Dentition

A number of studies have reported that chin cup treatment has several short-term orthopaedic effects [4, 47] such as:

backward repositioning of the mandible
redirection and possible retardation of mandibular growth
overjet correction by mandibular incisor retroclination
increased anterior facial height and the mandibular plane angle
remodelling of the temporomandibular joint **anterior morphogenetic rotation of the mandible**

16. Should Chin Cup Therapy be Considered for Mandibular Prognathic Class III Patients?

A great deal of clinical and cephalometric reports has witnessed a more favorable growth pattern and an improvement in the skeletal relationship after early orthopaedic approach to Class III malocclusion [47]. It seems that patients who began treatment at the pre-pubertal period showed a more posterior positioning of the mandible than those who entered treatment at the growth spurt period. However, the treatment effects of chin cup therapy may be offset by rapid mandibular growth during puberty [22, 49]. As a result, chin cup therapy should be limited to the mild to moderate skeletal Class III malocclusions which can be camouflaged by dento-alveolar compensation during the second phase of orthodontic treatment [36, 37].

CONCLUDING REMARKS

Once cephalometric radiography became a regular part of orthodontics, it became apparent that growth modification treatment with functional appliances or headgears is more dento-alveolar than previously thought. It seems that the functional active phase of treatment has a greater impact on the growth rate but not on the overall amount of mandibular growth. However, the functional phase of treatment improves the Class II convex facial profile, increases children's self-esteem issues due to their dental appearance and decreases the possibility of their having incisal trauma due to protruded incisors.

There is still a big controversy about treatment timing for patients with mandibular prognathism. Protraction facemask with maxillary expansion has been advocated as one effective treatment modality in the early treatment of Class III malocclusion in maxillary deficient individuals.

REFERENCES

[1] Angle EH. Treatment of Malocclusion of the Teeth 1907.

[2] McNamara JA Jr. Components of class II malocclusion in children 8-10 years of age. Angle Orthod 1981; 51(3): 177-202.
[PMID: 7023290]

[3] Moyers RE, Riolo ML, Guire KE, Wainright RL, Bookstein FL. Differential diagnosis of class II malocclusions. Part 1. Facial types associated with class II malocclusions. Am J Orthod 1980; 78(5): 477-94.
[http://dx.doi.org/10.1016/0002-9416(80)90299-7] [PMID: 6933855]

[4] Proffit WR, Fields HW, Sarver DM. Contemporary orthodontics. 4th ed., St. Louis, Mo.: Mosby Elsevier 2007.

[5] Brezniak N, Arad A, Heller M, Dinbar A, Dinte A, Wasserstein A. Pathognomonic cephalometric characteristics of Angle Class II Division 2 malocclusion. Angle Orthod 2002; 72(3): 251-7.
[PMID: 12071609]

[6] Peck S, Peck L, Kataja M. Class II Division 2 malocclusion: a heritable pattern of small teeth in well-developed jaws. Angle Orthod 1998; 68(1): 9-20.
[PMID: 9503130]

[7] Van der Linden. Development of the Human Dentition. Hanover Park, IL: Quintessence Publishing Co., Chandler Drive 2014.

[8] Mossey PA. The heritability of malocclusion: part 2. The influence of genetics in malocclusion. Br J Orthod 1999; 26(3): 195-203.
[http://dx.doi.org/10.1093/ortho/26.3.195] [PMID: 10532158]

[9] Mossey PA. The heritability of malocclusion: Part 1--Genetics, principles and terminology. Br J Orthod 1999; 26(2): 103-13.
[http://dx.doi.org/10.1093/ortho/26.2.103] [PMID: 10420244]

[10] Townsend G, Hughes T, Luciano M, Bockmann M, Brook A. Genetic and environmental influences on human dental variation: a critical evaluation of studies involving twins. Arch Oral Biol 2009; 54(1) (Suppl. 1): S45-51.
[http://dx.doi.org/10.1016/j.archoralbio.2008.06.009] [PMID: 18715551]

[11] Graber TM, Rakosi T, Petrovic AG. Dentofacial orthopedics with functional appliances. St. Louis: Mosby 1997.

[12] McNamara JA Jr. Functional determinants of craniofacial size and shape. Eur J Orthod 1980; 2(3): 131-59.
[http://dx.doi.org/10.1093/ejo/2.3.131] [PMID: 6935065]

[13] Klein ET. Pressure habits, etiological factors in malocclusion. Am J Orthod 1952; 38: 569-87.
[http://dx.doi.org/10.1016/0002-9416(52)90025-0]

[14] Kydd WL, Neff CW. Frequency of deglutition of tongue thrusters compared to a sample population of normal swallowers. J Dent Res 1964; 43: 363-9.
[http://dx.doi.org/10.1177/00220345640430030701] [PMID: 14159039]

[15] Bishara SE, Jakobsen JR, Vorhies B, Bayati P. Changes in dentofacial structures in untreated Class II division 1 and normal subjects: a longitudinal study. Angle Orthod 1997; 67(1): 55-66.
[PMID: 9046400]

[16] Bishara SE. Mandibular changes in persons with untreated and treated Class II division 1 malocclusion. Am J Orthod Dentofacial Orthop 1998; 113(6): 661-73.
[http://dx.doi.org/10.1016/S0889-5406(98)70227-6] [PMID: 9637570]

[17] Karlsen AT. Craniofacial morphology in children with Angle Class II-1 malocclusion with and without deepbite. Angle Orthod 1994; 64(6): 437-46.
[PMID: 7864465]

[18] Lau JW, Hägg U. Cephalometric morphology of Chinese with Class II division 1 malocclusion. Br Dent J 1999; 186(4 Spec No): 188-90.
[PMID: 10205956]

[19] Pancherz H, Zieber K, Hoyer B. Cephalometric characteristics of Class II division 1 and Class II division 2 malocclusions: a comparative study in children. Angle Orthod 1997; 67(2): 111-20.
[PMID: 9107375]

[20] Melsen B. Effects of cervical anchorage during and after treatment: an implant study. Am J Orthod 1978; 73(5): 526-40.
[http://dx.doi.org/10.1016/0002-9416(78)90242-7] [PMID: 277067]

[21] Melsen B, Dalstra M. Distal molar movement with Kloehn headgear: is it stable? Am J Orthod Dentofacial Orthop 2003; 123(4): 374-8.
[http://dx.doi.org/10.1067/mod.2003.72] [PMID: 12695763]

[22] Dugoni SA. Comprehensive mixed dentition treatment. Am J Orthod Dentofacial Orthop 1998; 113(1): 75-84.
[http://dx.doi.org/10.1016/S0889-5406(98)70278-1] [PMID: 9457021]

[23] Fidler BC, Artun J, Joondeph DR, Little RM. Long-term stability of Angle Class II, division 1 malocclusions with successful occlusal results at end of active treatment. Am J Orthod Dentofacial Orthop 1995; 107(3): 276-85.
[http://dx.doi.org/10.1016/S0889-5406(95)70143-5] [PMID: 7879760]

[24] Lima Filho RM, Lima AL, de Oliveira Ruellas AC. Longitudinal study of anteroposterior and vertical maxillary changes in skeletal class II patients treated with Kloehn cervical headgear. Angle Orthod 2003; 73(2): 187-93.
[PMID: 12725376]

[25] Clark WJ. The art of Orthodontic.Twin Block functional therapy application in Dentofacial

Orthopedics. London: Mosby-Wolfe Publication 2002.

[26] O'Brien K, Macfarlane T, Wright J, *et al.* Early treatment for Class II malocclusion and perceived improvements in facial profile. Am J Orthod Dentofacial Orthop 2009; 135(5): 580-5. [http://dx.doi.org/10.1016/j.ajodo.2008.02.020] [PMID: 19409340]

[27] O'Brien K, Wright J, Conboy F, *et al.* Effectiveness of early orthodontic treatment with the Twin-block appliance: a multicenter, randomized, controlled trial. Part 1: Dental and skeletal effects. Am J Orthod Dentofacial Orthop 2003; 124(3): 234-43. [http://dx.doi.org/10.1016/S0889-5406(03)00352-4] [PMID: 12970656]

[28] Snow MD, Turvey TA, Walker D, Proffit WR. Surgical mandibular advancement in adolescents: postsurgical growth related to stability. Int J Adult Orthodon Orthognath Surg 1991; 6(3): 143-51. [PMID: 1812179]

[29] Mihalik CA, Proffit WR, Phillips C. Long-term follow-up of Class II adults treated with orthodontic camouflage: a comparison with orthognathic surgery outcomes. Am J Orthod Dentofacial Orthop 2003; 123(3): 266-78. [http://dx.doi.org/10.1067/mod.2003.43] [PMID: 12637899]

[30] Firouz M, Zernik J, Nanda R. Dental and orthopedic effects of high-pull headgear in treatment of Class II, division 1 malocclusion. Am J Orthod Dentofacial Orthop 1992; 102(3): 197-205. [http://dx.doi.org/10.1016/S0889-5406(05)81053-4] [PMID: 1510043]

[31] Tulloch JF, Phillips C, Proffit WR. Benefit of early Class II treatment: progress report of a two-phase randomized clinical trial. Am J Orthod Dentofacial Orthop 1998; 113(1): 62-72. [http://dx.doi.org/10.1016/S0889-5406(98)70277-X] [PMID: 9457020]

[32] Petrovic A, Stutzmann JJ, Oudet CL. Control processes in the postnatal growth of the condylar cartilage of the mandible.Determinants of mandibular form and growth, monograph 4, craniofacial growth series. Ann Arbor: Center for Human Growth and Development, The University of Michigan 1975.

[33] Sankey WL, Buschang PH, English J, Owen AH III. Early treatment of vertical skeletal dysplasia: the hyperdivergent phenotype. Am J Orthod Dentofacial Orthop 2000; 118(3): 317-27. [http://dx.doi.org/10.1067/mod.2000.106068] [PMID: 10982934]

[34] Tulloch JF, Proffit WR, Phillips C. Outcomes in a 2-phase randomized clinical trial of early Class II treatment. Am J Orthod Dentofacial Orthop 2004; 125(6): 657-67. [http://dx.doi.org/10.1016/j.ajodo.2004.02.008] [PMID: 15179390]

[35] Woodside DG, Metaxas A, Altuna G. The influence of functional appliance therapy on glenoid fossa remodeling. Am J Orthod Dentofacial Orthop 1987; 92(3): 181-98. [http://dx.doi.org/10.1016/0889-5406(87)90411-2] [PMID: 3477085]

[36] Niu Y, Zhou H. Effect on functional appliances on mandibular growth on skeletal Class II malocclusion: a systematic review. West China J Stomatol 2011; 29(4): 384-8. [PMID: 21932659]

[37] Zhou J, Lu Y, Gao XH, *et al.* The growth hormone receptor gene is associated with mandibular height in a Chinese population. J Dent Res 2005; 84(11): 1052-6. [http://dx.doi.org/10.1177/154405910508401116] [PMID: 16246940]

[38] Yamaguchi T, Maki K, Shibasaki Y. Growth hormone receptor gene variant and mandibular height in the normal Japanese population. Am J Orthod Dentofacial Orthop 2001; 119(6): 650-3. [http://dx.doi.org/10.1067/mod.2001.114536] [PMID: 11395710]

[39] Litsas G. Effects of Gh application in Craniofacial Growth. Oral Dis 2013; 19: 559-67. [http://dx.doi.org/10.1111/odi.12041] [PMID: 23279133]

[40] Flores-Mir C, Major PW. A systematic review of cephalometric facial soft tissue changes with the Activator and Bionator appliances in Class II division 1 subjects. Eur J Orthod 2006; 28(6): 586-93. [http://dx.doi.org/10.1093/ejo/cjl034] [PMID: 17095741]

[41] Flores-Mir C, Major PW. Cephalometric facial soft tissue changes with the twin block appliance in Class II division 1 malocclusion patients. A systematic review. Angle Orthod 2006; 76(5): 876-81. [PMID: 17029526]

[42] Antonarakis GS, Kiliaridis S. Short-term anteroposterior treatment effects of functional appliances and extraoral traction on class II malocclusion. A meta-analysis. Angle Orthod 2007; 77(5): 907-14. [http://dx.doi.org/10.2319/061706-244] [PMID: 17902235]

[43] Küçükkeleş N, Ilhan I, Orgun IA. Treatment efficiency in skeletal Class II patients treated with the jasper jumper. Angle Orthod 2007; 77(3): 449-56. [http://dx.doi.org/10.2319/0003-3219(2007)077[0449:TEISCI]2.0.CO;2] [PMID: 17465652]

[44] de Almeida MR, Henriques JF, de Almeida RR, Weber U, McNamara JA Jr. Short-term treatment effects produced by the Herbst appliance in the mixed dentition. Angle Orthod 2005; 75(4): 540-7. [PMID: 16097222]

[45] de Almeida MR, Flores-Mir C, Brandão AG, de Almeida RR, de Almeida-Pedrin RR. Soft tissue changes produced by a banded-type Herbst appliance in late mixed dentition patients. World J Orthod 2008; 9(2): 121-31. [PMID: 18575306]

[46] Baccetti T, Reyes BC, McNamara JA Jr. Gender differences in Class III malocclusion. Angle Orthod 2005; 75(4): 510-20. [PMID: 16097218]

[47] Sugawara J, Mitani H. Facial growth of skeletal Class III malocclusion and the effects, limitations, and long-term dentofacial adaptations to chincap therapy. Semin Orthod 1997; 3(4): 244-54. [http://dx.doi.org/10.1016/S1073-8746(97)80057-6] [PMID: 9573886]

[48] Miyajima K, McNamara JA Jr, Sana M, Murata S. An estimation of craniofacial growth in the untreated Class III female with anterior crossbite. Am J Orthod Dentofacial Orthop 1997; 112(4): 425-34. [http://dx.doi.org/10.1016/S0889-5406(97)70051-9] [PMID: 9345155]

[49] Mitani H, Sato K, Sugawara J. Growth of mandibular prognathism after pubertal growth peak. Am J Orthod Dentofacial Orthop 1993; 104(4): 330-6. [http://dx.doi.org/10.1016/S0889-5406(05)81329-0] [PMID: 8213653]

[50] Moreno Uribe LM, Vela KC, Kummet C, Dawson DV, Southard TE. Phenotypic diversity in white adults with moderate to severe Class III malocclusion. Am J Orthod Dentofacial Orthop 2013; 144(1): 32-42. [http://dx.doi.org/10.1016/j.ajodo.2013.02.019] [PMID: 23810043]

[51] Delaire J. Maxillary development revisited: relevance to the orthopaedic treatment of Class III malocclusions. Eur J Orthod 1997; 19(3): 289-311. [http://dx.doi.org/10.1093/ejo/19.3.289] [PMID: 9239959]

[52] De Clerck HJ, Cornelis MA, Cevidanes LH, Heymann GC, Tulloch CJ. Orthopedic traction of the maxilla with miniplates: a new perspective for treatment of midface deficiency. J Oral Maxillofac Surg 2009; 67(10): 2123-9. [http://dx.doi.org/10.1016/j.joms.2009.03.007] [PMID: 19761906]

[53] Perillo L, Vitale M, Masucci C, D'Apuzzo F, Cozza P, Franchi L. Comparisons of two protocols for the early treatment of Class III dentoskeletal disharmony. Eur J Orthod 2016; 38(1): 51-6. [http://dx.doi.org/10.1093/ejo/cjv010] [PMID: 25770942]

[54] Alcan T, Keles A, Erverdi N. The effects of a modified protraction headgear on maxilla. Am J Orthod Dentofacial Orthop 2000; 117(1): 27-38. [http://dx.doi.org/10.1016/S0889-5406(00)70245-9] [PMID: 10629517]

[55] Ngan PW, Hagg U, Yiu C, Wei SH. Treatment response and long-term dentofacial adaptations to maxillary expansion and protraction. Semin Orthod 1997; 3(4): 255-64.

[http://dx.doi.org/10.1016/S1073-8746(97)80058-8] [PMID: 9573887]

[56] Merwin D, Ngan P, Hagg U, Yiu C, Wei SH. Timing for effective application of anteriorly directed orthopedic force to the maxilla. Am J Orthod Dentofacial Orthop 1997; 112(3): 292-9. [http://dx.doi.org/10.1016/S0889-5406(97)70259-2] [PMID: 9294359]

SUBJECT INDEX

A

B

George Litsas

C

D

E

F

G

H

I

L

M

N

O

P

Q

R

S

T

U

V

Made in the USA
Las Vegas, NV
03 November 2026

57422776R00145